Cardiology

CLINICAL CASES UNCOVERED

T0223944

To my wife, Mags, for her patience. TB

To my parents for their lifelong support. JD

To my father, for his constant love and support. SB

How to use this book

Clinical Cases Uncovered (CCU) books are carefully designed to help supplement your clinical experience and assist with refreshing your memory when revising. Each book is divided into three sections: Part 1, Basics; Part 2, Cases; and Part 3, Self-assessment.

Part 1 gives you a quick reminder of the basic science, history and examination, and key diagnoses in the area. Part 2 contains many of the clinical presentations you would expect to see on the wards or crop up in exams, with questions and answers leading you through each case. New information, such as test results, is revealed as events unfold and each case concludes with a handy case summary explaining the key points. Part 3 allows you to test your learning with several question styles (MCQs, EMQs and SAQs), each with a strong clinical focus.

Whether reading individually or working as part of a group, we hope you will enjoy using your CCU book. If you have any recommendations on how we could improve the series, please do let us know by contacting us at: medstudentuk@oxon.blackwellpublishing.com.

Disclaimer

CCU patients are designed to reflect real life, with their own reports of symptoms and concerns. Please note that all names used are entirely fictitious and any similarity to patients, alive or dead, is coincidental.

Preface

Although there are many books already published on the subject of cardiovascular medicine, we felt that there was nothing that offered medical students and junior doctors a practical, patient-based approach. This book has been written to fill that gap. It is suitable for students, trainees in general internal medicine, general practice and budding cardiologists.

It provides a concise resume of the key features of anatomy and physiology that have direct clinical applications when investigating and treating patients with cardiac disease. By presenting 'real world' examples in 26 case scenarios, all the common (and some uncommon) cardiac diagnoses are revealed. Particular emphasis is placed on history taking, the interpretation of physical signs and the appropriate use of non-invasive and invasive investigations. Arguments for and against differential diagnoses are discussed. Treatment options are explained in detail and the impact of cardiovascular disease on prognosis, lifestyle and genetic screening is explored. Throughout the text, key points and red flags are highlighted and learning points are summarized at the end of each case. High-quality reproductions of electrocardiograms, echocardiograms and other imaging modalities have been included to simulate the real patient encounter.

Three self-assessment sections have been written in the format of commonly-used examination methods. The questions stem from the clinical cases, yet add an additional layer of education and information for the reader.

We hope this book acts as a stepping stone from traditional cardiology texts to the application of knowledge in the clinical world. As well as being a reference and assessment tool, it should above all be an enjoyable read that can be dipped in and out of or read from cover to cover in one go. We hope it inspires the next generation of cardiologists!

Tim Betts
Jeremy Dwight
Sacha Bull
Oxford

(**Part 3**) **Self-assessment,** 208

Contents

This edition first published 2010, © 2010 by T. Betts, J. Dwight and S. Bull

Blackwell Publishing was acquired by John Wiley & Sons in February 2007. Blackwell's publishing program has been merged with Wiley's global Scientific, Technical and Medical business to form Wiley-Blackwell.

Registered office: John Wiley & Sons Ltd, The Atrium, Southern Gate, Chichester, West Sussex, PO19 8SQ, UK

Editorial offices: 9600 Garsington Road, Oxford, OX4 2DQ, UK
      The Atrium, Southern Gate, Chichester, West Sussex, PO19 8SQ, UK
      111 River Street, Hoboken, NJ 07030-5774, USA

For details of our global editorial offices, for customer services and for information about how to apply for permission to reuse the copyright material in this book please see our website at www.wiley.com/wiley-blackwell

Library of Congress Cataloging-in-Publication Data

Betts, Tim (Tim Rider)
  Cardiology / Tim Betts, Jeremy Dwight, Sacha Bull.
    p. ; cm. – (Clinical cases uncovered)
  Includes indexes.
  ISBN 978-1-4051-7800-6
1. Heart–Diseases–Case studies. I. Dwight, Jeremy. II. Bull, Sacha. III. Title. IV. Series: Clinical cases uncovered.
  [DNLM: 1. Cardiovascular Diseases–diagnosis–Case Reports. 2. Cardiovascular Diseases–diagnosis–Problems and Exercises. 3. Cardiovascular Diseases–therapy–Case Reports. 4. Cardiovascular Diseases–therapy–Problems and Exercises. WG 18.2 B565c 2010]
  RC682.B48 2010
  616.1′2–dc22
  2009035144

ISBN: 978-1-4051-7800-6

A catalogue record for this book is available from the British Library

Set in 9 on 12 pt Minion by Toppan Best-set Premedia Limited
Printed in Singapore by Markono Print Media Pte Ltd

4   2013

Cardiology

CLINICAL CASES UNCOVERED

Tim Betts

MD, MBChB, MRCP
Consultant Cardiologist and
Electrophysiologist
Department of Cardiology
John Radcliffe Hospital
Oxford, UK

Sacha Bull

MRCP
Cardiology Registrar
Department of Cardiology
John Radcliffe Hospital
Oxford, UK

Jeremy Dwight

MD, FRCP
Consultant Cardiologist
Department of Cardiology
John Radcliffe Hospital
Oxford, UK

⟨W⟩WILEY-BLACKWELL

A John Wiley & Sons, Ltd., Publication

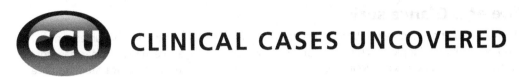

CLINICAL CASES UNCOVERED

Get the most from clinical practice, with *Clinical Cases Uncovered*

No other series is quite like *Clinical Cases Uncovered*, where you can rehearse for life in clinical practice with easy-to-use and well-instructed walk-through scenarios. Each case is presented as you would see it and the use of real-life experiences means the decisions and outcomes are factually based. Along the way to determining a diagnosis and identifying treatments, you learn about variable symptoms, danger signs and get overviews of all the common, classical and atypical presentations

Background to the subject and how to approach the patient are covered in an introductory section and once you have worked through the range of cases you can test yourself with a selection of MCQs, EMQs and SAQs. This distinct blend of learning means you will improve time and again, greatly enhancing your decision-making skills. With such a wide range of subjects covered you will soon see the benefit of the CCU approach

The series so far...

Acute Medicine: Clinical Cases Uncovered
978-1-4051-6883-0

Cardiology: Clinical Cases Uncovered
978-1-4051-7800-6

Endocrinology and Diabetes: Clinical Cases Uncovered
978-1-4051-5726-1

General Practice: Clinical Cases Uncovered
978-1-4051-6140-4

Haematology: Clinical Cases Uncovered
978-1-4051-8322-2

Infectious Disease: Clinical Cases Uncovered
978-1-4051-6891-5

Nephrology: Clinical Cases Uncovered
978-1-4051-8990-3

Obstetrics and Gynaecology: Clinical Cases Uncovered
978-1-4051-8671-1

Paediatrics: Clinical Cases Uncovered
978-1-4051-5984-5

Psychiatry: Clinical Cases Uncovered
978-1-4051-5983-8

Radiology: Clinical Cases Uncovered
978-1-4051-8474-8

Respiratory Medicine: Clinical Cases Uncovered
978-1-4051-5895-4

Surgery: Clinical Cases Uncovered
978-1-4051-5898-5

Coming soon...

Gastroenterology: Clinical Cases Uncovered
978-1-4051-6975-2

Neurology: Clinical Cases Uncovered
978-1-4051-6220-3

All content reviewed by students for students

Wiley-Blackwell Medical Education books are designed exactly for their intended audience.
All our books are developed in collaboration with students, which means our books are always published with you, the student, in mind.
If you would like to be one of our student reviewers, go to www.reviewmedicalbooks.com to find out more.

The *at a Glance* series

Written by experts and reviewed by students, the *at a Glance* series breaks complex subjects into short, easily digested topics. Each topic is presented as a double-page spread with a clear, easy-to-follow diagram supported by succinct explanatory text. Tens of thousands of medical students have passed their exams using the *at a Glance* approach. Why shouldn't you?

List of abbreviations

AICD	automated implantable cardioverter-defibrillator		Hb	haemoglobin
ACE	angiotensin-converting enzyme		HDL	high-density lipoprotein
ACS	acute coronary syndrome		HFNEF	heart failure normal ejection fraction
A&E	Accident & Emergency		HGV	heavy goods vehicle
AHA	American Heart Association		HIV	human immunodeficiency virus
ALT	alanine aminotransferase		HOCM	hypertrophic obstructive cardiomyopathy
AR	aortic regurgitation		ICD	implantable cardioverter defibrillator
AS	aortic stenosis		ICU	Intensive Care Unit
ASD	atrial septal defect		INR	international normalised ratio
AV	atrioventricular		IVAB	intravenous antibiotics
AVA	aortic valve area		JVP	jugular venous pressure
AVNRT	atrioventricular nodal re-entrant tachycardias		LAD	left anterior descending
			LBBB	left branch bundle block
AVRT	atrioventricular re-entrant		LCA	left coronary artery
BMI	body mass index		LCx	left circumflex
BNP	brain natriuretic peptide		LDH	lactate dehydrogenase
bpm	beats per minute		LDL	low-density lipoprotein
CCU	Coronary Care Unit		LMS	left main stem
COPD	chronic obstructive airways disease		LQTS	long-QT syndrome
CPAP	continuous positive airways pressure		LVEF	left ventricular ejection fraction
CPR	cardiopulmonary resuscitation		LVH	left ventricular hypertrophy
CT	computer tomography		MCV	mean corpuscle volume
CTR	cardiothoracic ratio		MEN	multiple endocrine neoplasia
CVP	central venous pressure		MIBG	metaiodobenzylguanidine
Cx	circumflex		MR	mitral regurgitation
CXR	chest X-ray		MRI	magnetic resonance imaging
DC	direct current		MS	mitral stenosis
DVLA	Driver and Vehicle Licensing Agency		MUGA	multi-gated acquisition
DVT	deep vein thrombosis		MCV	mean corpuscle volume
ESR	erythrocyte sedimentation rate		NICE	National Institute for Health and Clinical Excellence
FBC	full blood count			
FEV_1	forced expiratory volume in 1 s		NYHA	New York Heart Association
FVC	forced vital capacity		PCI	percutaneous coronary intervention
GFR	glomerular filtration rate		PDA	patent ductus arteriosus
GGT	gamma-glutamyl transpeptidase		PEA	pulseless electrical activity
GI	gastrointestinal		PFO	patent foramen ovale
GP	general practitioner		PV	pulmonary valve
GTN	glyceryl trinitrate		RBBB	right branch bundle block
			RCA	right coronary artery

rtPA	recombinant tissue plasminogen activator	TIMI	thrombolysis in myocardial infarction
rPA	reteplase	TNK	tenecteplase
SA	sinoatrial	TS	tricuspid stenosis
SCD	sudden cardiac death	TR	tricuspid regurgitation
STEMI	ST-elevation myocardial infarction (also non-STEMI)	tPA	tissue plasminogen activator
		TR	tricuspid regurgitation
SVT	supraventricular tachycardia	VPC	ventricular premature contraction
TB	tuberculosis	VSD	ventricular septal defect
TC	total cholesterol	VVIR	ventricular inhibited rate responsive
TIA	transient ischaemic attack	WCC	white cell count

Basic science

Anatomy

The primary function of the heart is to pump deoxygenated blood to the lungs and to return oxygenated blood to the rest of the body. The basic anatomy consists of:

- Pericardium (visceral and parietal): the fibrous sac containing the heart.
- Four cardiac chambers: the right and left atria and ventricles.
- Heart valves:
  - Two outflow valves: the aortic and pulmonary valves consist of three semi-lunar cusps.
  - Two atrioventricular (AV) valves: the mitral and tricuspid valves, which are attached by chordae tendinae to papillary muscles.
- Vascular system:
  - Great vessels: the pulmonary artery, pulmonary vein and aorta.
  - Three main coronary arteries: the left anterior descending (LAD) and circumflex (Cx) arteries, which originate from the left main stem (LMS) and the right coronary artery (RCA).
  - Venous system: the venous blood is drained via the great cardiac vein, small anterior cardiac vein and thesbian veins.
- Electrical conducting system, which consists of specialised cells that are able to depolarise spontaneously (*automaticity*) forming:
  - The sinoatrial (SA) node.
  - The atrioventricular node.
  - The Bundle of His (right and left) and terminal Purkinje fibres.

The foetal heart

A knowledge of basic cardiac embryology is helpful for understanding how lesions found in adult congenital heart disease develop.

Foetal atria and ventricles (Figure A)

The heart begins life as a primitive tube, which folds to produce early cardiac chambers: the sinus venosus, the primitive atrium, the ventricle and the bulbus cordis. Further separation of the chambers occurs as follows:

- A pair of septa, the *septum primum* and *septum secundum*, grow to separate the right and left atria. The septum primum fuses with the endocardial cushions, the septum secundum does not. The free edge of the septum primum and secundum form the *foramen ovale*.
- A muscular interventricular septum grows from the floor of the common ventricle to divide it into two chambers.

Foetal shunts (Figure B)

The lungs are bypassed in the foetal circulation by the following right to left shunts:

- *Foramen ovale*: oxygenated blood passes from the left umbilical vein to the right atrium via the *ductus venosus*. From the right atrium the blood is then shunted through the foramen ovale to the left atrium.
- *Ductus arteriosus*: the remaining oxygenated blood passes from the right atrium to the right ventricle and enters the pulmonary trunk. From here it passes via the ductus arteriosus directly to the aorta, bypassing the lungs.

Circulation changes at birth

As the newborn takes its first breath, the pulmonary vascular resistance drops and conversion from the foetal to adult circulation starts. The following changes occur:

- The *foramen ovale* closes by the mechanical effect of the reversal in pressure between the two atria, and forms the *fossa ovalis* in adult life.
- Changes in oxygen concentration of the blood and hormonal changes contribute to the closure of the *ductus arteriosus*.

Cardiology: Clinical Cases Uncovered. By T. Betts, J. Dwight and S. Bull. Published 2010 by Blackwell Publishing.

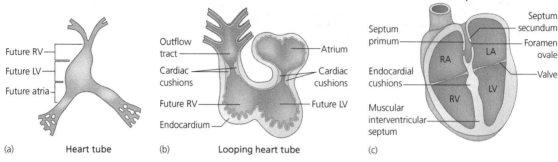

Figure A Development of the heart. LA, left atrium; LV, left ventricle; RA, right atrium; RV, right ventricle.

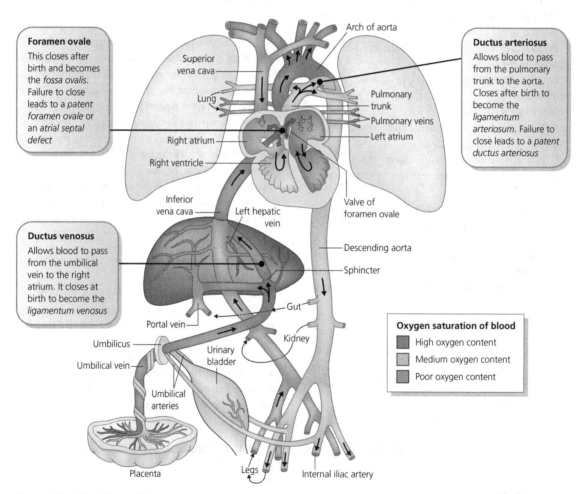

Figure B Foetal circulation and shunts.

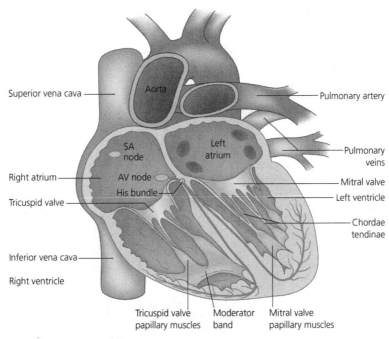

Figure C Adult heart. AV, atrioventricular; SA, sinoatrial.

The adult heart
Right atrium
This chamber is a low-pressure (0–7 mmHg), thin-walled receiving chamber for systemic and cardiac venous blood. It also contains the 'pacemaker' (SA node) and the AV node of the heart.

Right ventricle
This chamber receives the venous blood from the right atrium and ejects it into the pulmonary artery. Unlike the left ventricle, it is heavily trabeculated. It contains the moderator band, which contains part of the conduction system, and the papillary muscles of the tricuspid valve. The pressure in this chamber is 15–30 mmHg during systole.

Left atrium
This chamber receives oxygenated blood from the pulmonary veins. Clinically important structures are:
• *Pulmonary veins:* in normal hearts four pulmonary veins (two upper and two lower) drain oxygenated blood from the lungs into the left atrium.
• *Left atrial appendage:* a blind-ending sac related to the left atrium and a common site for thrombus formation in patients with atrial fibrillation.
The pressure in this chamber is slightly higher than in the right atrium (4–12 mmHg).

Left ventricle
This is a high-pressure (90–140 mmHg), thick-walled chamber, which reflects its greater contractile performance. It delivers oxygenated blood systemically. It contains the *mitral valve papillary muscles*. These are conical muscular projections from the walls of the left ventricle that attach to the chordae tendinae to support the two cusps of the mitral valve.

Vascular anatomy (Figure D)

Great vessels
• *Superior and inferior vena cava*: drain systemic deoxygenated venous blood into the right atrium.
• *Pulmonary artery*: carries *deoxygenated* blood to the lungs from the right ventricle. It has thinner walls than systemic arteries and subdivides many times into branches that carry blood to the network of 280 billion capillaries where it is oxygenated.

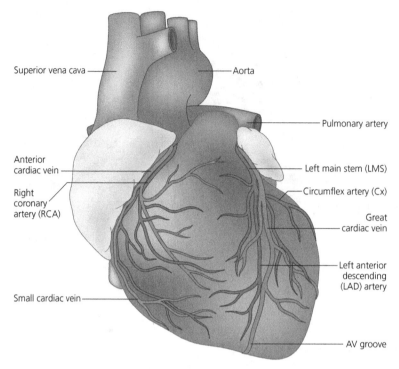

Figure D Vascular anatomy.

<table>
<tr><td>

Box A Clinical reasons to know cardiac embryology

- A *patent foramen ovale (PFO)* is found in up to 20% of the population. The majority of people with a PFO have no symptoms. In some patients emboli form in the venous circulation and pass via the patent foramen into the systemic circulation, causing a stroke. (This is known as paradoxical embolus.) In such patients and some other selected groups, closure of the PFO is recommended. This can be done percutaneously.
- Failure of the *ductus arteriosus* to close after birth leads to the congenital heart defect *patent ductus arteriosus (PDA)*. Surgical or percutaneous duct closure is recommended.
- Failure of the *interventricular septum* to fuse with the endocardial cushions gives rise to a *ventricular septal defect,* one of the most common congenital abnormalities.
- Failure of the atrial septum primum and septum secundum to fuse gives rise to the congenital defect known as *atrial septal defect.*

</td></tr>
</table>

- *Pulmonary veins:* there are four draining oxygenated blood from the lungs into the left atrium.
- *Aorta:* carries oxygenated blood from the left ventricle to supply the rest of the body.

Arteries

Three main coronary arteries supply blood to the myocardium and arise from the sinuses of Valsalva above the semi-lunar cusps of the aortic valve. These are the RCA, the LAD and the Cx artery. The latter two arteries arise from the LMS.

- The RCA:
  - Arises from above the anterior cusp of the aortic valve.
  - Runs down the AV groove.
  - Supplies the *SA node,* the *AV node* and *right ventricle.*
  - Is 'dominant' in 85–90% of the population. It is called a 'right dominant system' when it gives rise to the *posterior descending artery* to supply the *inferior wall of the left ventricle* and *the inferior third of the interventricular septum.*

- The LMS arises from the left coronary cusp and bifurcates into the LAD and Cx coronary arteries.
- The LAD:
  - Arises from the LMS.
  - Runs down the AV groove.
  - Supplies the *anteroapical* aspects of the *left ventricle*, septum and part of the lateral wall.
- The Cx artery:
  - Arises from the LMS.
  - Runs down the posterior AV groove.
  - Supplies the *posterolateral* aspect of the *left ventricle.*
  - Gives rise to the posterior descending artery in 10–15% of patients (known as a 'left dominant' system).

Cardiac veins
- Great cardiac vein: drains blood from the left ventricle into the right atrium via the coronary sinus.
- Small anterior cardiac vein: drains blood from the right ventricle into the right atrium.

> ### Box B Clinical reasons to know the vascular system
>
> #### Coronary arteries
> To understand the main infarct sites, associated complications and prognosis of myocardial infarction:
> - Acute occlusion of the LAD causes an anterolateral and anteroseptal territory infarct, which may result in extensive left ventricular impairment and increased morbidity and long-term mortality.
> - Acute occlusion of the Cx causes a posterolateral territory infarct in a non-left dominant system.
> - Acute occlusion of the RCA causes infarction of the inferior wall of the left and right ventricle and can lead to complete heart block because it supplies the SA and AV node.

- Thebesian veins: drain remaining blood directly into the cardiac chambers.

Valve anatomy
The normal valve anatomy is demonstrated in Figure E.

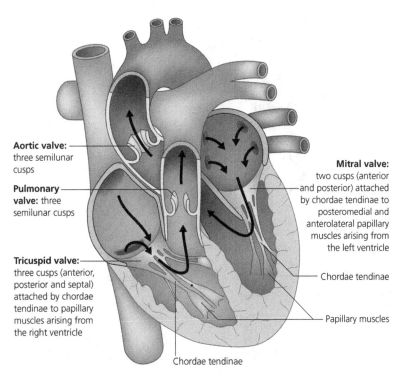

Aortic valve: three semilunar cusps

Pulmonary valve: three semilunar cusps

Tricuspid valve: three cusps (anterior, posterior and septal) attached by chordae tendinae to papillary muscles arising from the right ventricle

Mitral valve: two cusps (anterior and posterior) attached by chordae tendinae to posteromedial and anterolateral papillary muscles arising from the left ventricle

Chordae tendinae

Papillary muscles

Chordae tendinae

Figure E Valve anatomy.

Box C **Clinical reasons to know valve structure and function**

- 'Bicuspid' aortic valves have only two semi-lunar cusps and occur in 2% of the population. They are associated with coarctation of the aorta and can lead to development of early aortic stenosis (AS) or aortic regurgitation (AR).
- Dilatation of the aortic root and valve annulus can lead to AR due to failure of the aortic leaflets to coapt.
- The mitral valve may fail very suddenly if there is rupture of papillary muscle or chordae tendinae tethering the valve cusps (e.g. following an inferior or anterior myocardial infarction). This situation can be fatal.
- 'Functional' tricuspid regurgitation (TR) or mitral regurgitation (MR) occurs when there is dilatation of the right or left heart, respectively, resulting in failure of the valve leaflets to coapt due to stretching of the valve annulus.
- Valve lesions are a common cause of heart murmurs and can give rise to endocarditis.

Electrical conduction system anatomy (Figure F)

Specialised cardiac myocytes make up the cardiac electrical conducting system. It consists of the:

- SA node: this forms the 'pacemaker' of the heart and generates the electrical impulse. It consists of a collection of specialised cardiomyocytes in the right atrium with 'automaticity' (the ability to depolarise spontaneously and faster than other conducting tissue in the heart).
- AV node: located at the base of the right atrium, the AV node transmits the electrical impulse from the atria to the ventricles.
- The bundle of His descends from the AV node down the membranous interventricular septum. It is the only electrical connection between the atria and ventricles. It divides into left and right bundle branches.
- The bundle branches are specialised conducting fibres that conduct the impulse rapidly into the ventricular myocardium. The right bundle is a discrete structure. The left bundle further divides into:

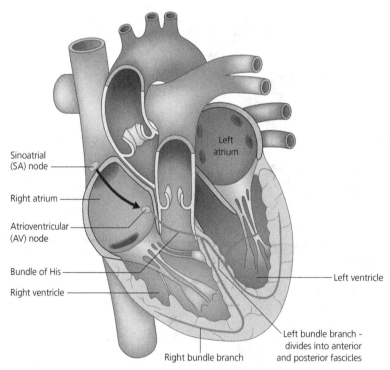

Figure F Electrical conduction system.

○ A smaller anterior and larger posterior fascicle.
○ Purkinje fibres: these distribute the impulse to the myocardial tissue.

Physiology
Cardiomyocytes
The myocardium is composed of specialised cardiac cells called *cardiomyocytes* that are characterised by:
• Electrical conduction: they are connected to each other via an *intercalated disc* containing *gap junctions*, which allow electrical conduction to neighbouring cells.
• Contraction: they can contract because of special contractile proteins that are arranged in a structural unit called a *sarcomere*, which consist of interlocking thin filaments (tropomysin) and thick filaments (myosin molecules).

• Excitation–contraction coupling: describes the process by which an action potential triggers a cardiomyocyte to contract. The process is divided into the following phases:
○ Phase 0: depolarisation of the cell membrane caused by an increase in sodium channel conductance.
○ Phase 1: repolarisation caused by opening of potassium channels.
○ Phase 2: calcium influx delays repolarisation. Calcium binding causes sarcomere shortening.
○ Phase 3: repolarisation.
○ Phase 4: return to resting membrane potential.

Cardiac cycle (Figure H)
The four phases of the cardiac cycle are:
• *Phase I: Isovolumetric contraction.* Tricuspid and mitral valves close as the ventricles contract. The aortic valve opens when left ventricular pressure exceeds aortic pressure.
• *Phase II: Ventricular ejection.* The aortic valve opens and blood is expelled into the aorta. The left ventricle begins to relax at the end of the T wave and the aortic valve closes after pressure falls.
• *Phase III: Isovolumetric relaxation.* All four cardiac valves are closed and the left ventricular pressure continues to fall.
• *Phase IV: Ventricular filling.* This occurs in two phases: 'rapid passive ventricular filling' happens when the mitral valve opens and 'active ventricular filling' happens at the end of diastole when the atrium contracts.

Cardiac output
Cardiac output (L/min) is the product of stroke volume (L) and heart rate (bpm).

Cardiac output = stroke volume × heart rate.

The normal value in an average healthy human at rest is around 5 L/min. During exercise, cardiac output increases 4-to-6-fold.

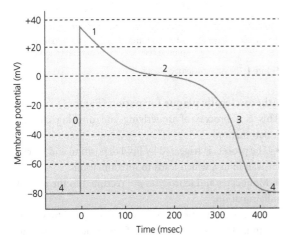

Figure G Action potential.

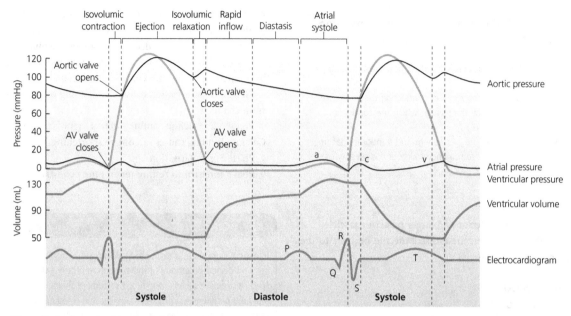

Figure H Cardiac cycle. AV, atrioventricular.

Cardiac output is influenced by:
• Preload: the filling pressure.
• Myocardial contractility.
• Afterload: this is also known as 'systemic vascular resistance'. This is the resistance to ejection of blood from the left ventricle. The majority of the resistance to flow comes from the small arterioles.

> **KEY POINT**
>
> Cardiac output can be measured invasively using a pulmonary catheter, thermodilution or, non-invasively, using an ultrasound Doppler probe. It is used to assess patients for cardiac transplantation and to monitor patients in cardiogenic shock.

Pathological processes affecting the cardiovascular system
Coronary artery disease
Coronary artery disease is one of the most common causes of death in the developed world. The atheromatous plaque underlines the pathophysiology of ischaemic heart disease (Figure I). Risk factors for development of atherosclerotic disease are described in Chapter 2.

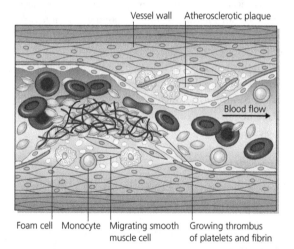

Figure I The atherosclerotic plaque.

Atherosclerotic plaque formation (Figure J)
This is a process of underlying and ongoing chronic inflammation:
• The process is triggered by lipid deposition and vascular wall injury, which leads to inflammation.
• Monocytes and leucocytes are recruited to the area of inflammation.
• 'Fatty streaks' are formed when inflammatory cells accumulate oxidised lipids to form macrophages and foam cells.

- Vascular smooth muscle cells are recruited to form a fibrous cap.
- The plaque expands further with ongoing inflammation and lipid deposition and encroaches on the vascular lumen.

Atherothrombosis formation

- Erosion or rupture of the fibrous cap overlying the atherosclerotic lesion may lead to thrombous formation.
- Thrombogenic material within the plaque is exposed, causing accumulation of platelets and formation of a thrombous within the vessel.
- The clinical course of the patient is largely determined by the nature and location of the thrombus formed on the atherosclerotic plaque.

Disruption of the atherosclerotic plaque

Erosion or rupture of the atherosclerotic plaque can result in three possible outcomes:

1. An acute coronary syndrome (ACS), where thrombus forms on the lesion causing obstruction to flow:

   a. Complete obstruction of the lumen by thrombus is associated with ST elevation on the ECG and characteristically gives rise to an ST elevation myocardial infarction (STEMI).

   b. Partial obstruction of the lumen by thrombus is associated with non-ST elevation ECG changes and either unstable angina or a non-ST elevation MI (non-STEMI).

The extent of myocardial damage is dependent upon the duration of occlusion of the infarct related vessel.

2. Resolution and healing of the plaque.

3. Plaque progression causing further occlusion of the vascular lumen and worsening of angina.

The reasons why some plaques rupture and others do not remain unclear.

Progression of the atherosclerotic plaque

When symptomatic this is associated with the development of angina. This is the syndrome of ischaemic chest pain occurring on exercise, which is associated with a mismatch between myocardial oxygen demand and supply.

Cardiac markers

Myocardial cell death can be recognised by the appearance in the blood of different proteins released into the circulation from the damaged myocytes. Cardiac

---

Box E Clinical situations: impact on cardiac output

Compensated

- *Sinus bradycardia*: cardiac output is maintained because the stroke volume is increased. There is a rise in pre-load (lower heart rate leads to increased filling time) and thus stroke volume is increased via the Frank-Starling relationship.
- *Rise in blood pressure*: the rise in systemic vascular resistance will initially reduce stroke volume. However the pre-load is increased because of incomplete left ventricular ejection leading to normalisation of cardiac output. These mechanisms maintain homeostasis.
- *Exercise and pregnancy*: cardiac output is increased in response to demand via an increase in venous return, stroke volume and heart rate.

Decompensated

High cardiac output states

These patients tend to have warm peripheries and a bounding pulse. Causes include:

- Anaemia.
- Thyrotoxicosis.
- Paget's disease.
- Sepsis.

Low cardiac output states

These patients have cool peripheries, low-volume pulse, prolonged capillary refill time and are hypotensive. Causes include:

- Hypovolaemia.
- Complete heart block.
- Tachyarrhythmia causing haemodynamic compromise.
- Poor left or right ventricular systolic function (e.g. ischaemic or dilated cardiomyopathy).
- Cardiac tamponade/ constrictive pericarditis
- Aortic stenosis (AS)
- Cardiogenic shock*

*This carries a high mortality rate of 80% with treatment. It normally occurs due to pump failure following a massive myocardial infarction. The definition of cardiogenic shock is: *'a state of hypotension (with systolic blood pressure <90 mmHg) with reduced end-organ perfusion due to low cardiac output'*.

> ### KEY POINT
>
> STEMI is a medical emergency and requires prompt treatment with reperfusion therapy. Prompt primary percutaneous coronary intervention is the gold standard treatment for STEMI.

> ### Box F **Myocardial infarction: definition and causes**
>
> The European Society of Cardiology definition of myocardial infarction is as follows: detection of a *rise and fall* of cardiac biomarkers (preferably troponin) *together* with evidence of myocardial ischaemia with at least one of the following:
> - Symptoms of ischaemia.
> - ECG changes indicative of new ischaemia (new ST changes, LBBB).
> - Development of pathological Q waves on ECG.
> - Imaging evidence of new loss of viable myocardium or new regional wall motion abnormality.
>   Atherosclerotic thrombosis causes the majority of myocardial infarcts. Other causes of myocardial infarction include:
> - Embolus (vegetation from infective endocarditis).
> - Spontaneous coronary artery dissection.
> - Intense spasm of the coronary arteries (e.g. cocaine).
> - Trauma.
> - Aortic dissection.
> - Iatrogenic due to coronary intervention.

troponin is the preferred marker used to measure myocardial necrosis because of superior specificity to other cardiac markers. It has the following properties:
- Exists as a contractile protein, mainly bound as part of the actin/myosin complex.
- Exists in three forms, of which T and I are used clinically.
- Highly sensitive and specific.
- Measurement 12 hours after onset of pain has 100% sensitivity for myocardial infarction.
- Levels rise within 12 hours of myocardial injury, peak at 24 hours and remain elevated for up to 14 days.
- Other less-specific markers of myocardial injury that can be measured include myoglobin, creatine kinase and lactate dehydrogenase.
- Myocardial necrosis and elevated troponin levels can occur for reasons other than myocardial infarction.

Pathology affecting the great vessels
Aortic dissection
Aortic dissection is a tear in the aortic intima through which blood enters and strips the media from the adventitia. Anterograde blood flow may cause the dissection to extend down the length of the aorta affecting the coronary, renal or femoral arteries.

Prognosis and management depend on the location of the tear.

Type A dissections (arising in the ascending aorta)
- Are a medical emergency and require immediate surgery.
- Carry a high mortality rate.
- May cause aortic root dilatation, AR, pericardial effusions or myocardial infarction (if the dissection extends to the coronary arteries).

Type B dissections (arising in the descending aorta)
- Carry a lower mortality rate than type A dissections and can be managed medically.
- May cause symptoms due to vascular compromise of other areas (e.g. acute limb ischaemia – iliac vessels; renal failure – renal ischaemia; paraplegia – spinal artery occlusion; and abdominal pain – mesenteric ischaemia) as the dissection extends.

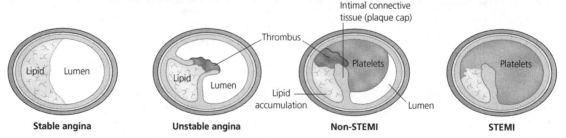

Figure J The fate of the atherosclerotic plaque. STEMI, ST-elevation myocardial infarction.

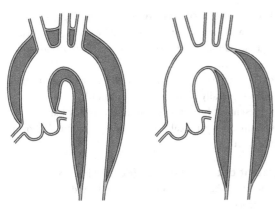

Type A aortic dissection   Type B aortic dissection

Figure K Aortic dissection classification.

> ### KEY POINT
>
> Emergency surgery is essential for type A dissections, which carry a mortality rate of up to 5% per hour.

Pulmonary embolism

- Is commonly caused by venous thromboembolism to the pulmonary artery.
- Most frequently occurs secondary to deep vein thrombosis.
- Air, fat, amniotic fluid and tumour fragments in the pulmonary artery are also possible embolic causes.
- Common risk factors for development of pulmonary embolism include major surgery, lower limb fracture, malignancy, prolonged hospitalisation and previous thromboembolism.
- Patients may present with chest pain, shortness of breath, haemoptysis or (in the case of a massive pulmonary embolism) cardiac arrest.
- Prognosis depends on the size and underlying cause of the pulmonary embolism.

> ### KEY POINT
>
> Patients presenting with pulmonary venous thromboembolism with no risk factors may have an underlying thrombophilia or malignancy.

Pulmonary hypertension

- Pulmonary hypertension is defined as *an increase in pulmonary arterial pressure >25 mmHg at rest or >30 mmHg with exercise.*

- Primary pulmonary hypertension is the diagnosis in patients with pulmonary arterial hypertension of unexplained aetiology.
- Secondary hypertension can be due to a number of causes, including multiple pulmonary emboli, connective tissue disease, congenital AV shunts and chronic left ventricular failure.
- Patients present with shortness of breath and symptoms of right-sided heart failure.
- Prognosis for primary pulmonary hypertension without treatment is very poor.

Congenital heart disease

Congenital heart disease is uncommon, affecting less than 1% of live births. However, increased numbers of patients survive into adulthood.

Atrial septal defects (ASD)

- ASD is a common congenital defect, more frequent in females.
- Direct communication between the atria, results in shunting of blood from left to right.
- Many patients with ASD are asymptomatic but symptomatic patients present with shortness of breath, stroke or heart failure.
- Larger ASDs associated with major shunting should be closed surgically or percutaneously.
- If the ASD is large and remains untreated, Eisenmenger's syndrome may develop (see p. 12).

Ventricular septal defect (VSD)

- Most common congenital abnormality.
- Incomplete separation of the ventricles allows blood flow between the ventricles (usually left to right).
- The direction of the shunt is determined by the size of the VSD and pulmonary vascular resistance. Large shunts can lead to heart failure and pulmonary hypertension causing reversal of shunt from right to left (Eisenmenger's syndrome).
- Patients with a small VSD may be asymptomatic and can be managed conservatively.
- Larger VSDs may require surgical repair.

Coarctation

- Coarctation is narrowing of the aorta in the region of the ligamentum arteriosum most commonly distal to the left subclavian artery.

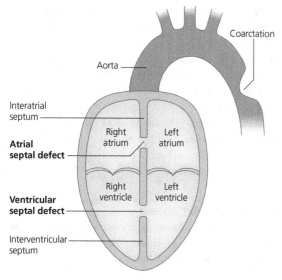

Figure L Congenital heart defects.

• 50% of patients with coarctation have a bicuspid aortic valve.
• Patients present with hypertension, radiofemoral delay, unequal upper limb pulses and a continuous murmur in the interscapular region.
• Surgical repair or stenting may be required if there is a significant gradient across the coarctation (>20 mmHg).

Cyanotic congenital heart disease
Cyanotic congenital heart disease is characterised by venous blood entering directly into the systemic circulation.

Eisenmenger's syndrome
• Eisenmenger's syndrome is a pathophysiological condition resulting from adult congenital heart disease. VSD, ASD and patent ductus arteriosus (PDA) are responsible for 80% of cases of Eisenmenger's syndrome.
• Uncorrected left-to-right shunting leads to the development of pulmonary hypertension.
• When pulmonary hypertension develops, the right-sided pressures in the heart exceed systemic pressure and cause *reversal* of the shunt.
• Deoxygenated venous blood is thus shunted from the right to the left side of the heart and enters the systemic circulation, causing the patient to develop chronic cyanosis and clubbing.
• The shunt reversal and resulting clinical consequences are known as Eisenmenger's syndrome.

Transposition of the great arteries (Figure M)
• The aorta arises from the morphological right ventricle and the pulmonary artery arises from the morphological left ventricle.
• The majority of patients have an associated PDA (physiologically corrected transposition).
• Presents at birth as a profoundly cyanotic baby.
• Immediate surgical intervention is required shortly after birth.

Patent ductus arteriosus (PDA) (Figure N)
Normally, the PDA closes after birth under hormonal influences.
• Failure of the PDA to close leads to persistent left-to-right shunting between the aorta and pulmonary artery.
• Long-term left-to-right shunting leads to increased blood flow to the pulmonary circulation, which can lead to pulmonary hypertension and Eisenmenger's syndrome.
• Closure of PDA (surgically or percutaneously) is recommended in almost all cases.

Tetralogy of Fallot (Figure O)
Is the most common cause of cyanosis in infancy after the first year of life and the long-term outcome without surgical intervention is poor. The four features of tetralogy are:

1. Overriding aorta.
2. Ventricular septal defect.
3. Pulmonary stenosis.
4. Right ventricular hypertrophy.

Pathology of the conduction system
Arrhythmias
Arrhythmia is a disturbance of the electrical rhythm of the heart. It may be described using the following terms:
• Heart rate:
  ○ *Bradycardia*: slow (heart rate <60 bpm).
  ○ *Tachycardia*: fast (heart rate >100 bpm).
• Anatomy:
  ○ *Supraventricular*: arises above the ventricles.
  ○ *Ventricular tachycardia*: arises from the ventricles.
• Time course:
  ○ *Paroxysmal*: happens intermittently and stops spontaneously.
  ○ *Persistent*: does not stop spontaneously but normal sinus rhythm can be restored with some form

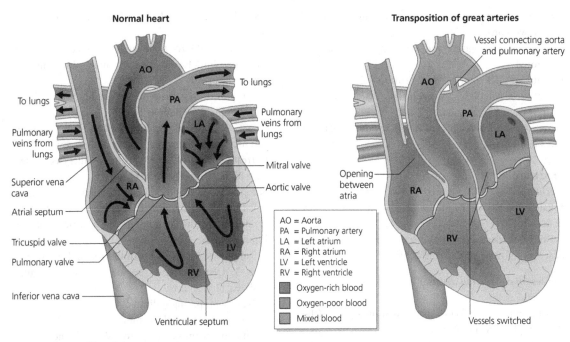

Normal heart

AO

PA

LA

To lungs

Pulmonary veins from lungs

To lungs

Pulmonary veins from lungs

Mitral valve

Aortic valve

Superior vena cava

RA

Atrial septum

Tricuspid valve

Pulmonary valve

LV

RV

Inferior vena cava

Ventricular septum

AO = Aorta
PA = Pulmonary artery
LA = Left atrium
RA = Right atrium
LV = Left ventricle
RV = Right ventricle

Oxygen-rich blood
Oxygen-poor blood
Mixed blood

Transposition of great arteries

Vessel connecting aorta and pulmonary artery

AO

PA

LA

Opening between atria

RA

LV

RV

Vessels switched

Figure M Transposition of the great arteries.

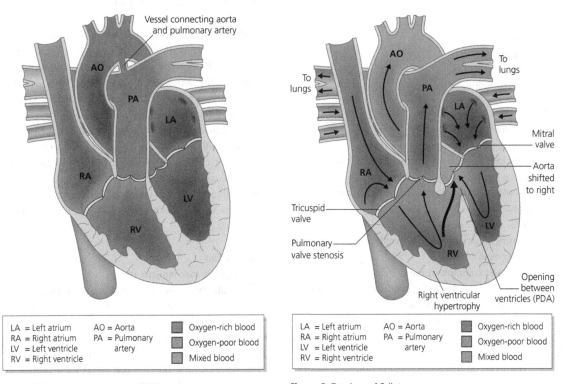

Vessel connecting aorta and pulmonary artery

AO

PA

LA

RA

LV

RV

LA = Left atrium   AO = Aorta
RA = Right atrium   PA = Pulmonary
LV = Left ventricle   artery
RV = Right ventricle

Oxygen-rich blood
Oxygen-poor blood
Mixed blood

Figure N Patent ductus arteriosus (PDA).

AO

PA

LA

To lungs

To lungs

Mitral valve

Aorta shifted to right

RA

Tricuspid valve

Pulmonary valve stenosis

LV

RV

Right ventricular hypertrophy

Opening between ventricles (PDA)

LA = Left atrium   AO = Aorta
RA = Right atrium   PA = Pulmonary
LV = Left ventricle   artery
RV = Right ventricle

Oxygen-rich blood
Oxygen-poor blood
Mixed blood

Figure O Tetralogy of Fallot.

of treatment (drugs or direct current [DC] cardioversion).

○ *Permanent*: ongoing and sinus rhythm cannot be restored.

- Width of QRS complex on the surface ECG:
  ○ Narrow-complex tachycardias (QRS width ≤120 msec; 3 small squares).
  ○ Broad-complex tachycardias (QRS width >120 msec; 3 small squares).

Bradycardias
Mechanism
- Failure of electrical impulse generation from the SA node.
- Failure of electrical impulse conduction through the heart via AV node and Bundle of His.

Causes (of conduction disease)
- Degenerative.
- Ischaemia, e.g. inferior myocardial infarction (the RCA supplies SA and AV nodes).
- Infiltrative: cardiac disease that cause infiltration of the conducting system (e.g. amyloid and sarcoidosis).
- Cardiac surgery.
- Antiarrhythmic drugs.

Presentation
- Blackouts.
- Breathlessness.
- Fatigue.
- Incidental finding.

Classification
- Sick sinus syndrome:
  ○ Incidence: common in the elderly.
  ○ Pathology: impaired SA node function. The SA node fails to generate and electrical impulse.
  ○ Symptoms: variable, ranging from no symptoms to blackouts.
  ○ ECG: sinus pauses.
  ○ Treatment: atrial pacing if symptomatic.
- First-degree AV block:
  ○ Incidence: common in the elderly.
  ○ Pathology: the AV node conducts sinus impulses more slowly to the ventricles.
  ○ Symptoms: most patients are asymptomatic.
  ○ ECG: shows a prolonged PR interval (>200 msec; 5 small squares).
  ○ Treatment: no treatment required unless associated with higher degrees of block.

- Second-degree AV block (Wenckebach or Mobitz type I):
  ○ Pathology: the AV node fatigues and conducts each successive impulse progressively more slowly until a beat is dropped.
  ○ Symptoms: most patients are asymptomatic. Some may complain of 'skipped beats'.
  ○ ECG: PR interval prolongs until an impulse fails to conduct to the ventricles and the node recovers.
  ○ Treatment: no treatment required unless associated with higher degrees of block.
- Second-degree AV block (Mobitz type II):
  ○ Pathology: intermittent failure of impulses to conduct from the AV node to the ventricles via the Bundle of His.
  ○ Symptoms: dizziness, breathlessness and syncope.
  ○ ECG: QRS complexes are dropped on a regular basis, e.g. 2:1, 3:1, etc.
  ○ Treatment: pacing indicated.
- Third-degree AV block (complete heart block):
  ○ Pathology: complete failure of AV nodal conduction.
  ○ Symptoms: syncope, breathlessness, dizziness.
  ○ ECG: complete dissociation between QRS complexes and P waves.
  ○ Treatment: pacing indicated.
- His–Purkinje disease:
  ○ Pathology: failure of conduction through the His–Purkinje system distal to the AV node. Conduction may fail through the right or left bundle branches or through the left anterior (associated with left-axis deviation) or posterior fascicles (associated with right-axis deviation).
  ○ ECG changes: variable. Right bundle branch block (RBBB), left bundle branch block (LBBB), or trifasicular block (RBBB, left-axis deviation and first-degree heart block)
  ○ RBBB and LBBB in isolation do not require pacing. Patients with trifasicular block should be considered for pacing.

Tachycardias
The two main mechanisms are:
- Automaticity: cells depolarise spontaneously. This is increased by sympathetic drive and decreased by parasympathetic drive.
- Re-entry (Figure T): occurs when there are two or more pathways of conduction within the heart that have different conduction properties (i.e. where there is an anatomical barrier such as scar tissue or pulmonary veins).

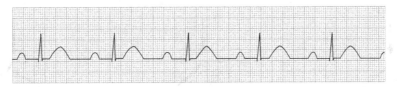

Figure P First-degree atrioventricular (AV) block. PR interval >200 mseconds.

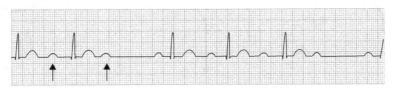

Figure Q Second-degree atrioventricular (AV) block Mobitz I. QRS complex dropped. Gradual prolongation of PR interval.

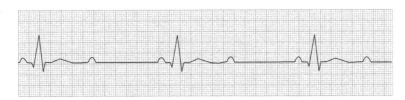

Figure R Second-degree atrioventricular (AV) block Mobitz II.

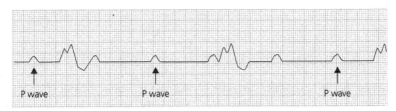

Figure S Third-degree atrioventricular (AV) block. Complete dissociation of P waves and QRS complexes.

• Patients with tachycardias of any description may present with palpitations and shortness of breath. If the tachycardia produces haemodynamic compromise (most commonly found with ventricular tachycardia and ventricular fibrillation) then patients may present with syncope or cardiac arrest.
• Tachycardias can be divided into:
  o Narrow complex (QRS ≤120 msec).
  o Broad complex (QRS >120 ms).

Narrow-complex tachycardias
Atrial fibrillation (Figure U)
• The most common arrhythmias presenting in hospital medicine and can be persistent, paroxysmal or permanent.
• Caused by *multiple* re-entry circuits in the atria.
• Triggered by ectopic beats originating in the pulmonary veins.
• Associated with enlarged or diseased atria.

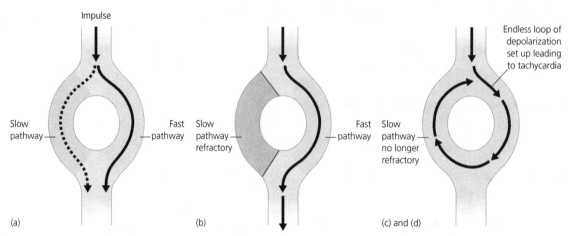

Figure T Tachycardiac re-entry mechanism. A, Conduction happens down both pathways in sinus rhythm. B, Premature early beat conduction may only be conducted down the fast pathway because the slow pathway remains refractory. C, The slow pathway is no longer refractory by the time the wave front reaches the distal aspect of the pathway and so conduction occurs down the slow pathway in the opposite direction. D, The wave front then travels down and re-enters the fast pathway setting up an endless loop of depolarisation and a tachycardia.

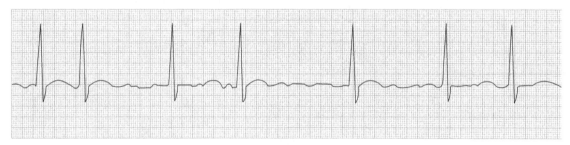

Figure U Atrial fibrillation.

• ECG is characterised by an irregularly irregular ventricular rhythm and by the absence of discrete P waves.

Atrial flutter (Figure V)

• Results from *one single* large re-entry circuit within the *right atrium.*

• Flutter circuit is centred around the tricuspid valve ring and strip of tissue in this vicinity can be targeted with ablation for curative treatment.

• The AV node limits the ventricular response to the atrial flutter. The atria normally depolarize at 300 bpm. Often a 2:1 or 4:1 block occurs, resulting in a ventricular rate of 150 or 75 bpm.

• ECG is characterised by a saw-tooth baseline.

Supraventricular tachycardias (SVTs) (Figure W)

• Can be divided into atrioventricular re-entrant (AVRT) and atrioventricular nodal re-entrant tachycardias (AVNRT).

• AVRT occurs when there is an accessory pathway between the atria and ventricles resulting in a re-entry circuit.

• AVNRT: there are two conduction pathways *within* the AV node and re-entrant tachycardia can be set up *within the node itself.*

Broad-complex tachycardias

Ventricular tachycardias

The underlying pathology is automatic activity or re-entry caused by:

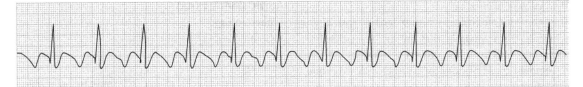

Figure V Atrial flutter. Saw tooth baseline with 2:1 block.

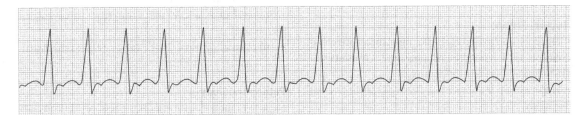

Figure W Supraventricular tachycardia.

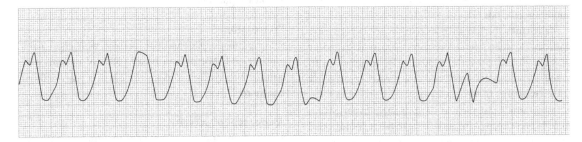

Figure X Ventricular tachycardia.

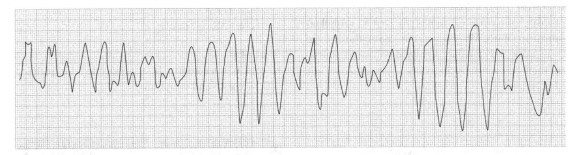

Figure Y Ventricular fibrillation.

- Ischaemic heart disease: re-entrant VT occurs around the infarct scar.
- Cardiomyopathies: can affect the His–Purkinje system and lead to re-entry.
- Normal heart VT: some patients have a structurally normal heart and present with VT during exercise. The mechanism is automatic and catecholamine driven. These patients have a good prognosis.

- Ion-channel defects: mutations affecting genes for cardiac ion channels can lead to unusual forms of VT. Examples include long QT syndrome (LQTS) and Brugada syndrome.
- Ventricular rate may range from 100 to 300 bpm with symptoms ranging from mild chest pain to complete cardiovascular collapse and cardiac arrest.

Ventricular fibrillation

The underlying mechanism is re-entry and automaticity.

• Results when multiple sites in the ventricles fire impulses rapidly in an uncoordinated fashion.

• Common mode of death in patients with ischaemic heart disease.

• Death follows within a few minutes, unless a normal rhythm is restored with immediate defibrillation.

Hypertension

• Hypertension is diagnosed after three successive measurements of a systolic blood pressure >140 mmHg or diastolic blood pressure >90 mmHg.

• Hypertension is a major risk factor for cardiovascular morbidity.

• 95% of cases are described as 'essential hypertension'.

• 5% of cases are described as 'secondary hypertension' and may be reversed with treatment of the underlying condition (see Box G).

• Malignant hypertension occurs in <1% of hypertensive patients (systolic blood pressure >200 mmHg and/or diastolic blood pressure >130 mmHg) together with grade 3 and 4 retinopathy and is a medical emergency with a mortality of 90% in 1 year.

• Long-term consequences of untreated hypertension include end-organs damage leading to heart failure, renal disease, vascular disease and hypertensive retinopathy.

Valvular heart disease

Valvular heart disease is commonly seen in cardiology outpatient clinics. Many patients are asymptomatic and are regularly monitored for signs and symptoms of deterioration. Assessment includes history, examination and echocardiography.

Aortic stenosis (AS)

Epidemiology

• Commonest valve lesion in the UK.

Aetiology

• Degenerative calcific disease is the most frequent cause in the elderly.

• Bicuspid aortic valves.

• Rheumatic valve disease.

• Supravalvular: above the valve (e.g. supravalvular membrane).

• Subvalvular: below the valve (e.g. subvalvular membrane).

Pathophysiology

Stenosis of the aortic valve leads to pressure overload and:

• Left ventricular hypertrophy.

• Left ventricular failure.

• Low output state.

Presentation

• Symptomatic patients may present with chest pain, syncope and shortness of breath; 50% of patients presenting with syncope and AS will die in 3 years without a valve replacement.

Assessment of severity

• Echocardiographic parameters for grading peak AS are:
  ○ Mild AS: 20–40 mmHg.
  ○ Moderate AS: 40–60 mmHg.
  ○ Severe AS: >60 mmHg.

Treatment

• Surgical intervention is recommended for patients with severe AS and symptoms.

Box G Secondary causes of hypertension

• Intrinsic renal disease (glomerulonephritis, polycystic kidneys, polyarteritis nodosa, etc.)
• Renovascular disease (renal artery stenosis).
• Endocrine causes (Cushing's syndrome, Conn's syndrome, phaeochromocytoma, acromegaly, hyperparathyroidism).
• Coarctation of the aorta.

KEY POINT

Percutaneous aortic valve replacement is currently available at some tertiary centres for elderly patients with critical AS who are unable to undergo open heart surgery. Further developments in this area are expected in the future.

Mitral stenosis (MS)

Epidemiology

Incidence of MS has significantly declined in developed countries due to reduction in the major cause – rheumatic fever.

Aetiology

MS may be caused by narrowing of the mitral valve orifice at the:

- Cusps (thicken and calcify).
- Commissures (fuse with the valve cusps but they are still mobile).

Pathophysiology

Narrowing of the mitral valve orifice leads to:

- A rise in left atrial pressures.
- Left atrial dilation.
- Pulmonary hypertension.
- Atrial fibrillation.

Presentation

- Breathlessness, fatigue, atrial fibrillation, peripheral embolism.

Specific medical treatments

- Anticoagulation is very important, the incidence of peripheral embolism is high.
- Rate control of atrial fibrillation.
- Diuretics for heart failure.

Indications for invasive intervention

- Severe MS.
- Poor symptom control.
- Progressive pulmonary hypertension.
- Recurrent peripheral embolism.

Interventions

- Percutaneous balloon valvotomy (offered only to carefully selected patients).
- Surgical mitral valve replacement.

Pulmonary stenosis

- Rare.
- Often associated with congenital heart disease.
- Can be treated by balloon valvotomy.

Tricuspid stenosis (TS)

- Rare.

- Carcinoid is the most common causes.
- Tricuspid valve replacement rarely required.

Aortic regurgitation (AR)

Epidemiology

- Accounts for 10% of all valvular heart disease.

Aetiology

- Onset may be acute (e.g. infective endocarditis) or chronic (e.g. secondary to bicuspid aortic valve).
- May be caused by destruction of the valve leaflets (e.g. infective endocarditis, rheumatic fever, bicuspid aortic valves, trauma and degenerative calcific AS), *or by*
- Dilation of the aortic root, leading to failure of the valve leaflets to coapt (aortic dissection, Marfan's syndrome and aortitis).

Pathophysiology

AR leads to:

- Increased volume load as blood leaks through the aortic valve back into the left ventricle.
- Increased stroke volume in the short term.
- Dilatation and failure of the left ventricle in the long term.

Presentation

- Shortness of breath, palpitations, fatigue.
- Chronic AR can be tolerated well for many years and is associated with a good prognosis.

Treatment

- Medical treatment includes good blood pressure control (afterload reduction) with calcium channel blockers and vasodilators (ACE inhibitors).
- Acute severe AR is associated with a high mortality and requires immediate intervention.
- Aortic valve replacement surgery is considered when patients develop symptoms of heart failure, deterioration in left ventricular function, or significant dilation of the left ventricle (based on echocardiographic criteria).

Mitral regurgitation (MR)

Epidemiology

- Common valve lesion.

Aetiology

- Onset may be acute (e.g. papillary muscle rupture) or chronic (e.g. mitral valve prolapse).

• May occur due to destruction or malfunction the valve leaflets or chordae (e.g. mitral valve prolapse, infective endocarditis, rheumatic fever), *or*
• Damage to the papillary muscles (e.g. post-myocardial infarction), *or*
• Dilation of the left ventricle, causing mitral annular dilatation and failure of mitral valve leaflet coaptation.

Pathophysiology

MR leads to:
• Increase in left atrial volume and size.
• Increase in left atrial pressure and pulmonary oedema.
• Increase in left ventricular size and left ventricular failure (volume overload).

Presentation

• Shortness of breath, palpitations, atrial fibrillation, fatigue.
• Prognosis is poor in severe MR, with 33% survival at 8 years without surgical intervention.

Treatment

• Medical treatment includes diuretic therapy. Patients in atrial fibrillation are treated with anticoagulation and rate-controlling medications.
• Surgical treatment is indicated in those with severe MR and symptoms or those with deteriorating left ventricular function. Surgical options include: mitral valve repair (preferred if technically feasible) or mitral valve replacement.

Tricuspid regurgitation (TR)
Epidemiology

TR is a common valve lesion.

Aetiology

TR may occur due to:
• Destruction of valve cusps (e.g. rheumatic fever, endocarditis, carcinoid).
• Dilatation of the right ventricle leading to tricuspid annular dilatation (e.g. right heart failure, pulmonary hypertension).

Presentation

• May present with symptoms of right heart failure (see p. 21).

Treatment

• Right heart failure symptoms are treated with diuretics.
• Surgical valve replacement is accompanied by a high operative mortality and is rarely indicated. Valve repair may be undertaken with tricuspid annuloplasty in conjunction with surgery for left-sided valvular disease.

Pulmonary regurgitation

• Mild regurgitation is often seen in normal individuals and is of no clinical consequence.
• May be secondary to pulmonary hypertension.
• Rarely requires surgical intervention.

General approach to treatment of valve pathology

Valve disease treatments include:
• Valvotomy:
  ○ Fused valve leaflets are divided surgically.
• Balloon valvuloplasty:
  ○ Fused valve leaflets are divided by inflating a balloon, which is passed percutaneously.
• Valve repair:
  ○ Preferable to valve replacement if possible, as native valve tissue is preserved (commonly carried out for isolated posterior mitral valve leaflet prolapse).
• Valve replacement with a:
  ○ Bioprosthesis (types: porcine or allograft). No need for anticoagulation, but shorter life span than mechanical valves (10 years).
  ○ Mechanical (types: ball and cage, tilting disc or bi-leaflet), require anticoagulation (target international normalised ratio [INR] 2.5–4.5, depending on valve prosthesis and position).

Infective endocarditis

• Incidence of 1500 cases/annum in the UK.
• Infection may settle on:
  ○ Native valves – diseased valves (e.g. AS, mitral valve prolapse) or the sites of vascular or myocardial abnormalities (e.g. coarctation, VSD or PDA).
  ○ Right-sided valves – commonly occurs in intravenous drug users.
  ○ Prosthetic valves – common in the immediate post operative period (1%) but declines thereafter.
• Patients may present with:
  ○ Fever, new murmur, malaise, weight loss and non-specific symptoms.
  ○ Diagnosis can be made using the Dukes classification (see Box H).
• Causative organisms include:
  ○ Streptococci (*S. viridens, S. pneumoniae*, Lancefield groups B, C and G, *S. bovis*), staphylococci (90% *Staph aureus*), enterococci, Gram-negative organisms and fungal infections (see Box 14.1 p. 133).

> **Box H Duke criteria for diagnosis of endocarditis**
>
> **Major criteria**
> - Positive blood cultures
>   - Typical microorganisms consistent with infective endocarditis from two separate blood cultures
>   - Persistent positive blood cultures of blood samples taken >12 hours apart
>   - Three or more positive cultures taken over more than 1 hour apart
> - Evidence of endocardial involvement noted on echocardiography
>   - New valvular regurgitation
>   - Abscess
>   - Vegetations
>
> **Minor criteria**
> - Predisposing valvular or cardiac abnormality
> - Fever: temperature >38°C
> - Vasculitic phenomena
> - Embolic phenomena
> - Microbiological evidence: positive blood culture but does not meet major criteria
> - Suggestive echocardiographic findings
>
> **Clinical diagnosis for infective endocarditis requires:**
> - Two major criteria, or
> - One major and three minor criteria, or
> - Five minor criteria

- There are multiple systemic complications.
- The associated mortality is high 10–20%.
- Treatment includes long-term intravenous antibiotics and surgery in complex cases (see Table 14.3, p. 134).

Heart failure

Heart failure is defined as a state in which the cardiac output is unable to match metabolic needs of the tissues. Prevalence of heart failure is around 3% of the general population, 20% in 70-to-80-year-olds.

Classification

- Anatomical – left, right and biventricular failure:
  - *Left-sided heart failure*: occurs when the left ventricle is predominantly affected. Patients present with left-sided heart failure symptoms (pulmonary oedema).
  - *Right-sided heart failure*: occurs when the right ventricle is predominantly affected. Patients present with right-sided heart failure symptoms (oedema, ascites, hepatomegaly).
  - *Biventricular failure*: both ventricles are affected. Patients present with a mixture of right- and left-sided heart failure symptoms and signs.
- Systolic and diastolic heart failure:
  - *Systolic.* Symptoms and signs of left heart failure with reduced left ventricular ejection fraction.
  - *Diastolic.* There are symptoms and signs of left heart failure with a preserved left ventricular ejection fraction. Also known as HFNEF (heart failure with normal ejection fraction).
- Pathology:
  - Cardiomyopathy:
    - Restrictive e.g. amyloid.
    - Dilated e.g. alcohol, post-viral, ischaemic.
    - Hypertrophic e.g. HOCM.

Presentation

May present as acute, chronic and acute-on chronic heart failure:
- *Acute heart failure*: sudden-onset of heart failure symptoms (shortness of breath and orthopnoea). May be due to 'de novo' causes (e.g. acute myocardial infarction, acute myocarditis, valvular rupture) or acute decompensation on the background of chronic heart failure (acute-on chronic)
- *Chronic heart failure*: gradual onset of symptoms of heart failure (e.g. due to cardiomyopathy).

Pathophysiology (Figure Z)

Heart failure pathophysiology is a vicious cycle which is initiated when there is a reduction in cardiac output leading to decreased blood pressure and reduced tissue perfusion or an increased demand (see Box E, p. 9).

Treatment

- Preload and afterload reduction with diuretics and nitrates.
- Disease-modifying drugs: prognostic benefit is gained from ACE inhibitors, aldosterone antagonists and beta blockers.
- Devices: cardiac resynchronization devices and intracardiac defibrillators can reduce mortality and improve symptoms in carefully selected patient groups.
- Transplantation: considered in patients with severe symptoms despite optimal medical treatments but is limited by shortage of donor organs.

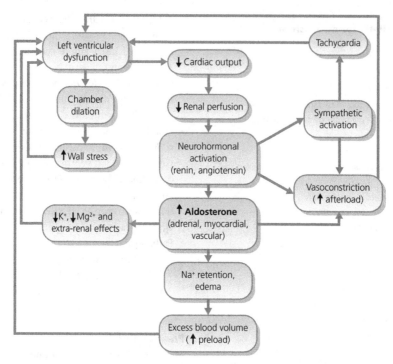

Figure Z The vicious cycle of heart failure.

• Prognosis: poor with median survival 3–5 years from time of diagnosis.

Pericardial diseases
Pericarditis
• Results from primary and secondary inflammation of the parietal and visceral pericardium.
• The majority of cases are viral or idiopathic.
• Patients present with sharp pleuritic chest pain, which is relieved on sitting forward.
• Outcome is largely benign. However, a minority of patients develop chronic relapsing pericarditis.

Pericardial effusion and tamponade
• There is normally a small amount of fluid (<50 ml) in the pericardial sac, which comes from the visceral pericardium.
• Large effusions can become life threatening and cause haemodynamic compromise because the heart is in a confined space and cannot fill properly.
• The most common causes of large pericardial effusions are malignancy, uraemia or tuberculosis (TB).
• Patients most commonly present with shortness of breath.
• Clinical signs of tamponade are tachycardia, pulsus paradoxus, muffled heart sounds and hypotension.

• Small pericardial effusions are harmless and can be managed conservatively.
• Treatment is based on the degree of haemodynamic compromise.

Constrictive pericarditis
• Pericardium becomes thickened and fibrotic and attaches to the myocardium; diastolic filling of the heart becomes restricted.
• Most cases are seen following acute viral or bacterial pericarditis, cardiac surgery or radiotherapy. TB is a likely cause in developing countries.
• Patients present with symptoms and signs of right heart failure.
• Diagnosis can be difficult and is aided by Doppler echocardiography, right- and left-heart catheterisation, cardiac CT and cardiac MR.
• Pericardectomy (stripping) of the pericardium can be carried out for relief of symptoms but carries a high mortality.

References
Durack DT, Lukes AS, Bright DK. New criteria for diagnosis of infective endocarditis: utilization of specific echocardiographic findings. Duke Endocarditis Service. *American Journal of Medicine* 1994: **96**(3);200–9.

Approach to the patient

History

This should be taken carefully and thoroughly, as most diagnoses are made from the patient history. You should always introduce yourself at the start of the consultation, giving your name and position, and ask for consent to take a history.

Presenting complaint

The consultation should start with an open question to determine the presenting complaint, e.g. 'What is your main health problem at the moment?'. The most common presenting complaints in cardiology are chest pain, palpitations, breathlessness and syncope. The aim of taking a history is to establish the cause of the symptoms and how they are affecting the patient's life.

Chest pain

Chest pain is a very common presenting complaint in the emergency room. It is essential that an accurate and complete chest pain history is taken rapidly to identify chest pain due to life-threatening causes such as acute coronary syndrome, aortic dissection or a massive pulmonary embolism. Once these life-threatening pathologies have been excluded, musculoskeletal, abdominal and respiratory causes of chest pain can be considered.

Cardiology: Clinical Cases Uncovered. By T. Betts, J. Dwight and S. Bull. Published 2010 by Blackwell Publishing.

> **KEY POINT**
>
> Time is of the essence when dealing with patients where the differential diagnosis includes MI because rapid, appropriate treatment can significantly improve mortality and morbidity rates in these patients – a principle summarised by Gibson as 'time is myocardium and time is outcome'.

Important points when taking a chest pain history

> **KEY POINT**
>
> The mnemonic 'SOCRATES' is helpful when taking a chest pain history.
> **S**ite
> **O**nset
> **C**haracter
> **R**adiation
> **A**ssociated features
> **T**iming
> **E**xacerbating/relieving features
> **S**everity of pain

It is important to remember that patients may refer to chest 'discomfort' rather than admitting to pain.

- Site:
  - The classic description of ischaemic cardiac pain is central.
  - Pain due to aortic dissection may be described as 'tearing'. A *posterior MI* can also present with inter-scapular pain.

- **Onset, trigger and frequency:**
  - Establish how quickly the pain started and what the patient was doing at the time.
  - Sudden onset of extremely severe chest pain is highly suggestive of aortic dissection.
  - In angina and ACS the pain often builds up to a maximum over a few minutes rather than reaching a maximum level instantly.
  - 'Crescendo angina' is characterised by increasing frequency and intensity of chest pain attacks.
- **Character:**
  - Ischaemic cardiac pain is often described as a 'chest heaviness' or as a 'crushing' central chest pain. It may be highly variable or absent in elderly or diabetic patients.
  - Pathology affecting the pleura or pericardium (pneumonia, pulmonary embolism, pericarditis). results in pleuritic chest pain (pain worse on inspiration) often described as 'sharp'.
- **Radiation:**
  - Ischaemic cardiac pain may radiate to the jaw and inner aspect of the left arm.
- **Associated features:**
  - Ischaemic cardiac pain may be associated with autonomic symptoms such as sweating, palpitations, breathlessness, vomiting and dizziness.
  - Respiratory causes of chest pain (pulmonary embolism/pneumonia) may be associated with haemoptysis, sputum, breathlessness and wheeze.
  - Syncope may occur in the case of a massive pulmonary embolism or secondary to an arrhythmia.
  - Aortic dissection may be associated with autonomic symptoms, neurological features (if the carotids are involved) abdominal pain or acute limb ischaemia (if the mesenteric artery or iliac vessels are involved).
- **Timing and duration.** It is important to establish the duration and time of onset of the worst episode of chest pain for the following reasons:
  - Timing of investigations. Troponin should be requested 8–12 hours after the worst episode of chest pain in patients with suspected myocardial infarction to maximise diagnostic accuracy.
  - May assist diagnosis. Pain from angina is relieved within a few minutes rest or by a GTN spray. Pain lasting for many hours is unlikely to be due to angina.
  - May influence treatment strategy, e.g. in a patient with a late presentation of STEMI (worst pain experienced >24 hours ago) the risks of immediate percutaneous intervention or thrombolysis may outweigh the benefits and a conservative management plan may be adopted.
- **Exacerbating and relieving factors. Chest pain is:**
  - Exacerbated by exertion and cold weather and relieved at rest or with GTN spray if it is due to angina pectoris.
  - Exacerbated by inspiration and relieved when sitting forwards if it is due to pericarditis.
- **Severity:**
  - Ask the patient to rate the severity of the chest pain on a scale 0–10, where 0 represents a pain free state and 10 is the worst pain they can imagine.
- **Assessment of risk.** In addition to taking an extensive chest pain history, it is important to assess the probability of atheromatous disease in patients on the basis of their cardiac risk profile. These are accepted risk factors for heart disease:
  - Smoking.
  - Hypercholesterolaemia.
  - Family history of premature cardiovascular disease (first-degree relatives – male aged less than 55 years or female less than 65 years).
  - Diabetes.
  - Hypertension.
  - Renal disease.
  - Male gender.
  - Ethnic group, i.e. Asian origin.

> **KEY POINT**
>
> The three main life-threatening differential diagnoses to consider when taking a history from a sick patient presenting with chest pain are myocardial infarction, pulmonary embolism and aortic dissection – these all require immediate and appropriate treatment.

Palpitations

The dictionary definition of palpitations is 'an unpleasant awareness of the heart beat'. Palpitations are generally a benign symptom unless associated with syncope or presyncope. It is important that a careful history is taken to differentiate between patients with benign and malignant arrhythmias.

Box I Causes of chest pain

- Cardiac:
  - Angina pectoris.
  - Acute myocardial infarction.
  - Arrhythmia.
  - Pericarditis.
  - AS.
  - Hypertrophic obstructive cardiomyopathy (HOCM).
- Aortic:
  - Aortitis.
  - Expanding aneurysm.
  - Aortic dissection.
- Respiratory:
  - Pulmonary embolism.
  - Pneumonia.
  - Pneumothorax.
  - TB.
  - Malignancy.
- Gastrointestinal (GI):
  - Oesophageal spasms/reflux.
  - Gall stones.
  - Mallory-Weiss tear.
- Musculoskeletal:
  - Costochondritis.
  - Trauma.
  - Prolapsed disc.
- Psychiatric:
  - Anxiety disorders.

KEY POINT

A useful technique to clarify the patient's symptoms is to ask the patient to tap out an example of their heart beat when they have 'palpitations'. This can give the clinician an idea of the speed and regularity of the heart beat when the patient experiences symptoms.

Important points when taking a history from a patient with palpitations

- Establish what the patient means by 'palpitations'. Is it:
  - A fast heart beat?(Sinus tachycardia, atrial tachycardias.)
  - A heart beat that is more 'forceful'? (Ventricular ectopics.)
  - Slower heart beat than normal? (Complete heart block, slow atrial fibrillation.)
  - Sensation of the heart having 'skipped a beat'? (Ventricular ectopics.)
  - Is the heart beat regular or irregular when the symptoms are experienced?
- Onset, duration and frequency of symptoms:
  - Gradual onset and resolution is more suggestive of a sinus tachycardia.
  - Sudden onset of symptoms and sudden termination make it more likely that the patient is experiencing a paroxysmal tachycardia.
  - Symptoms that last for seconds only are most likely to be due to ventricular ectopy.
  - Tachyarrhythmias can last anything from a few seconds to several minutes or hours.
  - It is important to establish the frequency of symptoms (several times a day/once a week/month/year?). This will influence investigation and treatment decisions (e.g. a 24-hour holter is most likely to aid diagnosis in patients who are symptomatic at least once a day).
- Establish whether there are any exacerbating or relieving factors:
  - If vagal manoeuvres can relieve/terminate symptoms, the most likely diagnosis is a supraventricular tachycardia.
  - Alcohol can trigger a sinus tachycardia, atrial flutter and fibrillation.
  - Caffeine can trigger sinus tachycardia and extrasystoles.
  - Exertion can induce ischaemic ventricular tachycardia, exercise-induced ventricular tachycardia or right ventricle outflow tract tachycardia and can reduce benign extrasystoles.
  - Anxiety or emotional stress can induce sinus tachycardia.
- Associated symptoms may include the following:
  - Pre-syncope and syncope; this suggests that the arrhythmia is causing significant haemodynamic compromise (limiting flow of blood to the brain and thus leading to syncope).
  - Breathlessness; may occur due to secondary cardiac failure.
  - Chest pain; a significant tachycardia may give rise to angina as a result of increased myocardial oxygen demand.

- Previous cardiac history:
  - Patients with a known structural abnormality of the heart or a previous cardiac history are predisposed to arrhythmias.
  - Patients with a past medical history of ischaemic heart disease are much more likely to suffer from ventricular tachycardia.
  - A history of hypertension and ischaemic heart disease predisposes patients to atrial fibrillation.
- Family history:
  - A family history of early sudden cardiac death may point to inherited causes of heart disease. Patients with Brugada, LQTS and HOCM may present with palpitations and syncope.

> **KEY POINT**
>
> Syncope associated with palpitations is a sinister symptom. It may result from an arrhythmia that carries a high risk of sudden cardiac death and causes haemodynamic compromise.

Breathlessness

Breathlessness is the sensation of not being able to get enough air. It is important to determine whether the breathlessness is cardiac, respiratory or psychogenic in origin. Breathlessness due to cardiac causes includes left ventricular failure, myocardial ischaemia and arrhythmias (tachycardias or bradycardias).

Important points when taking a history from a patient with breathlessness

- *Triggers*. It is important to establish in which situations the patient gets breathless:
  - Exertional dyspnoea is common to both cardiac and respiratory causes of breathlessness. If there is associated chest pain a diagnosis of ischaemic heart disease is more likely.
  - Orthopnoea is a feature of heart failure and chronic obstructive airways disease (COPD). The patient feels breathless when lying flat (increased venous return leads to pulmonary oedema) and better when sitting upright.
  - Paroxysmal nocturnal dyspnoea is a fairly specific symptom for diagnosis of heart failure. Characteristically, the patient wakes at night with breathlessness that is relieved with sitting or standing.

> **KEY POINT**
>
> Asking the patient how many pillows they sleep on is helpful in establishing whether they need to sleep upright due to orthopnoea (this is likely if they sleep on >3 pillows).

> **Box J Causes of palpitations**
>
> **Sinus tachycardias (augmented stroke volume)**
> - Anaemia.
> - Hyperthyroidism.
> - Fever.
> - Phaeochromocytoma.
> - Drugs.
>
> **Intermittent tachycardias**
> - SVTs (AV nodal re-entry tachycardia, atrial tachycardias).
> - Ventricular tachycardias.
> - Atrial fibrillation.
>
> **Bradycardia**
> - Sinus node disease or second- or third-degree AV block.
>
> **Extrasystoles**
> - Ventricular and atrial premature beats.
>
> **Non-cardiac**
> - Emotional stress, anxiety and hyperventilation syndrome.

- *Onset, duration and exercise tolerance*. It is important to establish when the symptoms started. When was the last time that the breathing was 'normal'?
  - Sudden onset of breathlessness is suggestive of massive pulmonary embolism, acute asthma, pneumothorax, flash pulmonary oedema and cardiac arrhythmias.
  - Gradual onset of symptoms may represent chronic respiratory pathology, e.g. COPD, pulmonary fibrosis.
  - Establish how far the patient can walk before they get breathless and how this compares to their exercise tolerance before they became unwell and the rate of deterioration of their symptoms.
- *Associated symptoms*:
  - Cough: a history of a cough may present in patients with COPD, asthma, interstitial lung disease, lung cancer and heart failure.

Box K Causes of ankle oedema

Local causes
- Impaired venous return – pregnancy, immobility.
- Obstruction of venous return – deep vein thrombosis (DVT), pelvic mass (ovarian cyst or malignancy).
- Calf muscle pump damage – paraplegia.
- Cellulitis.
- Lymphatic obstruction – filariasis, malignant involvement of inguinal nodes.
- Congenital – Milroy's disease.

Systemic causes
- Congestive cardiac failure.
- Hypoalbuminaemia, e.g. liver disease, malnutrition, nephrotic syndrome.

Box L Causes of breathlessness

- Cardiac:
  - Heart failure.
  - Myocardial ischaemia (angina).
  - Arrhythmias.
  - Congenital heart disease.
  - Pericardial disease.
  - Valvular heart disease.
- Respiratory:
  - COPD.
  - Infections – pneumonia, TB, bronchiectasis.
  - Pulmonary embolism.
  - Lung cancer.
  - Pneumothorax.
  - Pleural effusion.
  - Restrictive lung disease – pulmonary fibrosis and alveolitis.
- Anaemia.
- Renal failure:
  - Kussmaul's respiration secondary to metabolic acidosis.
- Hyperthyroidism.
- Deconditioning and obesity.
- Neuromuscular.
- Anxiety.

○ Haemoptysis: this is a red flag symptom for lung carcinoma. Other underlying causes include pulmonary embolism, COPD, bronchiectasis and heart failure.

○ Wheeze: can be a feature of asthma, COPD and heart failure ('cardiac asthma').

○ Ankle oedema: common incidental finding in the elderly. However, there are many causes and in conjunction with breathlessness it may support the diagnosis of heart failure.

Syncope

The dictionary definition of syncope is: *the temporary loss of consciousness (awareness of oneself and surroundings) with spontaneous recovery.* Dizziness and syncope are common in the elderly. These symptoms affect one third of people over the age of 65 years. The causes of these symptoms are multiple; however, cardiac pathology accounts for 15% of all episodes.

KEY POINT

Cardiac causes of syncope are associated with a 5-fold greater mortality than other causes. It is therefore important to take a detailed history to identify high-risk patients.

Important points when taking a history from a patient with syncope

• *Witnesses*. If a patient has blacked out, a history from a witness can be invaluable in helping establishing a diagnosis. Useful questions to ask a witness include:

○ Were there tonic–clonic movements? (Consistent with epilepsy.)

○ Was there urinary incontinence and tongue biting? (Epilepsy more likely.)

○ Was the patient pale prior to collapse? (Consistent with neurocardiogenic syncope.)

• *Prodrome and trigger*. It is important to establish what the patient was doing at the time and whether they had any symptoms prior to collapse:

○ No warning prior to collapse is typical for a 'Stokes Adams' attack (cardiac syncope), where collapse is due to a cardiac arrhythmia causing haemodynamic compromise.

○ Nausea or painful stimuli prior to collapse points to a more likely to a benign 'faint'

○ Syncope on exertion is more likely if it is due to outflow obstruction, e.g. AS or HOCM.

Box M Cardiac causes of syncope

Cardiac arrhythmia
- Bradycardia:
  - Sinus node dysfunction.
  - Atrioventricular block.
  - Drug induced (beta blocker, amiodarone).
- Tachycardia:
  - Paroxysmal atrial fibrillation.
  - SVTs.
  - Ventricular tachycardias.
  - Inherited (LQTS, Brugada syndrome).

Neurally mediated syncope
- Vasovagal syncope.
- Situational syncope.
- Carotid sinus hypersensitivity.

Orthostatic hypotension
- Autonomic failure.
- Drug induced.
- Volume depletion.

Other causes
- Atrial myxoma.
- Left ventricular outflow obstruction (e.g. HOCM).
- AS.
- Large pulmonary embolism.
- Cardiac tamponade.

- Collapse when the patient gets up from a seated position makes postural hypotension a more likely diagnosis.
- Epileptic seizures may be preceded by an aura.
- Syncope after neck rotation or neck pressure may be due to carotid sinus hypersensitivity and after neck extension may be due to basilar artery insufficiency.

- *Syncope and recovery*:
  - A prompt recovery time with return to normal conscious state is usual with cardiac syncope.
  - Prolonged recovery time with a period of reduced consciousness may occur with hypoglycaemia and epilepsy.

- *Injuries*:
  - Patients who suffer from cardiac syncope may present with severe injuries (broken limbs, broken nose, head injuries) because they collapse with no warning.

- *Frequency of episodes*:
  - Important to establish the frequency of syncope as this will be important when planning diagnostic tests and assessing the impact on the patient's quality of life.

- *Drug history*:
  - Diuretics and antihypertensive medication may lead to excessive BP reduction and cause postural hypotension, particularly in frail elderly patients.
  - Antiarrhythmic drugs (beta blocker, calcium-channel antagonists, amiodarone) can induce symptomatic bradycardias.
  - Hypoglycaemic medications may cause symptomatic hypoglycaemia.
  - Recreational drugs (cocaine) can cause arrhythmias.

Examination

You should obtain informed consent before starting the examination of the patient. Ensure that the patient is comfortable. Examination of the cardiovascular system ideally requires positioning of the patient in a seated position at an angle of 45 degrees.

Routine

Cardiac examination is best carried out and presented in a methodical fashion in the following order:
- General inspection.
- Hands and arms.
- Neck.
- Face.
- Precordium.
- Abdomen.
- Lower limbs.

General inspection

General observation should ideally be made from the end of the bed. The approach will vary slightly according to the setting. In an emergency setting the 'ABC' (Airway, Breathing, Circulation) approach will take priority.

The bedside

- *Telemetry*: is the patient being monitored for arrhythmias? Are the complexes on the monitor regular or irregular (sinus rhythm/atrial fibrillation)? Are there pacing spikes?
- *Medication*: is there a GTN spray or any other medication on the bedside table?
- *Oxygen*: is the patient able to achieve adequate saturations without oxygen supplementation?
- *Other equipment and devices*: is there an intravenous cannula (e.g. intravenous diuretics or antibiotics)?

• *Notices above the bed*: e.g. 'fluid intake restricted to 1 litre a day' are common in patients with decompensated heart failure.

The patient's demeanour
• Comfortable or in pain?
• Fully conscious and cooperative, or drowsy and confused?

Body habitus
• *Obese*? Associated with increased risk of ischaemic heart disease.
• *Cachectic*? Associated with chronic cardiac failure.
• *Marfanoid* (tall with long arm span)? Associated with aortic valve disease and aortic dissection.

Breathing
• Assess respiratory rate.
• Note use of accessory muscles (suggestive of COPD).
• Pattern:
  ○ *Kussmaul's respiration*: deep sighing breaths seen in metabolic acidosis.
  ○ *Cheyne Stokes respiration*: alternative deep rapid breaths and shallow slow breaths with periods of apnoea occurring in cycles. This is caused by damage to the respiratory centre in the brainstem (e.g. caused by stroke) or slow circulation time (heart failure).
• Breath sounds:
  ○ Wheeze (pulmonary oedema, asthma and COPD).
  ○ Basal crackles (pulmonary oedema).

Face
Note in particular if there is:
• Mitral facies or a malar flush indicative of possible mitral valve pathology.
• Dysmorphism.
• Central cyanosis.

Chest
Check the front and the back of the chest wall and lift the arms to check for surgical scars:
• A mid-line sternotomy scar is found in patients with previous cardiac surgery, e.g. coronary arterial bypass graft surgery or valve placement.
• A scar at the apex indicates that mitral valve surgery may have taken place.

Box N Dysmorphism and cardiac lesions

• *Hypertelorism* (wide set eyes): associated with pulmonary stenosis.
• *Elfin facies* (receding jaw, flared nostrils, pointed ears): associated with supravalvular AS.
• *Down's syndrome* (trisomy 21): associated with valve defects, atrial and VSDs.

• Look for scars over the right and left pre-pectoral area, suggestive of pacemaker or internal cardiac defibrillator implantation.

Legs and arms
• Veins for coronary artery bypass grafting are generally harvested from the medial aspect of the legs.
• The radial artery is sometimes harvested from the arms.

Hands and arms
Hands signs
During the cardiac examination the main signs to assess in the hands are:
• *Temperature*: assessment of peripheral perfusion:
  ○ A low cardiac output state may lead to cold clammy hands, prolonged capillary refill (>3 seconds).
  ○ A hyperdynamic circulation may lead to warm hands and normal capillary refill.
• *Nicotine staining*.
• *Finger clubbing*. Clubbing is swelling of the tissue of the terminal phalanx causing a loss of nail angle and increased bogginess of the nail bed. Cardiac causes include:
  ○ Cyanotic congenital heart disease.
  ○ Infective endocarditis.
• Vasculitic lesions associated with endocarditis:
  ○ Splinter haemorrhages on finger and toe nails (may also be caused by trauma).
  ○ Osler's nodes are painful pulp infarcts on fingers and toes or palms and soles.
  ○ Janeway lesions are painless flat areas of erythema on palms and soles.
• *Xanthomata*. These are yellowish deposits of lipids on tendons, skin and soft tissues:
  ○ Palmar xanthomata are found in skin creases of palms and soles (associated with type III hyperlipidaemia).
  ○ Tendon xanthomata are found on the extensor tendons and Achilles tendon (associated with type II hyperlipidaemia).

Radial pulse

- Check the radial pulse bilaterally and comment on rate and regularity (character and volume of the pulse should be assessed at the carotids).
- Check for radial–radial and radial–femoral delay (may be present in aortic dissection or coarctation).
- Absent radial pulses can occur where the radial artery has been harvested for coronary artery bypass grafting, aortic dissection, severe peripheral vascular disease, or where the pulse is of such low volume that it cannot be palpated, e.g. in patients with coarctation, severe AS or low-output heart failure.
- Check the pulse with the arm raised above the patient's head – there is a rapid downstroke in severe AR (known as a 'collapsing pulse').

Blood pressure

This should be measured with the patient in a relaxed sitting position and it is essential that the appropriate-sized blood pressure cuff is used.

- Check the blood pressure in both arms if aortic dissection is suspected.
- Take more than one blood pressure reading after some time has elapsed if the initial reading is surprisingly high or low.

Box O Blood pressure measurement by standard mercury sphygmomanometer or semi-automated device (British Hypertension Society Guidelines)

- Use a properly maintained, calibrated and validated device.
- Measure sitting blood pressure routinely: standing blood pressure should be recorded at least at the initial estimation in elderly or diabetic patients.
- Remove tight clothing, support arm at heart level, ensure arm relaxed and avoid talking during the measurement procedure.
- Use cuff of appropriate size.
- Inflate cuff to 20–30 mmHg above palpated systolic blood pressure.
- Lower mercury column slowly (2 mm/s).
- Read blood pressure to the nearest 2 mmHg.
- Measure diastolic blood pressure as disappearance of sounds (phase V).
- Take the mean of at least two readings; more recordings are needed if marked differences between initial measurements are found.
- Do not treat on the basis of an isolated reading.

Box P Auscultatory (Korotkoff) sounds (European Society of Hypertension Guidelines)

Phase I The first appearance of faint, repetitive, clear tapping sounds that gradually increase in intensity for at least two consecutive beats is the systolic blood pressure.

Phase II A brief period may follow during which the sounds soften and acquire a swishing quality. Auscultatory gap in some patients, sounds may disappear altogether for a short time.

Phase III The return of sharper sounds, which become crisper, to regain or even exceed the intensity of phase I sounds.

Phase IV The distinct, abrupt muffling of sounds, which become soft and blowing in quality.

Phase V The point at which all sounds finally disappear completely is the diastolic pressure.

The clinical significance, if any, of phases II and III has not been established.

Neck

Jugular venous pressure (JVP)

The JVP should be measure with the patient lying at 45 degrees and timed against the carotid pulse. It is an index of right atrial pressure (Figure AA).

Abnormalities of the JVP include:

- Large a-wave: occurs when there is right ventricular hypertrophy (e.g. pulmonary stenosis).
- Cannon waves: prominent waves occur when there is atrial contraction against a closed tricuspid valve, e.g. in complete heart block.
- Large v-waves: occur with TR (timing is simultaneous with carotid pulse).
- Fixed raised JVP with no wave form: occurs in superior vena cave obstruction.
- Kussmaul's sign: JVP increases with inspiration – a feature of cardiac tamponade.

Carotid pulse

Comment on pulse volume and character:

- High-volume pulse is associated with high-output states, e.g. pyrexia, AR.
- Low-volume pulse is associated with low-volume output states, e.g. hypovolaemia, severe AS.
- Pulsus paradoxus – this occurs when the pulse decreases or disappears on inspiration and occurs in cardiac tamponade.
- Slow rising pulse – in severe AS the upstroke of the pulse feels delayed.

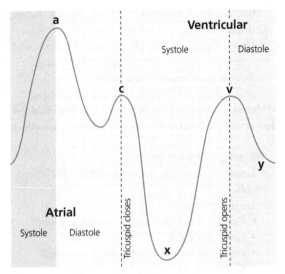

Figure AA A JVP wave form. a-wave, rise in JVP due to atrial contraction; c-wave, rise in JVP due to onset of systole (not seen in clinical practice); v-wave, rise in right atrium pressure due to filling against closed tricuspid valve in systole; x-descent, right atrial relaxation followed by descent of the tricuspid ring in systole; y-descent, pressure drop as the tricuspid valve opens at the start of diastole.

• Pulse bisferiens – this is associated with severe AR and sometimes HOCM and there is a double systolic peak.

Face

Note any dysmorphic features as described under the general inspection.

• Eyes:
  ○ Check for pallor of the conjunctivae.
  ○ Xanthelasma on the skin of the upper eyelids.
  ○ Corneal arcus is a yellow ring that is visible on the outside of the iris. It may be associated with hyperlipidaemia or can occur with increasing age.
  ○ Fundi should be examined for changes associated with hypertension and diabetes.
  ○ Roth spots are retinal haemorrhages with a central white spot and can be seen in patients with endocarditis.
• Mouth:
  ○ Check dentition (poor dentition associated with endocarditis).
  ○ Look for high-arched palate (associated with Marfan's syndrome).

  ○ Tongue: check for central cyanosis (associated with congenital cyanotic heart disease).

Precordium

Inspection

• Check scars (coronary artery bypass graft, valve replacements, congenital heart disease correction operations, pacemakers, defibrillator scars).
• Chest-wall deformity (pectus excavatum with Marfan's syndrome).
• Gynaecomastia associated with digoxin and spironolactone.

Palpation

Place the palm of the hand over the aortic and mitral area:
• Thrills are a 'palpable murmur' (a thrill may be felt in the aortic area with AS and over the mitral area with mitral valve disease).
Apply the flat of the palm parasternally over the right ventricular area:
• Heaves occur when there is right ventricular dilatation or hypertrophy (e.g. with mitral valve disease or cor pulmonale).

Apex position and character

Palpate the apex beat and check the location with respect to the mid-clavicular line and rib space.
• 'Normal' apex beat location is in the fifth intercostal space, mid-clavicular line.
• Displacement of the apex beat laterally occurs with cardiomegaly (congestive cardiac failure, AR, MR).
• Apex beat may be 'absent' or difficult to palpate in patients with emphysema, obesity or pericardial effusion.
• Forceful impulse may be found with left ventricular hypertrophy (LVH).
• 'Tapping' apex beat may be found in MS.

Auscultation routine

The bell of the stethoscope is best used for low-pitched sounds (e.g. mid-diastolic murmur of MS, third and fourth heart sounds). The diaphragm should be used for high-pitched sounds (e.g. high-pitched early diastolic murmur of AR). The heart sounds should be timed against the carotid or subclavian pulse:
• Listen individually to the first and second heart sounds and note any prosthetic heart sounds.

- Listen over the following areas with the diaphragm and the bell: apex, right and left lower and upper sternal borders, carotids and axilla.
- Listen over the apex with the patient lying on the left hand side – this is the best position to listen for mitral murmurs.
- Listen at the lower sternal edge with the patient sitting forwards at end expiration – this is the best position to listen to the murmur of AR.

Heart sounds
- The first heart sound:
  ○ Is caused by the closure of the mitral and tricuspid valve.
  ○ Loudness is determined the force of closure of the mitral and tricuspid valves.
  ○ Is loud in high cardiac output states, e.g. after exercise.
  ○ Is quiet when cardiac output is low, e.g. severe cardiac failure.
- The second heart sound:
  ○ Is caused by the closure of the aortic and pulmonary valves.
  ○ Is split when inspiration increases venous return, causing the pulmonary valve to close after the aortic valve (this is known as 'physiological splitting'). Wide splitting occurs with an atrial septal defect and RBBB, reverse splitting occurs in LBBB.
  ○ Loudness is increased with a high pressure beyond the valve, i.e. pulmonary or systemic hypertension.
  ○ Is quieter with stenosis of the semi-lunar valves, i.e. AS and pulmonary stenosis.
- Prosthetic heart sounds:
  ○ Occur due to mechanical valves.
  ○ If heard as the first heart sound are likely to be due a mitral valve replacement.
  ○ If heard as the second heart sound are likely to be due to an aortic valve replacement.
  ○ If absent in a patient with a known prosthetic valve are suggestive of valve dysfunction (e.g. thrombosis).
  ○ Bioprosthetic valves do not have prosthetic sounds.
- Added sounds:
  ○ *Third heart sound*: heard due to either rapid ventricular filling or left ventricular failure. Occurs shortly after the second heart sound in early diastole.
  ○ *Fourth heart sound*: heard in patients where there is atrial systole against a poorly compliant ventricle

(LVH, hypertension, heart failure). Occurs before first-heart sound.
  ○ *Opening snap*: heard after the second heart sound due to sudden opening of a stenotic mitral valve.
  ○ *Ejection click*: heard in bicuspid AS.
  ○ *Mid-systolic click*: heard in mitral valve prolapse.
- Murmurs (Box Q): these occur due to turbulent blood flow across the heart valves and are described according to:
  ○ Timing (systolic/diastolic).
  ○ Length of murmur (pan-systolic/late-systolic/early systolic).
  ○ Loudness:
    ▪ Grade 1 is only just audible in a quiet room.
    ▪ Grade 2 is quiet.
    ▪ Grade 3 is easy to hear but there is no thrill.
    ▪ Grade 4 is easy to hear with a thrill.
    ▪ Grade 5 is very loud with a thrill.
    ▪ Grade 6 is can be heard without a stethoscope.

Box Q Murmurs

Continuous murmurs
- Ruptured sinus of Valsalva.
- Patent ductus arteriosus.
- Arteriovenous fistula.

Systolic murmurs
- Ejection systolic: AS, outflow tract obstruction, pulmonary stenosis (radiates posteriorly to the pulmonary area), flow related (e.g. associated with AR and ASD)
- Pan systolic: MR, VSD, TR
- Mid systolic: MR, mitral valve prolapse, 'innocent flow murmur' (high-output states, e.g. anaemia and pregnancy)

Diastolic murmurs
- Early diastolic: AR, pulmonary regurgitation.
- Mid-diastolic: MS, TS, myxoma.

Graham Steel murmur
- The name given to the early diastolic murmur of pulmonary regurgitation

Austin-Flint murmur
- The name given to the mid-diastolic murmur that is heard due to the functional MS secondary to severe AR.

Chest
Check for:
• Pleural effusions (basal dullness and absent breath sounds)
Listen for added sounds in the chest:
• Basal inspiratory crackles (pulmonary oedema)

Abdomen
Check for:
• Pulsatile hepatomegaly (right heart failure with tricuspid incompetence).
• Ascites (heart failure).
• Splenomegaly (endocarditis).
• Listen for bruit over the renal arteries.
• Palpate abdominal aorta.

Lower limbs
Check for:
• Bilateral oedema or unilateral leg swelling (heart failure or DVT, respectively).
• Scarring.
• Ulcers (venous/ arterial).

Box R Example of an OSCE check list for examination of the cardiovascular system

Total possible marks 20.
• Introduction:
  ○ Student introduces themselves to patient.(*1 mark*)
• Attitude:
  ○ Student has professional attitude to patient and the examiner. (*2 marks*)
• Examination:
  ○ Peripheral pulses and peripheral oedema. (*1 mark*)
  ○ Blood pressure. (*1 mark*)
  ○ JVP and carotids. (*2 marks*)
  ○ Precordium. (*1 mark*)
  ○ Lung bases. (*1 mark*)
  ○ Liver and aortic abdominal aneurysm. (*1 mark*)
• Presentation:
  ○ Findings presented in an articulate and logical manner. (*2 marks*)
  ○ Positive and negative findings appropriately emphasised. (*1 mark*)
• Differential diagnosis:
  ○ Accurate differential diagnosis. (*4 marks*)
• Investigations:
  ○ Appropriate investigations in sequential order. (*3 marks*)

• Check the lower limb pulses (femoral, popliteal, dorsalis pedis and posterior tibial) and listen for femoral bruits.

Investigations
Most diagnoses are made by taking a careful history backed up by a thorough examination. The roles of investigations are:
• To confirm the clinical diagnosis.
• To exclude differential diagnosis.
• To monitor treatment response.

Some investigations have the potential to cause harm to the patient and so the benefits and risks of the investigations must be assessed. It is essential that patients are properly consented before they undergo any invasive investigations, such as coronary angiography.

It is usual to carry out low-risk non-invasive tests first and then use the results of these to direct further investigations.

Initial cardiac investigations
Electrocardiogram (ECG)
This is usually one of the first investigations to be carried out. It is important to carry out ECG interpretation in context of the patient history and examination.

Basic ECG interpretation
Confirm that the ECG has been taken at a paper speed of 25 mm/s and that the calibration indicates 1 cm = 1 mV.

A systematic approach is recommended, considering in turn the heart rate, rhythm and axis. Thereafter the individual components of the ECG complex can be assessed in more detail.

Heart rate
• Count the number of large squares (0.2 s) between successive QRS complexes.
• Divide this number into 300. This calculates heart rate in beats/ minute.
• Alternatively for a standard 12 lead ECG the number of recorded QRS complexes on the rhythm strip is multiplied by 5.

Heart rhythm
Ask the following questions:
• Are there P waves in front of every QRS complex (e.g. sinus rhythm)?
• Are the P waves directly related to the QRS complexes (they become dissociated in complete heart block)?

• Is the baseline regular or irregular (e.g. atrial fibrillation)?

Axis

The cardiac axis is the average vector of ventricular depolarisation in the frontal plane and is affected by anatomical and electrical factors (Figures BB and CC):

Normal axis:	−30 to 90 degrees	(QRS positive in leads I & II)
Left-axis deviation:	−30 to −90 degrees	(QRS negative in leads II & III)
Right-axis deviation:	90 to 180 degrees	(QRS negative in leads I & II)
Extreme-axis deviation:	180 to −90 degrees	

Assessment of individual aspects of the ECG complex (intervals and normal ranges) (Figure DD)

P waves

• Amplitude is normally <0.2 mV.
• If bifid (P mitrale), are suggestive of left atrial hypertrophy (e.g. MS).
• If negative in lead II, may reflect an ectopic focus or a SVT.
• Tall P waves (P pulmonale) in inferior leads indicate an enlarged or hypertrophied right atrium (e.g. pulmonary hypertension).

PR interval

• Represents normal conduction through the AV node.
• A prolonged PR interval indicates slow AV conduction and occurs in first-degree heart block.

• Short AV conduction occurs in the presence of an accessory pathway.

QRS complex

• Amplitude:
  ○ Large – in LVH (criteria: R wave lead I or aVL >12 mm, or R in I + S in III >25 mm).
  ○ Small – in patients with barrel chest, obesity or pericardial effusions.
  ○ Progression – the R wave usually increases in amplitude from V1–V5.
• Width:
  ○ Normal QRS is <0.12 s.

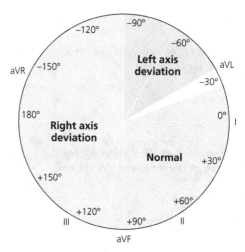

Figure BB Cardiac axis deviation.

	Normal axis 0 to 90	Left axis Physiological 0 to −30	Left axis Pathological −30 to −90	Right axis 90 to 180	Extreme axis −90 to 180	Indeterminate axis ?
Lead I	Λ	Λ	Λ	V	V	⌁
Lead II	Λ	⌁	V	Λ	V	⌁
Lead III	Λ	V	V	Λ	V	⌁

Figure CC ECG changes with axis deviation.

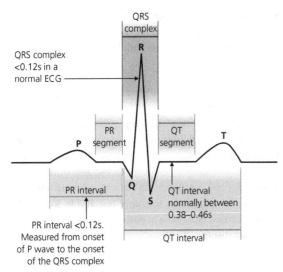

Figure DD Assessment of individual aspects of the ECG complex (intervals and normal ranges).

o Broad QRS complex represents a delay through the conduction system, leading to either LRBB or RBBB or a ventricular focus of origin.

ST segments
• Are measured from the ECG baseline.
• ST depression: caused by ischaemia, digoxin, left ventricular strain, cardiomyopathies or metabolic disturbances.
• ST elevation: caused by myocardial infarction, pericarditis and left ventricular aneurysms.

QT interval
• Represents duration of ventricular repolarisation.
• Varies according to the heart rate.
• Calculated according to Bazett's formula (R-R interval is the time between R waves):

$$QTc = QT \text{ interval (s)}/\sqrt{(\text{R-R interval (s)})}.$$

• May be prolonged due to LQTS, metabolic disturbances and drugs.
• Prolongation predisposes individuals to developing polymorphic ventricular tachycardia.

T waves
• Represent ventricular repolarisation.
• Normally in the same direction as the R wave.
• Tall T waves occur in acute ischaemia, hyperkalaemia, LVH, acute pericarditis.

• Inverted T waves occur in ischaemia, hyperventilation, stroke and other conditions.

Chest radiograph (CXR)
• Pulmonary oedema and cardiomegaly may be present in a patient with heart failure.
• A widened mediastinum is suggestive of dissection and wedge-shaped infarcts is suggestive of pulmonary embolism.

Blood tests
• Electrolytes, urea and creatinine. Patients with renal impairment are at greater risk of ischaemic heart disease. The contrast used for cardiac angiography can cause contrast nephropathy, which in severe cases can lead to renal failure.
• Full blood count (FBC). Severe anaemia can lead to patients presenting with high output cardiac failure and chest pain.
• Total cholesterol and lipid profile.
• Fasting glucose.
• Troponin measurement.

Exercise tolerance test
The Bruce protocol is the most commonly used exercise protocol for assessment of patients with suspected coronary artery disease. It is used for risk stratification purposes. The patients should be encouraged to reach 85% of their target heart rate (220 – age of the patient) to maximise the sensitivity (68%) and specificity (77%) of the test. Indications for carrying out an exercise test are:
• Diagnosis of coronary artery disease.
• Risk assessment in patients with established coronary artery disease.
• For risk stratification post-myocardial infarction (pre-discharge day 4–7 to assess prognosis- modified Bruce protocol).
• For evaluation of arrhythmias (exercise-induced arrhythmias).
  The criteria for a positive exercise test are:
• ST depression of >1 mm/80 ms after the J point.
• Chest pain/provocation of symptoms.
• ST elevation.
• Failure of blood pressure to increase during exercise.
• Ventricular arrhythmias.
  False-positive exercise tests are more common in women or in the context of non-specific symptoms and can occur in cardiomyopathies, hypertension and mitral valve prolapse.

Cardiac imaging
Ultrasound imaging
Transthoracic echocardiogram
This is a quick, non-invasive, safe and easily accessible cardiac investigation that provides instant information regarding:
- Size and function of the left and right ventricle.
- Regional wall motion abnormalities.
- Valvular pathology and intracardiac shunts.
- Pericardial effusion.

Transoesphageal echocardiogram (Figure EE)
This involves placing an ultrasound in the patient's oesophagus and is normally carried out under light sedation. The resolution is better than in a transthoracic echocardiogram and the cardiac valves can be examined in greater detail. Some indications for transoesophageal echocardiogram are:
- Suspected aortic dissection.
- Poor transthoracic echocardiogram windows in a sick ventilated patient.
- Infective endocarditis.
- Mitral valve pathology that requires assessment for repair.
- Detection of thrombus in the LA appendage.
- Congenital heart defects.

Stress echocardiography
- Pharmacological or physical stress is used to increase the patient's heart rate. Simultaneously, echocardiography is carried out to identify myocardial regional wall motion abnormalities.

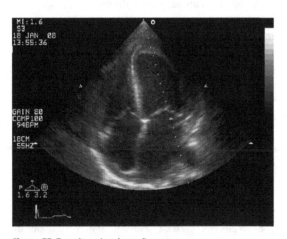

Figure EE Transthoracic echocardiogram.

- Useful for risk assessment in patients who are not able to carry out an exercise tolerance test and to assess myocardial variability in patients with known ischaemic heart disease.

Nuclear imaging
- Myocardial perfusion imaging estimates the regional myocardial blood flow at rest and after stress by assessing the relative distribution of radiopharmaceutical at stress and rest.
- Used for risk assessment in patients who are not able to carry out an exercise tolerance test and to locate the areas of cardiac ischaemia in patients with known ischaemic heart disease.

Angiography
- Cardiac catheterisation is carried out for assessment of coronary artery disease.
- It can be carried out electively in outpatients complaining of stable angina or in an emergency in patients with STEMI or NSTEMI.
- Catheterisation is most commonly carried out via the right femoral artery or radial artery.
- The right and left coronary arteries can be visualised by injection of contrast agent and fluoroscopy.

Cardiac magnetic resonance imaging (MRI) (Figure FF)
MRI has emerged as a recent important investigative tool in cardiac imaging.
- *Advantages*: it has high spatial resolution, is non-invasive and can give anatomical, haemodynamic and functional information from the same scan.
- *Disadvantages*: limited availability and is unsuitable for claustrophobic patients and patients with a permanent pacemaker or intracardiac defibrillator.

Cardiac computer tomography (CT) (Figure GG)
Electron beam CT
This is used to detect coronary artery calcification. Its value is debatable in patients with a history of angina. Its use is primarily to detect patients at higher risk from coronary vascular events who may be suitable for more aggressive preventative therapy.

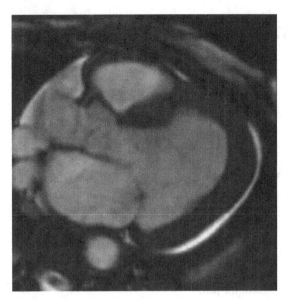

Figure FF Cardiac MRI scan.

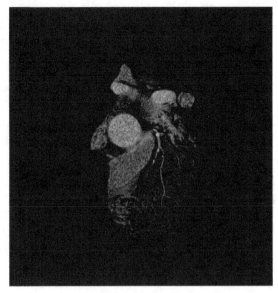

Figure GG Cardiac CT scan.

Multislice CT

Multislice CT is now available to detect coronary disease; however, this technique is currently more valuable in excluding coronary disease than in accurately quantify-ing the nature of coronary disease. Unlike tests that involve stressing the myocardium, it is not possible to correlate symptoms with the development of myocardial ischaemia.

Case 1   A 47-year-old man with chest pain

A 47-year-old plumber rings his general practitioner's (GP's) surgery and speaks to the receptionist asking for an urgent appointment. He gives a 2-day history of intermittent central chest pain culminating in a 30-minute episode of chest pain at rest. His GP is currently on a home visit.

What advice should the receptionist give?

Even in the context of this brief history there is a significant probability that the pain is cardiac in origin. The patient should be advised to ring for an ambulance immediately. Most patients are now told to ring for an ambulance in the context of chest pain that may be cardiac in origin in order to minimise delay to treatment.

In the ambulance he continues to complain of chest pain. His pulse is 110 bpm. His blood pressure is 190/100 mmHg.

What action can be taken by the paramedics?

The initial treatment of patients with chest pain is usually undertaken by paramedics. Most ambulances have the facility to perform an ECG and the capacity to transmit the recording to the local Coronary Care Unit (CCU). Patients with ST-elevation myocardial infarction (STEMI) may be candidates for pre-hospital thrombolysis with a bolus thrombolytic such as reteplase or tenecteplase. All patients receive oxygen, aspirin and glyceryl trinitrate (GTN) if the pain is thought to be cardiac in origin.

On arrival in Accident & Emergency (A&E) he is pain free.

What is the differential diagnosis for a patient presenting in this way and what features may help to establish that the pain is cardiac in origin?

Chest pain is a common presentation in the A&E department and has a broad differential diagnosis (Table 1.1). The usual principles apply in trying to characterise the cause of the pain.

- Site.
- Onset.
- Character.
- Radiation.
- Associated symptoms.
- Timing/duration.
- Exacerbating factors.
- Severity.

It is important to try to elicit a prior history of angina. Many patients will describe exertional chest pain in the weeks preceding presentation. With angina or an acute coronary syndrome (ACS) the pain usually builds to a maximum over a few minutes rather than reaching its maximal intensity instantaneously. The distribution of the pain is important. It is usually retrosternal and encompasses an area greater than the palm of the hand.

Table 1.1 Chest pain – common differential diagnoses

Angina pectoris
Acute myocardial infarction
Oesophageal pain (reflux, spasm, inflammation)
Musculoskeletal
Pulmonary embolic disease
Cervical root compression
Aortic dissection
Chest wall pain
Pancreatitis
Cholecystitis
Anxiety disorders

Cardiology: Clinical Cases Uncovered. By T. Betts, J. Dwight and S. Bull. Published 2010 by Blackwell Publishing.

The pain may radiate to the neck, jaw, shoulder and inner aspect of the arm and forearm (usually left sided). Pain that is very localised (less than 5 cm in radius), or that is localised to the submammary region, is unlikely to be ischaemic cardiac pain. Pain may be felt between the shoulder blades (especially in the case of posterior myocardial infarction) and therefore mimic an aortic dissection. Presentation with epigastric pain can occur and may be confused with the pain of biliary disease, peptic ulceration or pancreatitis.

A description of the character of the pain is highly variable and often not helpful; indeed, it may be absent in the elderly or diabetic patient. However, the classic description is of heaviness or a crushing sensation ('elephant sitting on my chest'). Pain that is clearly pleuritic in nature is unlikely to be due to an ACS. During the pain the patient may feel apprehensive; although this may not be the worst pain they have had, it is usually the most worrying. It is unusual for the patient to continue with any physical exertion during symptoms. It may be difficult to distinguish the pain from an ACS from that of angina; however, the pain is usually more severe and is either rapidly progressive (occurring with minimal exertion) or occurs at rest. Pain from angina is usually relieved within a few minutes by rest or with GTN. Associated symptoms of sweating nausea or vomiting and a duration of pain of >15 minutes increase the likelihood of myocardial infarction. Pain lasting for many hours is unlikely to be due to a myocardial infarction.

Pain due to myocardial infarction may be associated with the following features:

• Sweating.
• Nausea.
• Vomiting.
• Breathlessness.
• Dizziness.

What other features in the history help to assess the probability of coronary artery disease?

In all cases, it is important to assess the probability of atheromatous disease in the patient on the basis of their risk-factor profile (Table 1.2). A past medical history of stroke, claudication, angina or previous myocardial infarction greatly increases the probability that the pain is cardiac in origin. Even when the pain is not entirely typical for ischaemia, it should be taken seriously when there is an adverse risk-factor profile or prior history of coronary disease.

Table 1.2 Risk factors for ischaemic heart disease

Hypertension
Diabetes
Hypercholesterolaemia
Smoking
Family history
Chronic renal disease
Physical inactivity
Obesity
Gender
Age

He reports pain of 8/10 severity radiating to the left arm and associated with breathlessness and sweating lasting 45 minutes, which has now resolved. Over the previous 2 months he has experienced exertional chest tightness relieved after a few minutes' rest. There is a history of hypertension, for which he has been treated with ramipril 10 mg daily. There is a history of mild chronic obstructive airways disease; however, this has not required treatment recently. He smokes 10 cigarettes a day. There is no prior history of peripheral vascular disease, ischaemic heart disease or stroke. His father died of a myocardial infarction at the age of 40 years. His lipid profile, measured by his GP 2 years previously, was reported as follows: low-density lipoprotein (LDL) cholesterol 8.2 mmol/L; high-density lipoprotein (HDL) cholesterol 0.8 mmol/L; triglycerides 5.1 mmol/L.

Observations are as follows: O$_2$ saturation 100% on 40% O$_2$; pulse 90 bpm; blood pressure 180/80 mmHg.

What features on examination help to confirm a cardiac cause of his pain?

The presence of a tachycardia and hypertension are not particularly helpful if the patient is in pain or anxious. The clinical examination in patients with angina or ACS is often normal. The following should be looked for:

• Arcus senilis – hypercholesterolaemia (in patients under 50 years).

• Fundoscopy – hypertensive changes.

• Xanthelasma – hypercholesterolaemia.

• Elevated JVP – heart failure.

• Carotid bruits – high probability of coexisting coronary disease.

• Cardiomegaly – heart failure.

• Hypertrophied apex beat – hypertension or aortic stenosis (AS).

• Systolic murmur – AS or hypertrophic cardiomyopathy (HOCM) can give rise to angina.
• Diastolic murmur – aortic regurgitation (AR) associated with a type A dissection.
• Pericardial friction rub – pericarditis.
• Abdominal aorta – aortic bruit or aneurysm associated with generalised vascular disease.
• Femoral arteries/foot-pulses, evidence of peripheral vascular disease associated with coronary disease.

On examination the only abnormal finding is of a soft systolic murmur.

His ECG is shown in Figure 1.1. What abnormalities are shown? How specific are these abnormalities for coronary artery disease?

The ECG demonstrates T-wave inversion in the anteroseptal leads and downsloping ST depression in the lateral chest leads (I, aVL and V4–V6). There is minor ST elevation in a single chest lead (V2). The most specific ECG finding for reversible ischaemia is ST depression. The ECG must always be interpreted in the context of the clinical history and is most sensitive when performed during pain. Downsloping ST depression can also occur in left ventricular strain and following digoxin therapy; however, where there is ST depression at the J point there is usually additional coronary disease (Figure 1.2). T-wave inversion is rather less specific and can be seen in a number of conditions (stroke, subarachnoid haemorrhage, HOCM); however, when symmetrical, greater that 2 mm in depth and present in the anteroseptal leads, it is a marker of severe disease in the left anterior descending (LAD) artery. When present in a single chest lead, it is not specific for myocardial infarction.

What other routine investigations should be arranged on admission?

The following standard investigations would be helpful:
• Full blood count (FBC).
• Electrolytes.
• Blood glucose.
• Renal function.
• Thyroid function.
• Troponin/creatinine kinase.
• Fasting lipid profile and glucose.
• Chest X-ray (CXR).
• Echocardiogram.

In practice, most analysers will automatically provide electrolytes, renal function and liver function tests. To

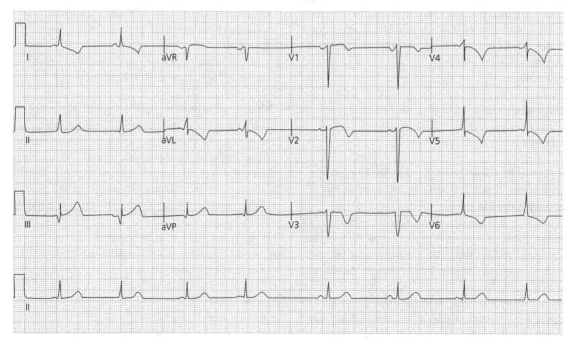

Figure 1.1 ECG showing ST depression.

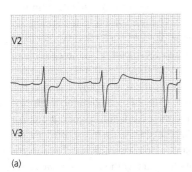
(a)

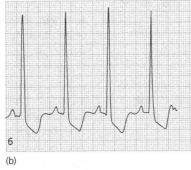
(b)

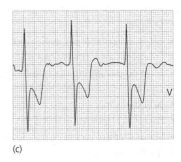
(c)

Figure 1.2 ST segment depression. (a) Horizontal ST depression. (b) Downsloping ST depression with left ventricular hypertrophy. (c) Downsloping ST depression.

these, thyroid function tests are often added, although the yield of positive results is low in the absence of clinical features in this age group (in the elderly, thyroid disease is more common and the usual clinical features are often absent). The CXR may help to exclude important differential diagnoses. The presence of a systolic murmur raises the possibility of AS, HOCM or mitral valve prolapse, all of which may give rise to symptoms of chest pain. Echocardiography is essential to exclude these differential diagnoses and may give further useful information, e.g. a regional wall motion abnormality pointing to a diagnosis of ischaemic heart disease.

The initial results are as follows: FBC normal; sodium 135 mmol/l; potassium 3.1 mmol/L; renal function normal; blood glucose 12.6 mmol/L; troponin I 0.7 µg/L (normal range 0–1 µg/L). CXR normal.

What is the significance of the troponin result?

The cardiac marker troponin is released from cardiac muscle only and is therefore much more specific than creatinine kinase, which it has now replaced. There are two measureable forms, T and I. There is some debate concerning the relative merits of the two forms. There is a single assay available for troponin T, allowing for comparison of values between laboratories. There are a number of troponin I assays and each laboratory has a separate reference range. Troponin I is not elevated in renal failure, which is one of the advantages of this marker.

Any form of myocardial damage will cause a troponin release and therefore a troponin rise is not specific for myocardial infarction (Table 1.3). The rise in cardiac troponin is delayed and therefore a myocardial infarction can only be reliably excluded when the measurement is

Table 1.3 Causes of an elevated serum troponin

Acute myocardial infarction
Myopericarditis
Pulmonary embolism
Direct current (DC) cardioversion
Post-cardiac surgery
Direct myocardial trauma
Renal failure (troponin T)
Severe intercurrent illness (e.g. septic shock) in the context of pre-existing coronary disease

Table 1.4 Characteristics of troponin as a marker for myocardial damage

Mainly bound as part of the actin/myosin complex
Exists in three forms, of which T and I are used clinically
Highly sensitive and specific
Measurement 12 hours after onset of pain has 100% sensitivity for acute myocardial infarction
Release occurs for up to 100 hours after myocardial damage

made 12 hours after the onset of pain. Troponin exists in two forms, a free form in the cytoplasm and a form that is bound to the contractile apparatus. The free form accounts for the early release of troponin; however, there is a prolonged (up to 100 hours) release of troponin that occurs from the bound form. Troponin is therefore a useful marker for patients presenting late following an episode of chest pain a few days previously (Table 1.4).

After a diagnosis of ACS is made, what treatments would be indicated?

- Oxygen.
- Aspirin 300 mg orally, followed by 75 mg daily.
- Sublingual or intravenous GTN if in pain.
- Clopidogrel 300 mg orally, followed by 75 mg daily.
- Low-molecular-weight heparin (weight adjusted).
- Beta blockade.
- IIb/IIIa antagonists.
- Statin therapy.
- Insulin infusion.

By the time they arrive in the A&E department, most patients will already have been given aspirin 300 mg by mouth and a trial of GTN. Oxygen is given routinely. Treatment is primarily based on the use of antiplatelet and antithrombin agents, which help to prevent embolisation and occlusion by the intracoronary thrombus. The antiplatelet agents aspirin, clopidogrel and the IIb/IIIa antagonists and the low-molecular-weight heparins, (which are antithrombin agents), have all been shown to be beneficial in non-ST elevation ACSs (non-STEMIs), although the benefits of the IIb/IIIa antagonists and low-molecular-weight heparins appear to be limited to the troponin-positive subgroup. Beta blockers are used routinely; although this patient has a history of mild chronic obstructive pulmonary disease this is not an absolute contraindication to beta blockade and a cardioselective beta blocker is often well tolerated. A nitroglycerine infusion may be required in those with ongoing chest pain. Statin therapy is also beneficial when given early; the effects are partly related to the anti-inflammatory and antithrombotic actions of these agents. Patients presenting with acute myocardial infarction are often found incidentally to have diabetes. There is some evidence that this should be treated aggressively in the first 24–48 hours with an insulin infusion although the majority of patients will subsequently be managed with diet or oral hypoglycaemic agents.

> *The 12-hour troponin value is 5 µg/L. The fasting lipid profile is as follows: LDL cholesterol 8.8 mmol/L; HDL cholesterol 0.8 mmol/L; triglycerides 2..0 mmol/L.*

How would you interpret the lipid profile?

Total cholesterol is often used as a screening test for patients with hyperlipidaemia; however, it is less reliable than the full lipid profile in assessing cardiovascular risk. The cardiovascular risk is determined by the ratio of the LDL cholesterol to HDL cholesterol. A high ratio is indicative of increased risk. The relationship is less strong for triglycerides; however, a very high triglyceride level should prompt further investigation for a cause, e.g. hypothyroidism, alcohol abuse, nephrotic syndrome, diabetes mellitus. This patient probably has familial hypercholesterolaemia. The LDL cholesterol levels are high (>8 mmol/L) and there is a family history of premature atherosclerosis. The disease is transmitted as an autosomal dominant. Homozygotes rarely survive beyond the age of 20 years without treatment. This patient is heterozygote and has a 10–50-fold risk of coronary disease. Current practice is to treat all patients with proven coronary disease with a statin, regardless of their cholesterol level (secondary prevention). This is supported by evidence that there is a reduction in cardiovascular event rates with statin therapy, even at low levels of cholesterol.

What is the pathology that gives rise to this clinical presentation?

Almost all acute coronary syndromes are due to plaque rupture or erosion with overlying thrombus formation (see Chapter 1, p. 9). One exception is in cocaine intoxication, where an acute coronary syndrome may be precipitated by coronary artery spasm.

How would you describe this ACS?

This patient has a non-STEMI. The classification of ACS is given in Figure 1.3. This is largely a practical classification, which determines management. The ECG determines those patients who have ST elevation and who therefore require treatment with thrombolysis or primary percutaneous coronary intervention (PCI). Those without ST elevation are divided into those with a troponin rise (non-STEMI) and those without (unstable angina).

| *The patient settles with medical therapy.*

What factors decide whether this patient should undergo coronary angiography?

The factors that indicate the need for angiography in a non-STEMI: are as follows

- Occupation.
- Age.
- Continuing symptoms of angina.
- ECG findings indicating high risk:

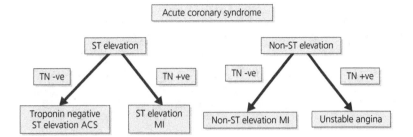

Figure 1.3 Acute coronary syndrome (ACS). STEMI, ST-elevation myocardial infarction; TN, troponin.

○ Widespread ST depression, particularly with ST elevation in aVR.

○ Anterior T wave inversion (Wellens' syndrome).

• Presentation with left ventricular failure.

• Troponin level.

• Thrombolysis in myocardial infarction (TIMI) risk score.

• Coexistent valvular heart disease requiring surgery.

It is a common misconception that the prognosis from non-ST-elevation ACS is better than that for STEMI. This is not the case. The in-hospital mortality is greater for STEMI than for other ACSs, largely because of the greater extent of myocardial damage. However, event rate following discharge with a non-ST-elevation ACS is higher and approximately one third of these patients will suffer a further myocardial infarction, death or readmission with an ACS within a year. The simplest approach would be to perform angiography in all patients admitted with ACS and this is the practice in some centres. However, this is not always appropriate. Those patients with ongoing symptoms of angina on medical therapy will automatically qualify for further intervention. The greatest benefit of coronary intervention (angioplasty or bypass grafting) in asymptomatic patients with ACS is in those patients with the highest risk of subsequent events. The evidence is largely in patients under the age of 75 years, and although the benefit is maintained, if not greater in the elderly, some account should be taken of the patient's life expectancy before intervening. Clearly, advanced age or serious comorbidity would favour a more conservative approach. Account should be taken of the patient's occupation. Angiography is likely to be necessary where the patient's occupation is at risk without evidence of complete revascularisation, e.g. airline pilots or patients holding an heavy goods licence (HGV); the same applies with those patients with a very physical occupation.

Table 1.5 ECG criteria for left anterior descending (LAD) syndrome (Wellens' syndrome)

Symmetric and deeply inverted T waves in V2 and V3 (occasionally V1, V4–V6), *or*

Biphasic T waves in leads V2 and V3, *plus*
• Isoelectric (<1 mm) ST segment
• No precordial Q waves
• History of angina
• Pattern present in pain-free state
• Normal or slightly elevated serum markers

Certain findings on the ECG indicate extensive coronary disease, which places the patient at high risk. These findings may indicate a high probability of left main coronary artery disease, triple-vessel disease or involvement of the LAD artery. The ECG in this patient demonstrates extensive T-wave inversion in the anterior chest leads. This is characteristic of an LAD syndrome also known as Wellens' syndrome (Table 1.5). An ECG demonstrating widespread ST depression with ST elevation in aVR is suggestive of triple-vessel or left main stem disease (Figure 1.4).

The presence of a troponin rise is indicative of a high-risk ACS. Although the patient's risk of adverse cardiac events is related to the height of the troponin rise, even a small rise is sufficient in some centres to qualify patients for automatic angiography.

The TIMI risk score (Table 1.6) is a more sophisticated method of estimating the risk of myocardial infarction or death following admission with a non-ST-elevation ACS.

The patient's TIMI risk score is 4 (multiple risk factors, ST depression on ECG, troponin rise and cardiac sounding chest pain). He is considered to be at a high risk of further infarction and is therefore referred for coronary angiography.

PART 2: CASES

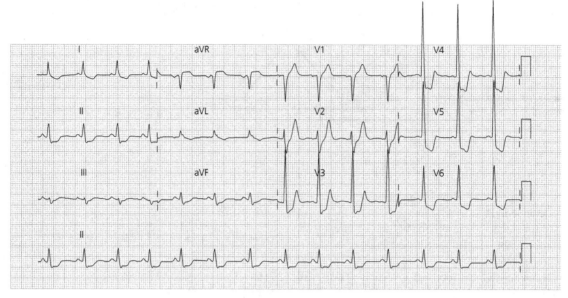

Figure 1.4 ECG demonstrating widespread ST depression and ST elevation in aVR, suggesting triple-vessel disease or left main stem disease.

RISK SCORING

Historical	Points	Presentation	Points
Age ≥65 years	1	Recent ≤24 hours severe angina	1
≥3 CAD risk factors*	1	Increased cardiac markers	1
Aspirin in past 7 days	1	ST deviation ≥0.5 mm	
Known CAD (stenosis ≥50%)	1		

Table 1.6 Thrombolysis in myocardial infarction (TIMI) risk score for non-ST-elevation acute coronary syndromes (ACSs). CAD, coronary artery disease; MI, myocardial infarction

*Family history, hypertension, hypercholesterolaemia, diabetes, active smokers.

Risk of cardiac events (%) by 14 days in TIMI IIB

Risk Score	Death or MI	Death, MI or urgent revscularisation
0/1	3	5
2	3	8
3	5	13
4	7	20
5	12	26
6/7	19	41

CONSIDER AUTOMATIC REFERRAL TO CARDIOLOGY IF RISK SCORE ≥3.

What is the role of exercise stress testing in this patient?

Early-risk stratification is based on information on admission and is not dependent on the result of an exercise test. The TIMI risk score provides a guide for deciding which patients should be referred to cardiology. Lower-risk patients may be further assessed with an exercise test. A strongly positive exercise test with ECG changes or the early onset of angina would prompt referral for angiography. In this patient, an exercise test is not required since he is considered to be high risk without additional risk stratification with an exercise test.

This patient's coronary angiogram is shown in Figure 1.5. The findings are of a critical LAD artery stenosis, which is treated with coronary angioplasty and a stent is inserted (Box 1.1).

What medication should this patient be discharged on and for how long should this be continued?

- Aspirin – indefinitely.
- Statin – indefinitely.
- Angiotensin-converting enzyme (ACE) inhibitor – indefinitely.
- Clopidogrel – for 1 year.
- Beta blocker – variable.

Most patients with coronary disease will end up on an ACE inhibitor, aspirin and a statin for life. Clopidogrel is recommended for a year after admission with ACS (the same applies for all patients with drug-eluting stents). The early beta-blocker trials were performed in patients with STEMI and therefore practice varies; in cases where there has been significant myocardial damage it is reasonable to continue beta blockers indefinitely. ACE inhibitors have a dual role. They prevent remodelling of the ventricle after myocardial infarction and reduce the incidence of heart failure. In addition, in the post-myocardial infarction trials of ACE inhibitors, a reduction in further myocardial infarction was observed due to a protective effect on the vascular endothelium and reduction in thrombotic events.

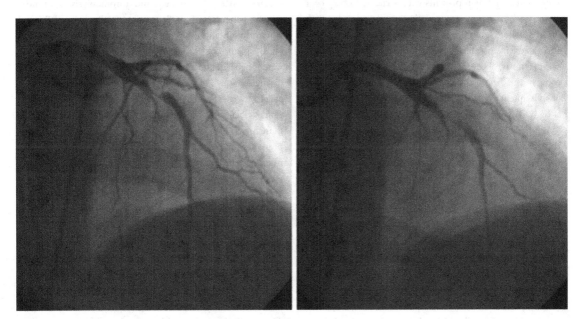

Figure 1.5 Angiographic findings of critical left anterior descending (LAD) artery stenosis.

Box 1.1 Coronary angioplasty and stenting

The preparation and access to the circulation for coronary angioplasty are the same as for coronary arteriography (see p. 69); however, all patients should be pre-treated with clopidogrel (usually a loading dose of 300–600 mg). In straightforward cases the patient may undergo angioplasty for a suitable lesion directly after angiography. The coronary ostium is engaged with a guide catheter and a wire passed across the lesion requiring angioplasty. A balloon is passed over the wire and inflated at the site of the stenosis; angiography is performed to establish that the lesion has been adequately treated. In over 90% of cases angioplasty is now accompanied by the insertion of a metal stent. This is essentially a cylindrical wire mesh, which is expanded at the site of the lesion using an angioplasty balloon. In most cases the lesion is pre-treated with a balloon procedure prior to stenting but occasionally the stent is inserted without pre-treatment (direct stenting). The main problem with angioplasty is restenosis caused by proliferation of endothelial cells and smooth muscle cells at the site of the stent; this usually occurs within 3 months. Restenosis may be reduced by the use of a drug-eluting stent (a stent coated with an antiproliferative agent, e.g. sirolimus or paclitaxel). Thrombosis in the stent is prevented by the use of clopidogrel, heparin and aspirin at the time of the procedure and afterwards with long-term antiplatelet therapy (aspirin and clopidogrel).

The primary indication for angioplasty is the treatment for the symptoms of angina and in the treatment of high-risk patients presenting with an ACS. Single-vessel or two-vessel disease and recurrent disease following coronary artery bypass surgery is nearly always treated with angioplasty (except where the vessels are chronically occluded). The standard therapy for triple-vessel disease or left main stem disease is surgery; however, when the risk of surgery is high angioplasty provides an alternative in most cases.

CASE REVIEW

This 47-year-old man presents with a classic history of a myocardial infarction. The pain is central and radiates to the arm. There is a preceding history of exertional angina and an adverse risk-factor profile, which support the clinical diagnosis. The ECG findings and raised troponin confirm the diagnosis of a non-STEMI. The patient's risk of subsequent events as determined by the TIMI risk score is high. Therefore, despite the absence of further symptoms, he was referred for angiography, which demonstrated disease of the left anterior descending artery; this was treated with angioplasty and stenting.

Chest pain is a very common cause of presentation to the A&E department. The diagnosis of an ACS is made on the basis of a characteristic history of cardiac chest pain, ECG changes and raised cardiac markers (troponin). A normal ECG and troponin does not exclude an ACS, and a good history in the presence of an adverse risk-factor profile is a reason for admission and further risk stratification. The pathology of all ACSs is similar, the rupture or erosion of an atheromatous plaque with the development of an overlying thrombus. The plaque may previously have been small and therefore 50% or more of patients do not have a history of preceding angina. The absence of ST elevation on the ECG classifies these patients as non-ST elevation ACSs and in these patients total occlusion of the coronary artery is unlikely and thrombolysis is of no benefit. Patients with ACSs require monitoring and ECGs when in pain and daily if pain free. Routine treatment is with aspirin, beta blockade, clopidogrel, low-molecular-weight heparin and a beta blocker. The decision to proceed to angiography is based on the risk of further events. The event rate (death and myocardial infarction revascularisation) per annum for non-STEMI is as high, if not higher, than for STEMI. Most of these events occur early after presentation and therefore the patient requires aggressive management and risk stratification on admission to hospital. An invasive strategy, i.e. early angiography and angioplasty, if required, has been shown to be more effective at reducing adverse events (death and myocardial infarction) than a conservative approach with angiography only for those with pain that does not settle or a strongly positive exercise test. The most commonly used scoring system to establish the need for angiography is the TIMI risk score. ST-segment depression and a troponin rise are the most useful risk factors that help to identify those patients who are likely to receive the most benefit from an early invasive approach. Those patients at low risk should undergo some form of stress testing prior to discharge, first to confirm the diagnosis and second to establish if they are likely to have further symptoms or events.

KEY POINTS

- All patients with cardiac sounding chest pain should be admitted to hospital as an emergency.
- An ECG should be performed as soon as possible to identify those patients with ST-elevation ACSs from those with non-ST-elevation ACSs.
- Patients with a supportive history and ECG changes should be treated with antiplatelet agents (aspirin, clopidogrel, IIb/IIIa antagonists), low-molecular-weight heparin, beta blockers and a statin.
- The need for coronary angiography and coronary

intervention is then established using information from the history, ECG and troponin results.
- Indications for angiography include continuing chest pain, an elevated troponin and a high TIMI risk score.
- For those patients not requiring intervention on the basis of the above, further risk stratification with an exercise test is recommended. A negative exercise test indicates a good prognosis and the patient can be treated with medical therapy alone.

Case 2 A 60-year-old heavy goods vehicle (HGV) driver with chest pain

A 60-year-old heavy goods vehicle (HGV) driver presents to A&E with a 6-hour history of crushing central chest pain associated with breathlessness and sweating. He is a smoker of 20 cigarettes a day and has a past history of hypertension and insulin-dependent diabetes mellitus. Ten years ago he had a bleeding duodenal ulcer diagnosed; he remains on a proton pump inhibitor and has had no recent symptoms of dyspepsia or bleeding since. Two months previously a deep vein thrombosis (DVT) was diagnosed for which he is on warfarin. On arrival in A&E he is still in pain. His ECG is shown in Figure 2.1.

What are the abnormal findings on the ECG? What is the diagnosis and which coronary artery is likely to be involved?

The ECG in this patient demonstrates ST elevation in the chest leads V1–V6, indicative of an anterior myocardial infarction. The anterior wall of the left ventricle is supplied by the left anterior descending (LAD) artery.

The site of ST-elevation myocardial infarction (STEMI) can be derived in most cases from the ECG leads involved:

- Anterior: V1–V6.
- Anteroseptal: V1–V4.
- Anterolateral: V3–V6.
- Lateral: aVL and aVF, V5 and V6.
- Inferior: II, III and aVF.

The LAD artery supplies the anterior wall of the left ventricle and the majority of the left ventricular myocardium in most individuals. The right coronary artery (RCA) supplies the inferior wall in all except approximately 15% of cases where the RCA is non-dominant and the inferior territory is supplied by the circumflex (Cx) coronary artery. Posterior wall infarction presents with ST depression and an increase in R wave amplitude in V1–V3, i.e. an inverse image of the usual infarction pattern of ST elevation and Q-wave formation. Posterior infarction is one of the causes of a dominant R wave in V1. The lateral wall of the left ventricle has a variable supply from all three coronary arteries and therefore infarcts are often inferolateral, anterolateral or posterolateral.

What other possible causes are there for ST elevation in the anterior chest leads?

- Left bundle branch block (LBBB).
- Early repolarisation / high take off.
- Hyperkalaemia.
- Brugada syndrome.
- Cocaine intoxication.
- Acute massive pulmonary embolism.
- Afro-Caribbean variant.
- Pericarditis.
- Myocarditis.

KEY POINT

A major difficulty in interpreting the ECG in myocardial infarction can be in distinguishing high take off/ early repolarisation from acute anteroseptal myocardial infarction. The ST segments in a case of early repolarisation are characteristically concave upwards, as opposed to the convex elevation seen in myocardial infarction. There is often slight splintering after the QRS complex, particularly in the lateral chest leads. This is particularly common in young men. An example is shown in Figure 2.2.

Features that suggest ST elevation due to myocardial infarction as opposed to other causes are defined by QRST:

- Q – the development of pathological Q waves.
- R – associated loss of R wave.
- ST – ST depression in reciprocal leads.

Cardiology: Clinical Cases Uncovered. By T. Betts, J. Dwight and S. Bull. Published 2010 by Blackwell Publishing.

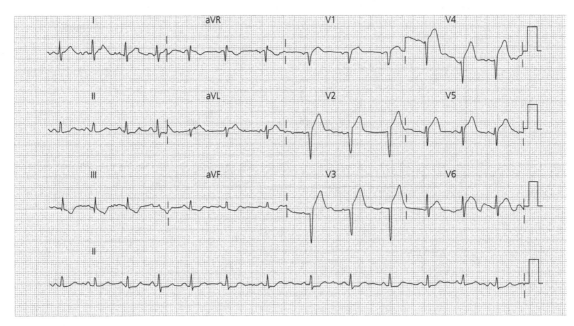

Figure 2.1 ECG on presentation.

Table 2.1 Contraindications to thrombolysis

Absolute:
- Any prior intracranial haemorrhage
- Known intracranial structural lesions
- Known intracranial neoplasm
- Ischaemic stroke within 3 months
- Active bleeding diathesis
- Significant head trauma within 3 months
- Aortic dissection
- Recent symptoms suggesting active peptic ulcer
- Coma
- Oesophageal varices

Relative:
- Severe hypertension (systolic >180 mmHg, diastolic >110 mmHg) despite treatment
- Traumatic or prolonged cardiopulmonary resuscitation
- Major surgery within 3 weeks
- Non-compressible vascular punctures
- Recent (within 2–4 weeks) internal bleeding
- Pregnancy
- Active peptic ulcer
- Current anticoagulant use
- Pain for >24 hours
- Abdominal aortic aneurysm

On examination his blood pressure is 200/100 mmHg, pulse 90 bpm. There is clinical evidence of left ventricular failure.

Is this patient a candidate for immediate thrombolysis?

The criteria for thrombolysis are:
- Typical ischaemic pain with an onset within the previous 12 hours, and an ECG showing:
  - ST elevation ≥2 mm in a minimum of two adjacent chest leads (V1–V6), *or*
  - ST elevation of ≥1 mm in two or more of the limb leads (I, II, III, aVL and aVF), *or*
  - New-onset LBBB.

Although the patient fulfils the ECG criteria for thrombolysis, his blood pressure is too high for immediate thrombolytic therapy and there are additional concerns since the patient is on warfarin.

For a patient to be a candidate for thrombolysis the presentation should be within 12 hours of the onset of the pain. After this period, there is no benefit from thrombolysis. The ideal time is very early following the onset of pain (the golden hour) when the mortality benefits are greatest. The rapid assessment and triage of patients presenting with chest pain is essential to reduce the time to thrombolysis (call to needle and door to needle times).

Thrombolysis is contraindicated in patients predisposed to bleeding and in those with uncontrolled hypertension (Table 2.1). There is an increased risk of bleeding

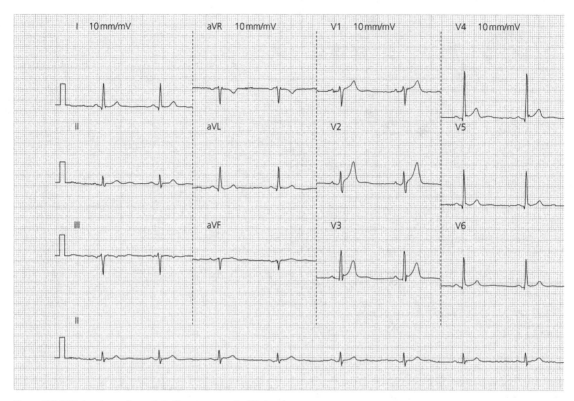

Figure 2.2 ECG showing early repolarisation as a cause for ST elevation.

Table 2.2 Advantages of primary angioplasty vs thrombolysis

- Improved vessel patency
- Reduced intracerebral bleeding
- Improved mortality
- Reduced incidence of post-infarction angina
- Improved outcome in cardiogenic shock
- Identification of non-infarct-related coronary disease

with thrombolysis in patients with an active duodenal ulcer. However, in this case, it is reasonable to assume thta the ulcer is adequately healed with medical therapy and that thrombolysis can be given. Uncontrolled hypertension should be treated prior to thrombolysis with intravenous beta blockade or intravenous nitrates. In this case it is preferable to use intravenous nitrates since the patient has evidence of left ventricular failure.

Anticoagulation with warfarin is a relative contraindication to thrombolysis and the international normalised ratio (INR) should be less than 2.5 if thrombolysis is to be considered.

What alternative treatment is available for this condition and what are the potential benefits?

Coronary angiography with primary angioplasty (Table 2.2). Although thrombolysis is an effective treatment for myocardial infarction, only a quarter of patients achieve adequate myocardial perfusion in the infarct related territory. This is due to a variety of factors including failure to open the occluded vessel, reocclusion, residual critical coronary narrowing and microvascular damage. Primary angioplasty is capable of achieving vessel patency with normal coronary flow in over 95% of cases. The risk of haemorrhage in particular cerebral haemorrhage (incidence approximately 1% after thrombolysis) is reduced. Coronary angiography also provides detailed information of the state of the other coronary vessels. Primary angioplasty has a marked benefit in patients presenting in cardiogenic shock where the mortality is high (80–90%) and thrombolysis is less effective.

The benefits of primary angioplasty are only maintained with the availability of skilled operators and rapid intervention (a door to balloon time of less than 90 minutes). Patients may be require to be transferred to an intervention centre for treatment; however, the delay involved does not appear to diminish the benefits of this therapy over thrombolysis.

The INR is 1.2. A decision is made to give thrombolysis since there are no angioplasty facilities available. Aspirin 300 mg, morphine and an infusion of GTN are commenced and the blood pressure falls to 120/70 mmHg.

What thrombolytic agent would you use?

The options are (Table 2.3):
- Streptokinase.
- Accelerated recombinant tissue plasminogen activator (rtPA).
- Anistreptase.
- Reteplase (rPA).
- Tenecteplase (TNK).

Streptokinase is only suitable for use in those patients who have not had previous exposure to the drug. There is trial evidence that rtPA is superior to streptokinase. This is most evident in younger patients with anterior myocardial infarction presenting early or in patients with a systolic blood pressure of <100 mmHg. TNK and rtPA have the advantage of being bolus agents and are often used for thrombolysis by ambulance teams. TNK and rtPA appear to be equivalent in efficacy to rtPA.

An infusion of streptokinase is commenced; however, shortly afterwards the patient becomes profoundly hypotensive (blood pressure 80/40 mmHg) with a pulse of 90 bpm.

Table 2.3 Thrombolytic regimens

Streptokinase	1.5 million units over 1 hour
Accelerated recombinant tissue plasminogen activator	15 mg bolus then 0.75 mg/kg over 30 minutes then 0.5 mg/kg over 60 minutes.
Anistreptase	30 units over 5 minutes
Reteplase	10 units over 2 minutes repeated After 30 minutes
Tenecteplase	500–600 μg/kg over 10 seconds (max. 50 mg)

What causes would you consider for the hypotension in this patient and what clinical features would you look for on examination?

- Bleeding.
- Cardiogenic shock.
- Pericardial tamponade.
- Adverse reaction to streptokinase.
- Other drug therapy (e.g. nitrate infusion, morphine, antihypertensive agents).
- Drug allergy.

The most important complication to exclude is bleeding. If this is acute gastrointestinal (GI) haemorrhage there may not be evidence of blood per rectum this early; however, the abdomen may be distended and the bowel sounds hyperactive if there has been a recent GI bleed. Examine for an abdominal aortic aneurysm that may have bled. Retroperitoneal bleeding may be very difficult to identify but the patient may complain of pain in the back or pain radiating down the anterior aspect of the thigh, the leg may be flexed due to pain from blood surrounding the psoas muscle. With blood loss, the venous pressure will be low and the patient will be tachycardic with cold peripheries. In cardiogenic shock and tamponade the venous pressure is usually markedly elevated and there is evidence of pulmonary oedema. Drug allergy may be associated with a skin rash or wheezing.

The jugular venous pressure (JVP) is low, the patient appears warm and well perfused and there is no evidence of heart failure or rectal bleeding and the abdominal examination is normal.

What action would you take?

Stop the streptokinase and GTN infusion and give a bolus of normal saline (200 ml). Monitor the patient carefully for GI haemorrhage. If the blood pressure responds rapidly and there is no evidence of bleeding, then commence a non-streptokinase-based thrombolytic (rtPA, rPA or TNK) or, if available, consider primary angioplasty.

The blood pressure improves rapidly once streptokinase and GTN have been discontinued and rtPA is commenced.

What additional treatments would be appropriate?
Aspirin
This is given in a dose of 300 mg initially followed by 75 mg daily. Aspirin and thrombolytic agent each reduce

the relative mortality from myocardial infarction by approximately 25%. Contraindicated if there is a history of allergy or evidence of active GI bleeding.

Beta blockade

Oral beta blockade is prescribed to all patients excluding those with asthma, cardiogenic shock or a bradycardia (<60 bpm). Chronic obstructive airways disease (COPD) is not an absolute contraindication to beta blockade, many of these patients will tolerate beta blockade perfectly well. The choice of beta blocker varies; however, the most commonly used are atenolol (25–50 mg daily) and metoprolol (25– 50 mg tds). Metoprolol has the advantage of a shorter half life if there is an adverse reaction.

The role of intravenous beta blockade is more controversial. In patients who are not in acute left ventricular failure or cardiogenic shock they are probably beneficial and they are particularly useful in controlling hypertension in patients prior to thrombolysis, e.g. i.v. metoprolol 5 mg over 2 minutes, repeated every 5 minutes up to 15 mg.

Statins

These agents reduce mortality by approximately a third after myocardial infarction. All patients are prescribed statins regardless of their cholesterol. They are usually started on admission. The agent most commonly used is simvastatin 40 mg orally daily.

Clopidogrel

Two recent trials have demonstrated the benefit of additional antiplatelet therapy with clopidogrel after myocardial infarction. A loading dose of 300 mg daily followed by 75 mg daily is prescribed.

Angiotensin-converting enzyme (ACE) inhibitors

These agents reduce the risk of heart failure and reinfarction following myocardial infarction. This appears to be a class effect. The agents are effective when given early after myocardial infarction; however, they should be delayed if the patient is unstable or in cardiogenic shock. A number of agents have been shown to be effective in clinical trials and should be titrated to the maximum tolerated dose, e.g. ramipril (starting dose 2.5 mg daily titrating to 10 mg daily if tolerated). Where ACE inhibitors are not tolerated due to cough, an angiotensin II blocker may be substituted.

Heparin

With the exception of streptokinase, either low-molecular-weight or unfractionated heparin is prescribed in conjunction with a thrombolytic agent to reduce the risk of reocclusion of the vessel.

Insulin

Careful management of diabetic control is beneficial. Most patients will be prescribed a sliding-scale insulin regimen in the first 48 hours.

Warfarin is discontinued and the patient is commenced on clopidogrel 75 mg od, simvastatin 40 mg daily and a heparin infusion. You are asked to review him after his thrombolytic infusion has been completed.

How would you assess whether the treatment with the thrombolytic drug had been successful?

The re-establishment of flow down the coronary artery is one of the most important factors in determining the outcome from myocardial infarction. The ideal way to assess vessel patency after thrombolysis is to perform coronary angiography; however, this is not practical in most cases in the acute setting and is associated with a risk of bleeding at the femoral puncture site. A surrogate is the ECG. Early ST segment resolution is a powerful predictor of reperfusion and prognosis (mortality rates are double in patients without ST resolution). An ECG is taken 90 minutes after the commencement of thrombolysis. Resolution of ST elevation of 50% or more is taken as an indication of reperfusion. In some centres patients who show no sign of reperfusion on the ECG would then undergo angiography and angioplasty to the infarct-related artery (rescue angioplasty).

The resolution of pain is not a reliable guide to reperfusion although it is often mistakenly taken as such. This is particularly the case in those patients who have received morphine analgesia and in the elderly and diabetics where pain may not be the predominant feature of myocardial infarction.

Following thrombolysis there is resolution of the ST segments and his ECG the following day shows T-wave inversion in the anterior chest leads with Q waves from V2 to V5. His troponin I is 50 μg/L (normal <1 μg/L). Routine bloods including electrolytes, FBC, thyroid and liver function tests are normal.

What other investigations/factors may be helpful in determining the prognosis in this patient?

Echocardiography

The most important factor in long-term prognosis is left ventricular function. Patients with more severely impaired left ventricular function have a relatively poor prognosis.

Brain natriuretic peptide (BNP)

BNP (see Chapter 10, p. 108) is elevated in acute myocardial infarction and is related to prognosis. A high BNP level indicates more extensive myocardial damage, giving rise to left ventricular failure.

Stress testing /coronary angiography

The presence of additional coronary disease and/or symptomatic angina increases the risk of further cardiac events. Stress testing is usually in the form of an exercise test although stress perfusion scanning or stress echocardiography are alternatives. The decision regarding coronary angiography is, in part, dependent upon the amount of myocardium felt to be at risk from the coronary disease and the amount of myocardium that has been lost following the infarction. With a very large infarct, with complete loss of function on echo of the territory supplied by the infarct-related artery, there may be little point in performing angiography since there is little myocardium left to be salvaged.

Comorbidities

Mortality rates amongst diabetics following myocardial infarction are approximately double those of non-diabetics.

An echocardiogram is performed the day following presentation and shows extensive anterior myocardial damage, predominantly in the septum and apex. There is clinical evidence of left ventricular failure. The patient is commenced on an ACE inhibitor and furosemide 40 mg daily. In the presence of a completed anterior infarction, it is decided that angiography is not indicated. You are asked to arrange an exercise test.

When would it be appropriate to arrange the exercise test and what factors may make it difficult to interpret?

The value of exercise testing after myocardial infarction is relatively limited. Ideally, the exercise test should be performed prior to discharge in order to identify patients at high risk and to guide cardiac rehabilitation. In uncomplicated myocardial infarction, a submaximal exercise test may be performed as early as 72 hours after the presentation. A symptom-limited early exercise test at 14–21 days is an alternative.

Contraindications to exercise testing would include:
- Uncontrolled atrial fibrillation.
- Complete heart block.
- Overt cardiac failure.
- Unstable angina.
- Physical disability, e.g. arthritis, severe claudication or COPD.
- Age (there is little to be gained in performing a post-myocardial infarct exercise test in patients over 80 years)
- ECG abnormality that renders the ST-segment shifts difficult to interpret e.g. LVH with strain, LBBB.

In patients with extensive anterior myocardial infarction and Q wave formation the ST segments in the anterior leads cannot be interpreted. It is not uncommon to see ST elevation in these leads on exercise testing post-myocardial infarction; this does not add any prognostic value to the test.

Three days later you are called urgently to the Coronary Care Unit as the patient has become acutely unwell with breathlessness.

What is your differential diagnosis for the cause of this man's sudden deterioration and what investigations would you request?

The complications of myocardial infarction are given in Table 2.4.

The most likely cause of this deterioration is the development of is *pulmonary oedema. Pulmonary embolism* is much less common this early following myocardial infarction, particularly in patients who have received thrombolysis and anticoagulation. A chest X-ray will be particularly helpful and should show evidence of pulmonary oedema.

Pulmonary oedema post-myocardial infarction is most commonly due to pump failure from extensive myocardial damage; however, pulmonary oedema may also be precipitated by dysrhythmias, a ventricular septal defect (VSD) or papillary muscle rupture. Dysrhythmias will be easy to identify on the ECG. However, the murmur of a ventricular septal defect or mitral regurgitation may be obscured by noisy breath sounds. If the patient is in

Table 2.4 Complications following myocardial infarction

Left ventricular failure

Cardiogenic shock

Acute renal failure

Dysrhythmias, e.g. atrial fibrillation, ventricular tachycardia, ventricular fibrillation, heart block

Mitral valve papillary muscle rupture

Myocardial rupture and tamponade

Ventricular septal defect (VSD)

Pericarditis

Dressler's syndrome (pericarditis and fever presenting after 4–6 weeks)

Stroke or other peripheral embolism secondary to mural thrombus

Ventricular aneurysm formation

Pulmonary embolism

---

sinus rhythm, an echocardiogram is essential to confirm the cause of the patient's deterioration. A ventricular septal rupture or papillary muscle rupture is an indication for urgent cardiac surgery since the prognosis without intervention is extremely poor.

The patient's ECG demonstrates atrial fibrillation at a rate of 180 bpm; there are no other changes. Echocardiography demonstrates an intact ventricular septum; there is no evidence of papillary muscle rupture. The ejection fraction is reported at 15%. The patient deteriorates rapidly with a blood pressure of 70/50 mmHg with oxygen saturations of 80% and is unresponsive.

How would you manage this patient?

The cause of the patient's deterioration is acute pulmonary oedema due to the onset of fast atrial fibrillation in the context of impaired left ventricular function. The estimation of ejection fraction is unreliable in patients with fast dysrhythmias and is usually an underestimate. There is probably no alternative to emergency cardioversion under general anaesthesia. Intravenous diuretics, digoxin and continuous airways pressure could be tried but are unlikely to act sufficiently rapidly to restore an adequate circulation. Amiodarone, even intravenously, takes several hours to act and is poor at controlling the ventricular rate.

The patient is cardioverted under general anaesthesia. Sinus rhythm is restored and the patient is ventilated overnight on the Intensive Care Unit (ICU); there is no requirement for inotropic support. An intravenous furosemide infusion produces a good diuresis. The following morning the patient is extubated. Over the course of the next 5 days the patient is stabilised on an ACE inhibitor and diuretics and is prescribed amiodarone to prevent recurrent episodes of atrial fibrillation. A repeat echocardiogram shows an ejection fraction of 25% with anterior, septal and apical akinesia.

What further interventions should be considered for this patient?
Angiography

This patient has had a complicated course following a large myocardial infarction. Even though it is unlikely that there is any recoverable myocardium in the infarct territory, any additional coronary disease should be identified and where appropriate treated.

Automated implantable cardioverter-defibrillator (AICD) implantation

This patient is at high risk of ventricular dysrhythmias. Although there is little evidence for benefit in the acute phase following myocardial infarction, further assessment with echocardiography at 6 months and referral for AICD implantation may be necessary (see Case 16, pp. 145–6).

Eplerinone

There is evidence from a single randomised control trial that the introduction of this aldosterone antagonist has mortality and morbidity benefit in patients with an ejection fraction <35% following myocardial infarction.

Beta blockade

In the context of a patient in frank pulmonary oedema or cardiogenic shock, beta blockade is contraindicated. However, it should be considered once the patient has stabilised. In the context of severe left ventricular impairment, beta blockers known to be of benefit in patients with heart failure should be used and titrated to appropriate doses over a number of weeks (see Case 9, p. 103).

What advice should this patient be given regarding driving and returning to work?

In the UK, patients are advised not to return to driving for 1 month after myocardial infarction. An HGV license cannot be regained until 3 months after completing 9 minutes of a standard Bruce protocol exercise test, off antianginal medical without angina or ST-segment changes, and providing the ejection fraction returns to >40%.

Most patients with non-physical jobs will return to work 4–6 weeks after myocardial infarction. For more physical jobs, assessment with an exercise test at 6 weeks may help guide advice.

CASE REVIEW

This 60-year-old diabetic smoker presents with a classical history of cardiac chest pain. An ECG confirms that he has an anterior STEMI. Streptokinase is administered and considered justified, despite the history of a previous bleeding duodenal ulcer and the use of warfarin, because of the 10-year interval from the gastrointestinal bleed and the low admission INR. Hypotension occurs with the use of streptokinase and rtPA is commenced once other causes of hypotension have been excluded.

Despite successful resolution indicated by ST segment reperfusion, there has been major myocardial damage. The onset of atrial fibrillation triggers pulmonary oedema and hypotensive shock and the patient requires cardioversion as an emergency procedure. Long-term treatment is required with beta blockade, ACE inhibitors, a statin and aspirin. With current treatments the in-hospital mortality for myocardial infarction has fallen to less than 10% (less than 5% in clinical trials performed on a selected population). However, in the context of major myocardial damage, the prognosis is poor. Late mortality following myocardial infarction is often due to malignant ventricular arrhythmias and where there has been major myocardial loss, implantation of an AICD should be considered.

KEY POINTS

- Patients presenting with ischaemic chest pain and ST elevation on the ECG form a subgroup of patients with acute coronary syndromes where there is a high probability that the coronary artery has occluded.
- Other causes of ST elevation need to be excluded prior to treatment, in particular pericarditis where the ST elevation is more widespread and concave as opposed to convex, the systemic disturbance less, and the troponin is usually normal or only mildly elevated.
- The loss of cardiac muscle in an STEMI is dependent upon the duration of occlusion and most of the damage is complete within the first few hours of the onset of pain. It is therefore important to identify and treat these patients rapidly.
- An assessment of the ECG as soon as the patient presents helps to identify those patients who are candidates for thrombolysis or primary angioplasty.
- All patients should receive aspirin and clopidogrel on presentation, unless these agents are contraindicated.
- The decision whether to thrombolyse or perform primary angioplasty is dependent upon the facilities available;

however, patients treated promptly with primary angioplasty have a better outcome than those treated with thrombolysis.
- Thrombolysis is less effective for those patients presenting late due to organisation of the coronary thrombus and more extensive myocardial damage and should not be given to those patients presenting more than 12 hours after the onset of pain.
- Beta blockade, ACE inhibitors and statins all improve survival in patients with myocardial infarction and should be prescribed unless contraindicated.
- Common early complications are left ventricular failure, cardiogenic shock and arrhythmias.
- Prognosis following myocardial infarction is dependent upon left ventricular function, which is best assessed with echocardiography.
- Stress testing +/– angiography should be considered on all patients following STEMI treated with thrombolysis to establish the extent of residual coronary disease.

An 85-year-old man with collapse

An 85-year-old man with maturity-onset diabetes and a history of hypertension is admitted to A&E after being found on the toilet floor by his neighbour. He reports feeling well that morning but felt slightly giddy and nauseated mid-morning and fell when passing urine. He was unable to get up because of pain in his right hip. He has a past history of hypertension and diabetes. His current medical therapy is: glibenclamide 10 mg od; diltiazem 60 mg po tds; aspirin 75 mg od.

What are the possible causes of his collapse and what further questions would you ask to try to confirm the diagnosis in each case?

Postural hypotension

Postural hypotension is a very common cause of dizziness and collapse in the elderly. The problem is more common in the diabetic population where it is associated with an autonomic neuropathy. Antihypertensive drugs (in this case diltiazem) may also contribute.

The patient should be asked for symptoms of dizziness when rising from a chair, when getting out of bed in the morning, or when getting out of a hot bath. The patient may have symptoms of a peripheral neuropathy (pain or numbness) or retinopathy, which may make the diagnosis of an autonomic neuropathy more likely. The symptoms of postural hypotension are relieved by lying down. When severe, the patient may lose consciousness. The symptoms may be brought on by intercurrent infection, which should be excluded.

Micturition syncope

The patient may report dizziness or syncope when straining to pass urine. There may be a history of prostatic disease.

Cardiology: Clinical Cases Uncovered. By T. Betts, J. Dwight and S. Bull. Published 2010 by Blackwell Publishing.

Arrhythmias

Rapid tachyarrhythmias (ventricular tachycardia or atrial fibrillation) may give rise to dizziness or syncope. They are more likely in the context of a history of preceding heart disease, e.g. ischaemic heart disease. The patient may be aware of palpitations prior to the attack. Heart block (usually complete heart block or Mobitz type 2 atrioventricular block) may present with syncope without any warning (Adam Stokes attack) and the patient may injure themselves as a result. This patient is on a rate-slowing agent (diltiazem), which may make this more likely.

Silent myocardial infarction

In diabetic patients, pain is not always a feature of myocardial infarction. They may present with syncope secondary to hypotension or arrhythmias secondary to an ischaemic event. The patient may not complain of chest pain but may admit to chest tightness or breathlessness.

Hypoglycaemia

Oral hypoglycaemic agents in the elderly are a common cause of hypoglycaemia, which the patient interprets as dizziness. When severe this may cause the patient to become disorientated and collapse. Features of sweating and other hypoglycaemic symptoms are not always present. The patient may present with neurological features suggestive of a stroke.

Seizure

A common differential diagnosis. A witness to the event is very helpful. There may be a history of a preceding aura. The period of loss of consciousness is prolonged and therefore not consistent with a cardiac cause. The patient may be confused or drowsy (post-ictal) afterwards and there may be evidence of tongue biting, incontinence or focal neurological signs.

Vasovagal syncope (see Case 15, p. 141).

Stroke/transient ischaemic attack

This is a common cause of collapse in the elderly. There are usually neurological signs or symptoms; however, these may be quite subtle with brain-stem and posterior fossa strokes. It is important to look for nystagmus and cerebellar signs, which are often not well assessed in a brief neurological examination. Loss of consciousness is extremely uncommon in the context of a stroke, unless it is very severe or when the stroke has been complicated by a seizure. If there has been loss of conscious and there are no residual neurological signs, an alternative cause should be sought.

> On arrival he appears well but is hypotensive with a blood pressure of 80/50 mmHg and has a bradycardia (pulse 40 bpm), his JVP is elevated and there is evidence of bilateral basal crepitations. His O$_2$ saturations are 92% on room air. He does not complain of chest pain but feels breathless since his collapse and has a painful right hip. There is no focal neurology. There is no evidence of external bruising.
> His ECG is shown in Figure 3.1.

What abnormalities are shown in his ECG?

- Complete heart block.
- Old anterior myocardial infarction.
- New inferior myocardial infarction.

The ECG shows a bradycardia of 50 bpm in complete heart block. The axis is normal. There is an acute inferior myocardial infarction with ST elevation in leads II, III and aVF. The patient has suffered a previous anterior myocardial infarction since there are Q waves in the anterior leads with loss of R-wave progression and T-wave inversion. The QT interval is prolonged at 480 ms; however, this has to be corrected for the slow heart rate, the QTc (Q-T/√R-R interval) is 424 ms, which is just within the normal range.

KEY POINT

It is sometimes difficult to identify complete heart block on an ECG where the P-wave rate is almost exactly double the QRS rate and the patient may appear to be in sinus rhythm. If the patient has bradycardia always look at the point on the ECG half way between the P waves to see whether a further P wave is present.

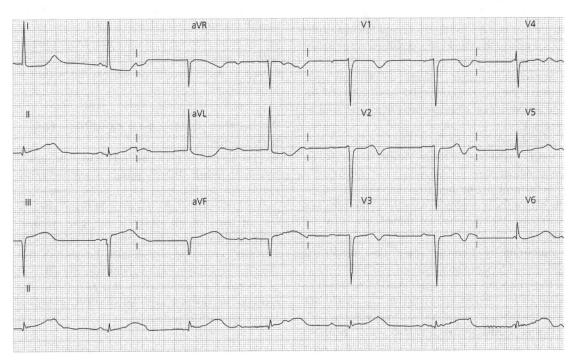

Figure 3.1 The patient's ECG.

What initial management steps should be instituted?

• **ABC.** The usual protocol of ABC (airway, breathing, circulation) is appropriate in the initial assessment of the patient. In addition the following should be considered.

• **Oxygen.** All patients with acute coronary syndromes are given oxygen on admission in order to achieve oxygen saturations of 98–100% where possible.

• **Pain relief.** There is often reluctance to give morphine in the context of hypotension; however, there is no evidence that this has a detrimental effect on outcome and, if the patient is in pain, morphine can be administered in low dose (2.5 mg intravenously).

• **Cardiac monitoring.** All patients with acute coronary syndromes should be monitored on admission.

• **Access to external pacing.** Complete heart block following an inferior myocardial infarction is often well tolerated and may not need intervention; however, it is important to be prepared. Most units are equipped with external pacing units. Although the patient may not require pacing immediately, the external pacing pads should be applied particularly in a patient who is haemodynamically unstable.

• **Portable chest X-ray (CXR).** This is not essential but will help to confirm the diagnosis of left ventricular failure that is suspected on the clinical findings. If the CXR is delayed this should not delay definitive treatment of the myocardial infarction.

• **Intravenous diuretics.** Although the patient is hypotensive there is evidence of left ventricular failure. The administration of intravenous furosemide will be beneficial.

• **Clopidogrel.** Now routinely administered to acute coronary syndrome patients where there is no contraindication.

• **Assessment of the hip.** It is important to assess the hip for the possibility of a fracture. Where this is a possibility, the decision to thrombolyse may be affected.

• **Admission to Coronary Care Unit (CCU).** All patients with ST elevation myocardial infarction (STEMI) or high-risk acute coronary syndromes (ACSs) should be admitted to coronary care; however, this should not delay thrombolysis, which may be administered in A&E.

• **Urgent cardiology review.** Myocardial infarction complicated by arrhythmias, cardiogenic shock or heart failure, or where the decision regarding thrombolysis versus angioplasty needs to be made, should be referred to a cardiologist.

Beta blockade is contraindicated in the context of heart block. Intravenous nitrates are contraindicated in view of the systolic hypotension. Full-dose low-molecular-weight heparin is only indicated if the patient undergoes thrombolysis. Pressor agents such as adrenaline, noradrenaline, dobutamine, isoprenaline and dopamine should be avoided if at all possible.

Which coronary artery is likely to be involved in the acute event?

In most cases, inferior myocardial infarction is caused by occlusion of the right coronary artery (RCA). A smaller proportion are due to the occlusion of the circumflex (Cx) coronary artery (where the Cx artery is dominant and gives rise to the posterior descending artery, which also supplies the inferior wall).

Why has this patient developed complete heart block?

Sinus bradycardia and AV block are frequently associated with inferior myocardial infarction since this artery commonly supplies the SA and AV nodes. Complete heart block in the presence of an inferior myocardial infarction usually resolves over the course of 3–5 days. By contrast, heart block is uncommon in the context of an anterior myocardial infarction. It usually signifies major myocardial damage with extensive damage to the intraventricular septum and is likely to be permanent.

Would this patient be a candidate for thrombolysis?

Yes. The absence of chest pain with myocardial infarction in an elderly diabetic patient is well recognised and is not an indication to withhold thrombolytic therapy in the context of a qualifying ECG and a defined time of onset of the event (in this case syncope). Although there may be some concern in case a pacing wire may need to be inserted after thrombolysis, it is likely that reperfusion following thrombolysis will result in restoration of sinus rhythm. If a pacing wire then needs to be inserted after thrombolysis, a femoral venous approach is preferable.

While in A&E the patient experiences syncope with a period of asystole lasting 10 seconds.

Table 3.1 Indications for pacing in complete heart block following myocardial infarction

- Anterior myocardial infarction
- Heart rate ≤40 bpm
- Broad complex escape rhythm
- Asystolic episodes
- Bradycardia-related syncope
- Bradycardia-related episodes of ventricular tachycardia
- Heart rate <60 bpm with one or more of the following:
  - Poor tissue perfusion
  - Renal failure
  - Systolic blood pressure <80 mmHg
  - Persistent left ventricular failure following acute myocardial infarction therapy

What action can be taken for the management of his complete heart block?

- Restore coronary perfusion with thrombolysis or angioplasty.
- Atropine.
- Temporary pacing/external pacing.
- Withdraw rate-slowing agents.

Since the cause of complete heart block is an inferior myocardial infarction, the best treatment is to restore coronary perfusion with thrombolysis or primary angioplasty. If sinus rhythm is not restored following thrombolysis or angioplasty and the patient remains hypotensive and in left ventricular failure or has recurrent syncopal episodes, then a temporary pacing wire should be inserted. The use of atropine is only a temporary measure and can be used pending insertion of a pacing wire. The criteria for insertion of a pacing wire are base on the patient's cardiac output, underlying rate and escape rhythm (Table 3.1). It is important to remember to withdraw and cross off the drug chart any rate-slowing agents the patient may be on (in this case diltiazem).

In view of his hypotension and concern over his heart block he is transferred immediately to the angiography suite where a temporary pacing wire is inserted and angiography is performed. The angiographic findings are as follows: LAD artery, 75% stenosis in mid-portion; Cx coronary artery; normal; RCA; occluded proximally.

He undergoes angioplasty and stenting to the RCA and is transferred back to the CCU. Twelve hours later he remains hypotensive with blood pressure 80/40 mmHg, heart rate

70 bpm in sinus rhythm; his JVP is elevated. The remainder of the cardiac and respiratory examination is normal. O₂ saturations are 98% on room air.

What are the possible causes of his hypotension, how would you investigate this further?

- Cardiogenic shock.
- Acute stent thrombosis.
- Haemorrhage.
- Right ventricular infarction.
- Pericardial tamponade.
- Ventricular septal defect (VSD).
- Papillary muscle rupture/ dysfunction.

The most likely cause of hypotension in this situation is **cardiogenic shock** due to poor left ventricular function. The patient has had a previous anterior myocardial infarction and a recent inferior myocardial infarction and there has therefore been major myocardial damage.

The RCA commonly supplies blood to the right ventricle as well as the inferior surface of the left ventricle. Therefore **right ventricular infarction** may accompany inferior myocardial infarction. If the predominant damage is to the right ventricle the patient presents with right ventricular failure in the absence of left ventricular failure. The JVP is usually elevated but the chest is clear and a CXR does not demonstrate evidence of pulmonary oedema. Hypotension is due to reduced left ventricular filling as a result of right ventricular failure. If complete heart block accompanies right ventricular infarction, severe hypotension is common since the function of both right and left ventricles is very dependent on atrial transport (filling due to atrial contraction). This is one indication for temporary dual chamber pacing. The ECG in right ventricular infarction commonly shows evidence of inferior ST elevation and also involvement of the posterior wall (ST depression and the development of tall R waves in V1–V2); additional leads placed to the right of the sternum (V4–6R) may demonstrate ST elevation.

Pericardial tamponade usually occurs within the first 4 days of myocardial infarction and is more common in elderly and hypertensive patients. Deterioration is usually extremely rapid and hypotension is accompanied by an elevated JVP. Pericardial aspiration may be required if the patient is critically ill but should otherwise be avoided as decompression of the pericardial space may lead to further bleeding. This patient has had a temporary pacing wire inserted and therefore pericardial tamponade due to perforation of the right ventricle by the pacing wire needs to be considered.

Acute stent thrombosis. Stent thrombosis can occur within hours or days of an angioplasty (acute) or months later (chronic). Acute stent thrombosis is rare with the use of antiplatelet agents such as clopidogrel and IIb/IIIa antagonists. The patient presents with further pain and ECG changes (usually ST elevation).

Haemorrhage always has to be considered in the differential diagnosis. The JVP is usually not elevated and initially there may be no external evidence of bleeding.

VSD or papillary muscle rupture usually occurs a few days after the initial infarction. The presentation is similar in both cases, with hypotension, left ventricular failure and a systolic murmur. The VSD murmur is usually pansystolic and very loud but in acute mitral regurgitation (MR) the murmur can be very short and may be missed. Severe MR can occur in the absence of papillary muscle rupture, either due to severe ventricular dilatation and stretching of the mitral valve annulus or as a result of papillary muscle dysfunction due to ischaemia or left ventricular remodelling.

An **urgent CXR** will help to establish whether the patient is in pulmonary oedema. If the lung fields are clear then right ventricular infarction or haemorrhage should be considered. Cautious filling with 100–200 ml aliquots of either colloid or normal saline may be tried; however, the patient should be monitored very carefully for the development of pulmonary oedema. An **ECG** may show evidence of new ST elevation associated with stent occlusion. However, the key investigation is **echocardiography.** This will show a pericardial collection or evidence of right ventricular dysfunction and dilatation in the case of a right ventricular infarction and can identify a VSD or MR.

The CXR demonstrates pulmonary oedema. An echocardiogram is reported as showing, a moderately dilated left ventricle with an ejection fraction of 25%. The anterior and inferior walls are hypokinetic (contracting poorly) and there is severe MR but no evidence of papillary muscle rupture.

How would you manage this patient?

Cardiogenic shock in the context of myocardial infarction is associated with a mortality of 80–90%. The prognosis for recovery is poor in a man of this age with evidence of previous myocardial infarction and a history of diabetes. Therefore, the first consideration may be whether further

intervention should be undertaken. It is important to take into account the condition and circumstances of the patient prior to this event and this may involve a discussion with the family and, where possible, the patient. If the patient has other serious comorbidity, e.g. cancer, then further treatment may not be appropriate.

If further intervention is indicated, then the management is for cardiogenic shock (see Case26, p. 202). The most helpful intervention is likely to be the insertion of a balloon pump. This treatment is particularly effective in patients with acute severe MR or a VSD and acts as a bridge to surgery. The patient may require continuous positive airways pressure to maintain oxygen saturations and inotropes if an adequate systolic pressure cannot be achieved using a balloon pump. As the patient has already undergone a successful procedure to the infarct-related artery and there is no evidence of papillary muscle rupture, there is no place for urgent surgical intervention.

A balloon pump is inserted and the patient improves. After 2 weeks on the CCU the patient is stable. A repeat echocardiogram is performed. The MR is now reported as mild. The ejection fraction is 30%. There is an infero-apical left ventricular aneurysm.

What ECG changes might be expected in conjunction with the aneurysm formation? What additional treatment may be required?

An inferior aneurysm is commonly associated with MR. There is a substantial risk of thromboembolic events and the patient should be anticoagulated with warfarin, usually for a minimum period of 3 months. With a ventricular aneurysm, the ECG shows persistent ST elevation and Q-wave formation with loss of R wave.

A ventricular aneurysm post-myocardial infarction should be suspected in the following circumstances:

• Embolic events post-myocardial infarction.
• Bulge on the left heart border on CXR.
• Persistent ST elevation on the ECG.
• Late post-myocardial infarction ventricular dysrhythmias.

Ideally, what medications should this patient have prescribed on discharge?

• Statin.
• ACE inhibitor.
• Beta blocker (bisoprolol, carvedilol, metoprolol or nebivolol).

- Loop diuretic.
- Aldosterone antagonist.
- Clopidogrel.
- GTN spray.
- Warfarin.

The patient was discharged on the above medications after a 2-week period in hospital.

What advice would you give him concerning his medication?

This patient has had a large myocardial infarction associated with severe left ventricular damage and a left ventricular thrombus and therefore the medication list is a long one. It is inadvisable to prescribe aspirin, clopidogrel and warfarin to a patient this age, the risk of haemorrhage being up to 25% in the first year. If warfarin is essential, then either clopidogrel or aspirin are not prescribed. In patients with a coronary stent, clopidogrel is given rather than aspirin.

Hypotension is a common problem in the elderly prescribed ACE inhibitors, beta blockers and diuretics. The patient should be warned of the **symptoms of postural hypotension** and to seek advice if they are present. If the patient develops **diarrhoea or vomiting** then the patient should see their GP so that the diuretic dosage may be adjusted or discontinued temporarily. Over-the-counter **non-steroidal anti-inflammatory drugs** or agents containing **aspirin** should be avoided (increased risk of bleeding on warfarin, increased risk of renal dysfunction on ACE inhibitors). The specific side-effects you might warn the patient about would include:

- Statins – muscle pain.
- Beta blockers – wheezing, cold peripheries and fatigue.
- ACE inhibitors – dry cough in 10% of cases.
- Aldosterone antagonists – gynaecomastia.
- Clopidogrel – GI disturbances.
- GTN – headache, postural hypotension.

The patient should be asked to seek advice before commencing any new medications in view of the risk of drug interactions.

PART 2: CASES

CASE REVIEW

This 85-year-old man has had an inferior myocardial infarction presenting with a syncopal episode due to complete heart block. Pain was not a prominent feature. His ECG showed evidence of a previous anterior myocardial infarction, which may well have been painless. His inferior myocardial infarction was associated with heart block due to occlusion of the vascular supply to the AV node. Treatment for this was restoration of perfusion, in this case by angioplasty to the RCA. His course was complicated by cardiogenic shock and MR due to the formation of an inferior wall aneurysm. He was treated with primary angioplasty since patients with cardiogenic shock have a better chance of recovery when treated with angioplasty than with thrombolysis. As the patient had already suffered an anterior myocardial infarction the area of infarcted muscle was large and gave rise to an inferior wall aneurysm with a significant risk of intracardiac thrombus formation, requiring treatment with warfarin. Although the patient had MR on echocardiography, this was not due to papillary muscle rupture and therefore surgical intervention was not required.

KEY POINTS

- Silent myocardial infarction is not uncommon in elderly and diabetic patients.
- Silent myocardial infarction should be considered in patients presenting with syncope, heart failure, dysrhythmias and unexplained hypotension.
- Cardiac syncope is short lived (seconds), unless complicated by a head injury.
- The complications that are specifically associated with inferior myocardial infarction are heart block and right ventricular infarction.
- Heart block secondary to acute myocardial infarction is most appropriately treated by restoring perfusion by thrombolysis or angioplasty. These treatments should not be delayed by the insertion of a pacing wire, unless the patient is very haemodynamically unstable.
- The mortality from cardiogenic shock following myocardial infarction is 80–90%.
- In patients with cardiogenic shock following myocardial infarction, an echocardiogram is essential to assess left ventricular function, mitral valve function, integrity of the ventricular septum and to exclude pericardial tamponade.
- When cardiogenic shock occurs in the context of an inferior myocardial infarction it is important to consider right ventricular infarction. In cases of right ventricular infarction the JVP is high but the patient is not in pulmonary oedema and an echocardiogram does not show severe left ventricular damage.
- In cardiogenic shock due to myocardial infarction, positive inotropic agents may increase the size of the infarction and therefore should only be used as a last resort. If the blood pressure is not restored by revascularising the myocardium then a period of balloon pump support may be required.
- Hypotension is a common complication of multiple drug therapies following myocardial infarction and patients should be warned of this in advance, together with the common complications of their medications.

A 71-year-old man with exertion chest tightness

A 71-year-old man presents to the outpatient clinic with breathlessness and chest tightness on climbing a single flight of stairs over the past 3 months. His GP has measured his electrolytes and creatinine and reports an estimated glomerular filtration rate (GFR) of 25 mL/min and a fasting blood glucose of 11 mmol/L. He has a mild normochromic, normocytic anaemia (10 g/dL). He is an ex-smoker with a 30-pack year history. His father died of a myocardial infarction at the age of 80 years and his mother (who was a heavy smoker) of a myocardial infarction age 50 years. His low density lipoprotein (LDL) cholesterol is known to be 5.0 mmol/L with a high density lipoprotein (HDL) cholesterol of 0.7 mmol/L. Urine testing shows protein + and glucose ++. Pulse is 70 bpm and regular with normal character and volume. His blood pressure is 170/95 mmHg lying and 160/95 mmHg standing. He has a soft systolic murmur at the left sternal edge but the rest of the examination of the heart and lungs is normal. There are bilateral femoral bruits and his foot pulses are absent. His ECG is shown in Figure 4.1.

What is the most likely cause of his symptoms and what other medical conditions does this patient have that may predispose to this presentation?

- Class II angina predisposed to by:
  - Mild aortic stenosis (AS).
  - Diabetes mellitus.
  - Chronic renal failure.
  - Peripheral vascular disease.
  - Anaemia.

This patient has numerous risk factors for ischaemic heart disease. It is highly likely that he has angina.

A fasting glucose >7.0 mmol/L is sufficient to make a diagnosis of diabetes and substantially increases the patient's risk of coronary disease.

The normal GFR is 100 mL/min. This patient therefore has established renal disease. This constitutes a further risk factor for coronary disease and has an adverse effect on the prognosis of patients with coronary disease.

Peripheral vascular disease is a marker for generalised atheromatous disease. The most common cause of death for patients with peripheral vascular disease is ischaemic heart disease.

The severity of angina is based upon the Canadian Cardiovascular Society Scale (Table 4.1). Many patients with angina do not describe pain but rather describe a discomfort or tightness in the chest and patients with silent angina describe breathlessness or fatigue only. The presence of a systolic murmur raises the possibility of AS or hypertrophic cardiomyopathy. Both can be a cause of breathlessness, chest pain and fatigue. However, the normal pulse character, increased pulse pressure, absence of clinical left ventricular hypertrophy and a normal second sound make a diagnosis of AS that is severe enough to cause angina unlikely (See Case 13, p. 125). The diagnosis of hypertrophic cardiomyopathy is unlikely in the context of a normal ECG and absence of a family history. It is possible that this is a presentation of chronic obstructive airways disease (COPD) or asthma; however, even if this is the case, angina would have to be excluded.

What other aspects of the history would be important in confirming your suspicions?

Stable angina occurs on exertion and is relieved by rest (usually within minutes). The diagnosis is unlikely if the patient complains of rest pain without a history of exertional symptoms, unless the first manifestation of coronary disease is an acute coronary syndrome. The pain is usually central and has the characteristics of an acute coronary syndrome although usually less severe (crushing, heavy, tight band or burning) and radiates to the inner aspects of both arms, neck or jaw. Occasionally, pain may radiate through to the back. The patient will

Cardiology: Clinical Cases Uncovered. By T. Betts, J. Dwight and S. Bull. Published 2010 by Blackwell Publishing.

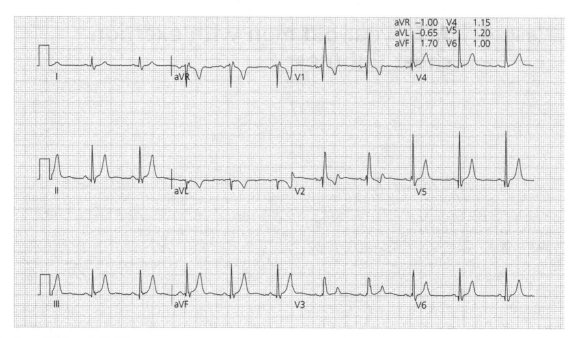

			aVR	−1.00	V4	1.15
			aVL	−0.65	V5	1.20
			aVF	1.70	V6	1.00

Figure 4.1 The patient's ECG.

Table 4.1 Canadian cardiovascular society classification of angina

Class I
Ordinary physical activity, such as walking and climbing stairs, does not cause angina
Angina with strenuous or rapid or prolonged exertion at work or recreation

Class II
Slight limitation of ordinary activity
Angina with walking or climbing stairs rapidly, walking uphill, walking or stair climbing after meals, in cold, in wind, or when under emotional stress, or only during the few hours after awakening. Walking more than two blocks on the level and climbing more than one flight of ordinary stairs at a normal pace and in normal conditions

Class III
Marked limitation of ordinary physical activity.
Angina with walking one to two blocks on the level and climbing more than one flight in normal conditions

Class IV
Inability to carry on any physical activity without discomfort
Anginal syndrome *may be* present at rest

have to stop what they are doing, although a small proportion of patients demonstrate 'walk though angina'. In these cases there is a classical description of angina when commencing a walk but this eases after a few minutes. Angina is usually worse in cold weather or after a heavy meal. A common presentation is with discomfort in the morning when the patient is having a shower or brushing their teeth. Pain that arises *after* exertion is unlikely to be angina. Where the patient has been prescribed GTN, it is useful to assess the response. The relief from GTN is usually within minutes. If a patient reports relief after 30 minutes or more this cannot be regarded as a response to GTN. It is important to establish whether the patient has symptoms of claudication or has a history of stroke, transient ischaemic attack (TIA) or amaurosis, since these conditions increase the likelihood of coronary disease and will affect the management of the patient's angina.

What is the significance of the family history?

A history of early coronary disease in first-degree relatives is an important risk factor for the development of coronary disease. A history of coronary disease in a first-degree relative is usually regarded as significant if it has arisen at an age of ≤60 years in a female relative and ≤55 years in a male relative.

The patient gives a history of a transient ischaemic attack 3 years previously. There are no symptoms of COPD or claudication.

What changes are shown on the ECG and what is the significance of these changes?

The ECG demonstrates sinus rhythm and a broad QRS complex (>120 ms). A broad QRS complex is caused by a bundle branch block or a focus arising below the AV node (usually ventricular). In this case the ECG shows sinus rhythm; therefore, the patient has left bundle branch block (LBBB) or right bundle branch block (RBBB). In V1 there is an rSR' complex and there is a deep S wave in V6. The morphology in the QRS complex in V1 is due to:
• Septal depolarisation from left to right, towards V1 (initial R wave).
• Left ventricular depolarisation away from V1 (S wave).
• Late depolarisation of the right ventricle (second R wave).
The S wave in V6 is due to late depolarisation of the right ventricle away from this lead.

In RBBB, the anteroseptal T waves can be inverted and therefore do not automatically reflect ischaemic heart disease. RBBB in the asymptomatic population is a common finding and is not associated with an adverse prognosis. New-onset RBBB may occur in the context of pulmonary embolism. In the context of ischaemic heart disease, RBBB indicates more severe coronary disease. It is associated with an adverse prognosis when occurring in the context of acute myocardial infarction. When RBBB is associated with ST elevation in the anterior leads in the absence of clinical features of myocardial infarction then Brugada syndrome should be considered (see p. 184).

What further non-invasive investigations can be performed to help to confirm the diagnosis of angina in this man and what factors determine which investigation is appropriate in the first instance?

• Stress electrocardiography:
  ○ Exercise.
  ○ Pharmacological (adenosine, dobutamine).
• Nuclear imaging:
  ○ Exercise isotope scan.
  ○ Pharmacological isotope scan (adenosine, dobutamine).
• Echocardiography:
  ○ Resting.
  ○ Stress (dobutamine).
• Contrast MRI.
• CT:
  ○ Electron beam CT.
  ○ Multislice CT.

There are a number of non-invasive investigations that may help to confirm the diagnosis. However, prior to performing any stress test it is important to exclude severe AS in this patient. A **resting echocardiogram** is therefore essential. The resting echocardiogram will also provide information regarding the patient's left ventricular function and any regional wall motion abnormalities, which may point to a diagnosis of coronary disease.

This patient has a high probability of coronary disease and does not have a disqualifying ECG, so it would be reasonable to start with a standard **Bruce protocol exercise test** (Box 4.1) providing the patient is not so limited by claudication to be unable to complete the test, in which case a pharmacological stress ECG can be performed.

In cases where an exercise test is contraindicated or uninterpretable there are a number of alternatives.

A **pharmacological stress ECG** is carried out during an infusion of an agent such as dobutamine or adenosine. Areas of ischaemia are identified by the development of new wall motion abnormalities during stress. It can be performed in patients with an abnormal resting ECG (although patients with LBBB present some problems) and does not require the patient to be able to exercise. A stress echocardiogram is more sensitive and specific than an exercise test and can identify more accurately regions of ischaemia and infarction. However, the test is labour intensive, dependent upon a skilled echocardiographer and is time consuming – it is therefore not a practical screening tool.

Box 4.1 Exercise electrocardiography

Standard exercise electrocardiography is the most widely used investigation for establishing a diagnosis of angina. The sensitivity and specificity of the exercise test for diagnosing coronary disease are 68% and 77%, respectively. There are inevitably a significant number of false positives and negatives. The predictive accuracy of the test depends on the pre-test probability of the patient having coronary disease (Bayesian theory). If the patient has a low probability of coronary disease then the false-positive rate is high and the test is effectively worthless.

In order to perform a standard exercise test, the patient must be mobile with a reasonable exercise tolerance on the flat. Patients with an exercise tolerance limited to 100 m or less are unlikely to manage a standard exercise test. The possible indications for exercise testing are given in Table 4.2.

ECG changes cannot be interpreted if the patient has LBBB and are difficult to interpret with RBBB, left ventricular hypertrophy and strain or in the presence of extensive changes from previous infarction. There are a number of important contraindications to exercise testing (see Case 2, p. 53).

The Bruce protocol is most commonly used and consists of graded exercise in stages. Each stage is 3 minutes in duration and there are up to 7 stages, although in practice most patients only exercise to stage 4. During the test the patient is monitored for symptoms, blood pressure response and ST-segment changes. The criteria for a positive test are:
- ST elevation.
- Planar ST depression of ≥1 mm, 80 ms after the J point (point at which the QRS complex crosses the baseline at the start of the ST segment).
- Failure of the blood pressure to rise or fall in blood pressure during the test.
- Ventricular arrhythmias.
- Typical symptoms of angina.
- Increase in QRS voltage (indicative of ischaemic dilatation).

A **stress isotope scan** can be performed with exercise or a pharmacological agent such as adenosine or dobutamine. A radioisotope (usually technetium) is injected at peak stress. The isotope is taken up by viable non-ischaemic heart muscle. Areas of infarction or ischaemia are identified on the initial scan. A resting scan is then performed later. The resting scan identifies areas of infarction. The difference in isotope uptake in each region of the heart between the resting and stress scans identifies areas of reversible ischaemia. This test is useful in patients with a grossly abnormal resting ECG. The sensitivity and specificity of a stress isotope scan are similar to stress echocardiography. The test is more expensive than an exercise test although less operator dependent than the stress echocardiogram.

Electron beam CT is used to detect coronary artery calcification. Its value is debatable in patients with a history of angina. Its use is primarily to detect patients at higher risk from coronary vascular events who may be suitable for more aggressive preventative therapy.

Multislice CT is now available to detect coronary disease; however, this technique is currently more valuable in excluding coronary disease than in accurately quantifying the nature of coronary disease. Unlike tests that involve stressing the myocardium, it is not possible to correlate symptoms with the development of myocardial ischaemia.

Contrast MRI. MRI is now available in most centres. MRI with a contrast agent (gadolinium) can be performed to show areas of infarction and pharmacological stress protocols are being evaluated. MRI provides detailed anatomical and some physiological data. However, the test is time consuming and expensive and tends to be restricted to those patients with severe left ventricular dysfunction who are being evaluated for revascularisation and where an accurate assessment of the amount of viable myocardium is important.

During the course of an exercise test the blood pressure is measured every 2–3 minutes. The normal blood

Table 4.2 Indications for exercise testing

Diagnosis of coronary artery disease

Risk assessment of patients with known coronary disease

After myocardial infarction

Exercise testing with ventilatory assessment (e.g. for transplantation or differentiation of cardiac and respiratory causes of breathlessness)

Prior to commencing rehabilitation programme

Evaluation of arrhythmias (e.g. exercise-induced arrhythmias, rate control of atrial fibrillation, etc.)

Table 4.3 Indications to terminate an exercise test

Symptoms:
- Worsening angina or breathlessness
- Dizziness
- Fatigue or at patient's request

Physiological:
- Achieved target heart rate (220 minus age for men, 210 minus age for women)
- Fall, or failure to rise, of blood pressure
- Exaggerated hypertensive response to exercise (systolic blood pressure >220 mmHg)

ECG:
- Atrial arrhythmias other than ectopic beats
- ST-segment elevation
- ST depression >3 mm
- Frequent ventricular ectopics or ventricular tachycardia
- New high-grade AV block or bundle branch block

pressure response is a rise in systolic blood pressure (the diastolic blood pressure may fall). Symptoms correlating with horizontal or downsloping ST-segment changes in multiple leads are most specific. Upsloping ST changes (J-point depression) that recover rapidly (<1 minute) after the cessation of exercise in the absence of symptoms are likely to be spurious. The ST segments should be monitored at least 3 minutes after the test is completed for late ischaemic changes. The patient is exercised if possible to the target heart rate. The exercise test should be terminated if conclusively positive (Table 4.3). The workload is estimated by calculating the oxygen consumption compared to that at rest (metabolic equivalent or MET; 1 MET = resting metabolic rate).

An echocardiogram shows mildly impaired left ventricular function. The aortic valve is calcified. There is no significant aortic valve gradient. The remainder of the echocardiogram is within normal limits. An exercise test is performed and is positive with anginal pain and 3 mm of ST depression in V4–V6 at 3 minutes of the Bruce protocol and a workload of 4 METS. The ST segments resolve after 1 minute into the recovery period. The blood pressure rises from 170/90 mmHg to 200/80 mmHg during the test.

Which findings are indicative of a poor prognosis on this exercise test?

- Failure to exercise for more than 6 minutes or a workload greater than 5 METS.

- More than 2 mm ST depression.

Failure to complete stage 2 of the Bruce protocol or to achieve a workload of 5 METS and ST depression ≥2 mm is indicative of a high risk of subsequent coronary events in this test. Other poor prognostic factors would be failure of the blood pressure to rise, a fall in systolic blood pressure during the test, ventricular dysrhythmias or prolonged ST depression in the recovery phase. It is important to identify the poor prognostic features on the exercise test since these will prompt further investigation with coronary angiography, even in the presence of a good response to medical therapy.

What classes of agents may be effective in controlling this patient's symptoms?

The classes of antianginal agents and their mechanism of action are shown in Table 4.4. Beta blockers, calcium-channel blockers and oral nitrates are all standard therapies for angina. Other agents including nicorandil or ivabradine may be used in patients unresponsive to, or intolerant of, the standard agents.

What are the most probable causes of his renal failure and how would you investigate this further?

Hypertension, diabetes, obstruction and renovascular disease are the most likely causes of the renal impairment in this man. Renovascular disease should always be considered in a patient with peripheral vascular disease. Urine dipstick may be helpful; in the absence of proteinuria, diabetic renal disease is unlikely. A renal ultrasound may show asymmetrical kidneys in patients with renal artery disease or small kidneys in chronic renal disease due to hypertension. A normal renal ultrasound does not exclude renal artery stenosis and if there is a high index of suspicion then magnetic resonance renal arteriography, aortography or a captopril renal perfusion scan can be performed.

The patient is commenced on bisoprolol 5 mg daily, aspirin 75 mg daily, simvastatin 40 mg at night, ramipril 2.5 mg daily and provided with a GTN spray. Satisfactory diabetes control is achieved with diet alone. A renal ultrasound shows normal-size kidneys with no evidence of obstruction. Arrangements are made for the patient to have coronary angiography.

Table 4.4 Antianginal agents, their mechanism of action and common side-effects

Agent	Mechanism of action	Side-effects
Beta blockers, e.g. atenolol, bisoprolol, metoprolol	Blockade of beta receptors Negatively inotropic, negatively chronotropic	Fatigue, bradycardia, cold peripheries, impotence, wheeze
Calcium antagonists, e.g. nifedipine, amlodipine, diltiazem, verapamil	Calcium-channel blockade Smooth muscle dilatation Negatively chronotropic –(diltiazem and verapamil only) Negatively inotropic – (verapamil, diltiazem, nifedipine)	Flushing. Peripheral oedema. Constipation (verapamil) Bradycardia (negatively chronotropic agents)
Nitrates, e.g. Glyceryl trinitrate (GTN) isosorbide mononitrate	Release of nitric oxide causing vasodilatation	Headache
Potassium-channel openers, e.g. nicorandil	Vasodilatation	Headache

What risks should be quoted to the patient and what precautions should be taken prior to performing his angiogram?

The risks of coronary angiography vary with each individual patient. A guide is given in Table 4.5. In this patient there is a risk of renal failure as a result of the use of radiographic contrast media. Although the risk is low and the deterioration in renal function is usually reversible, non-ionic contrast media should be used and the patient should be pre-hydrated with normal saline.

His coronary angiogram is performed and shows severe triple vessel disease with an occluded proximal left anterior descending (LAD) artery and disease of the left main coronary artery.

How should this patient be managed?

The options for treatment of stable angina are medical therapy, angioplasty and coronary artery bypass grafting. Most patients will receive a trial of medical therapy and, in cases where this fails to relieve symptoms, further intervention will be required. However, in certain cases the severity of the coronary disease indicates that the patient is at high risk of myocardial infarction or death. The findings on angiography reveal that there is a prognostic indication for coronary artery bypass grafting (see Table 4.6).

Table 4.5 Risks of coronary angiography

Local arterial access site complications (bleeding, etc.)	<0.1%
Cardiac arrhythmias	<0.2%
Coronary artery occlusion	<0.2%
Stroke	<0.2%
Death	<0.1%
Renal failure	<0.1%
Contrast reaction	<0.3%

With disease of the left main coronary artery and the proximal LAD artery a large amount of myocardium is at risk and therefore treatment may be appropriate, even in the absence of significant symptoms. Patients with involvement of all three main coronary arteries, and in particular where there is left ventricular impairment due to a previous myocardial infarction, will have a better prognosis with surgery than with medical therapy. With the advent of coronary angioplasty and coronary artery stenting (see Case 1, p. 46) more patients are managed with percutaneous intervention than with surgery. However, in patients with vessels that are completely occluded, angioplasty is less successful. Patients with left main stem disease are still treated with coronary artery bypass surgery in most cases; however, angioplasty can be a highly successful treatment in those who are not suitable or who are at high risk for surgery.

Box 4.2 Coronary angiography

Coronary angiography is the gold standard for assessing the coronary anatomy in patients with angina. Other indications include cardiac failure of unknown aetiology, pre-operative assessment of valvular heart disease and the investigation of ventricular dysrhythmias. The procedure is usually performed as a day-case procedure. The patient should be nil by mouth for 4 hours prior to the procedure. A pre-med of a benzodiazepine, either orally or intravenously, may be given. The patient is awake during the procedure and local anaesthesia is used for the arterial puncture. Access to the circulation is usually via the femoral artery but brachial and radial approaches are also used. A contrast agent is injected into the left coronary artery (LCA) and right coronary artery (RCA) using pre-shaped catheters (usually Judkins catheters). Usually five views are taken of the LCA and three of the RCA using an image intensifier. Images are stored digitally and can be reviewed instantly. A stenosis on a coronary artery is regarded as significant, i.e. has an effect on coronary flow if the artery is narrowed to 50% or more of the luminal diameter on angiography. The procedure lasts approximately 15 minutes.

After removal of the catheter the puncture site is compressed for 10 minutes, or alternatively a collagen plug is inserted to seal the artery (angioseal). With brachial arteriography using a cut-down approach, the arteriotomy is closed under direct vision with fine sutures. After the procedure the patient is required to lie flat for 4 hours with a femoral puncture and compression, or for 30 minutes to 1 hour with an angioseal closure. Prior to angiography it is important to check:
- That the patient can lie flat.
- The peripheral pulses and check for femoral bruits.
- Any history of a previous contrast reaction.
- History of diabetes.
- Drug history for the use of anticoagulants.
- Electrolytes and FBC.
- That there is a recent ECG for comparison.

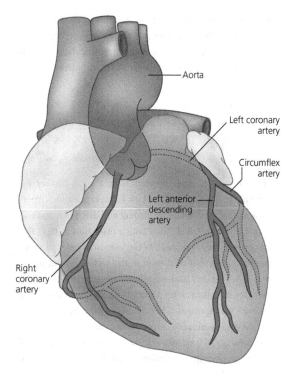

Figure 4.2 A diagrammatic representation of the coronary circulation.

Table 4.6 Prognostic indications for coronary artery bypass grafting based on coronary angiographic findings

Left main stem stenosis
Proximal LAD disease
Triple vessel disease and impaired left ventricular function

The patient is referred for coronary artery bypass surgery. What further investigation is appropriate prior to surgery?

One of the major risks of coronary artery bypass surgery is stroke. This man is at increased risk as a result of the history of a previous TIA. A **carotid duplex scan** will reveal the extent of any carotid disease. Symptomatic carotid stenoses of >75% are usually treated prior to bypass surgery. Carotid endarterectomy can be performed safely under local anaesthetic with a risk of stroke of <1%.

> A carotid duplex scan reveals a 90% stenosis of the right internal carotid. The patient undergoes right carotid endarterectomy under local anaesthesia. Successful bypass surgery is performed 5 days later. The patient returns for follow-up in the cardiology outpatient clinic.

What medications should be continued long term following bypass surgery?

Long-term treatment with aspirin, a statin and an angiotensin-converting enzyme (ACE) inhibitor would be appropriate. ACE inhibitors reduce the cardiovascular event rates of patients over 55 years with documented coronary disease. Although ACE inhibitors should be used with caution in patients with documented renal disease, this is not an absolute contraindication. In this patient the presence of left ventricular impairment con-stitutes another indication for ACE inhibition. Despite the absence of symptoms of angina the patient should continue on beta blockers if an echocardiogram con-tinues to show significant left ventricular impairment.

CASE REVIEW

This 71-year-old man presents with a good history for angina. He has a number of risk factors including hyper-tension, diabetes, renal impairment and dyslipidaemia and is an ex heavy smoker, all of which place him at high risk for coronary artery disease. As is common in older patients, there are a number of comorbidities (renal disease, previ-ous TIA, diabetes and peripheral vascular disease) that have to be taken into account when considering the patient's management. The evidence of peripheral vascular disease on examination supports the diagnosis of angina. The presence of a systolic murmur raises the possibility of AS or hypertrophic cardiomyopathy, which may also present with angina; however, the absence of other clinical features and the findings on echocardiography rule out these as the cause.

The diagnosis is confirmed with an exercise test. He develops ECG changes and symptoms at an early stage of the test, raising the possibility of severe coronary disease. He is commenced on antianginal medication and aspirin and his risk factors are addressed with the introduction of a statin and a diabetic diet. He is referred for angiography on the basis of persistent angina and a strongly positive exercise test. The angiographic findings are of triple vessel coronary disease, including the presence of left main stem disease for which he is referred for coronary artery bypass grafting. However, in view of the prior history of a TIA, he has carotid duplex scans performed to assess the need for carotid endarterectomy prior to his bypass operation. The duplex scans confirm the presence of severe carotid disease and he undergoes carotid endarterectomy prior to bypass surgery.

KEY POINTS

- The diagnosis of angina is made primarily on the history. The most important feature is the relationship of symptoms to exertion and their relief with rest. Most patients present with chest discomfort on exertion; however, a proportion will complain only of breathlessness.
- Establishing the risk-factor profile for ischaemic heart disease is very important since this will determine the likelihood that the patient has angina and also direct preventative therapy once the diagnosis has been established.
- The clinical examination and ECG are frequently entirely normal in patients on their first presentation. However, it is important to look for evidence of vascular disease elsewhere and establish that the symptoms have not been triggered by a dysrhythmia, anaemia, valvular heart disease or uncontrolled hypertension.
- Exercise testing is the most commonly used non-invasive investigation for establishing the presence of coronary artery disease. However, it is only useful in patients who have typical symptoms or a risk-factor profile that points to a high probability of coronary disease.
- Where an exercise test is not possible due to physical disability, or cannot be interpreted due to abnormalities in the resting ECG, other non-invasive tests such as dobutamine stress echocardiography or pharmacological stress isotope scanning of the heart may be appropriate.

- Management of the patient involves the relief of symptoms and treatment of the underlying disease process.
- The most important aspect of the treatment of patients with angina is risk-factor modification. Aggressive control of blood pressure, diabetes and cholesterol and life-style measures (weight loss, diet and exercise) will reduce the incidence of death and myocardial infarction. Aspirin and ACE inhibition also have a beneficial impact on long-term prognosis.
- Symptomatic treatment with beta blockers and nitrates may be sufficient in some patients; however, in most patients further intervention is required.
- Interventional therapy with balloon angioplasty is used where the coronary anatomy is suitable. However, the treatment is for symptoms and does not affect prognosis in patients presenting with stable angina.
- Where the coronary anatomy is not suitable for angioplasty, coronary artery bypass grafting is indicated. Coronary artery bypass surgery is of prognostic benefit in patients with triple vessel or left main stem coronary artery disease and may be indicated even in the absence of significant symptoms in some patients.
- With appropriate treatment most patients can be rendered asymptomatic and lead a normal life.

Case 5 A 50-year-old man with sudden-onset severe central chest pain

A 50-year-old man is admitted via A&E with a history of a sudden onset of central chest pain. On examination pulse is 110 bpm, blood pressure is 200/130 mmHg, heart sounds are reported as normal, and there is evidence of mild left ventricular failure. Oxygen saturations are 100% on room air. The ECG shows left ventricular hypertrophy and strain. During the course of the clinical examination the patient reports increasingly severe pain, travelling through to the back.

What is the differential diagnosis?

The history of a sudden onset of central chest pain radiating to the back is suggestive of aortic dissection but the differential diagnosis include those conditions given in Table 1.1 (see p. 38) The features in the history that are particularly suggestive are the almost instantaneous onset of the pain, its immediate severity (the pain does not increase over time as with a myocardial infarction) and the radiation or travelling of the pain to the back. However, the pain may also radiate to the neck, throat, jaw or abdomen. The most common differential diagnosis is of an acute myocardial infarction. Unfortunately, aortic dissection can be associated with ECG abnormalities of ischaemia (ST depression and T-wave inversion), left ventricular hypertrophy and strain or of an inferior ST-elevation myocardial infarction (STEMI) (1–2% of cases). In the latter case, the dissection involves the aortic root and the origin of the RCA. Anterior infarction is extremely rare. This would require the dissection to involve the left main coronary artery which is almost universally fatal. It is therefore reasonable to assume that when the patient presents with chest pain and anterior ST elevation that an aortic dissection is not the cause.

What additional findings on examination may help to determine the cause of his pain?

The clinical examination findings that point specifically to an aortic dissection are:

- Presence of a focal neurological deficit (due to involvement of the carotid vessels).
- Pulse deficits.
- A blood pressure difference of >20 mmHg between the arms.
- An aortic diastolic murmur indicating involvement of the aortic valve. (The patient is usually hypertensive; however, this feature does not appear to add to the diagnostic accuracy in the presence of other suggestive clinical features.)

It is important to look for features of Marfan's syndrome, which is strongly associated with aortic dissection. These include:

- High arched palate.
- Anterior lens dislocation.
- Joint hypermobility.
- Increased height.
- Increased arm span.
- Arachnodactily.

The useful clinical features pointing to an aortic dissection are summarised in Table 5.1.

The only additional finding on examination is dullness at the right lung base on percussion.

What further investigations would you consider?

- The **CXR** is abnormal in approximately 90% of cases of aortic dissection and a normal CXR therefore helps exclude the diagnosis. The most characteristic finding is of a widened mediastinum; however, irregularities of the aortic contour or a pleural effusion may also be present.

Cardiology: Clinical Cases Uncovered. By T. Betts, J. Dwight and S. Bull. Published 2010 by Blackwell Publishing.

Table 5.1 Clinical features pointing to a diagnosis of aortic dissection

History of hypertension

Sudden chest pain

Tearing or ripping pain

Migrating pain

Pulse deficit

Horner's syndrome

Marfanoid habitus

Focal neurological deficit

Diastolic murmur

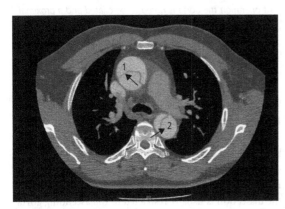

Figure 5.1 Contrast CT demonstrating aortic dissection flap. 1, aortic dissection 2, flap.

• **Contrast CT aortography** is the most frequently performed further investigation and has the advantage of being readily available in nearly all centres. The findings are of a false lumen containing contrast. The site of origin can usually be identified and complications such as a leak into the pericardium maybe demonstrated. An example is shown in Figure 5.1.

• **Transthoracic echocardiography** may identify an aortic dissection involving the proximal aorta and may identify complications such as AR and pericardial tamponade but a normal echocardiogram does not exclude a dissection.

• **Transoesophageal echocardiography** has a high sensitivity and specificity (>98%).

• **MRI** gives both anatomical information and will identify complications such as AR and a pericardial collection, but it is not available in the emergency setting in some centres

How would you classify this dissection?

A type A aortic dissection:

• Type A dissections involve the aortic root.

• Type B dissections arise after the origin of the left subclavian artery.

What would be your immediate management of this patient?

• Intravenous access.

• Analgesia.

• Blood pressure control.

• Transfer to ITU or CCU.

• Arterial line.

The mortality from aortic dissection is approximately 1% per hour. Patients should have two large-bore intravenous catheters inserted and analgesia given (usually morphine). For both type A and B dissections the key to the initial management is the control of blood pressure. The systolic blood pressure should be maintained at between 100 and 120 mmHg. Intravenous beta blockade is particularly useful, since it reduces pulse pressure and wall stress.

Labetalol 20 mg, administered i.v. over a 2-minute period, followed by additional doses of 40–80 mg every 10–15 minutes (up to a maximum total dose of 300 mg) is a standard regimen. Alternatives are intravenous nitrates or sodium nitroprusside. An arterial line is usually inserted for blood pressure monitoring and the patient is transferred to ITU or CCU.

The patient is transferred to the CCU and commenced on an intravenous labetalol infusion. However, 15 minutes later the blood pressure is reported at 80/30 mmHg and the patient becomes acutely breathless. His jugular venous pressure (JVP) is elevated and examination of the chest reveals bibasal crepitations consistent with pulmonary oedema.

What complications may have occurred that would account for this deterioration and how would you investigate this further?

- Rupture into the pleural cavity.
- Pericardial tamponade.
- Acute aortic regurgitation (AR).
- Inferior myocardial infarction.

An aortic dissection may leak into the pleural cavity with rapid haemodynamic deterioration and evidence of an enlarging pleural effusion. A type A dissection may extend proximally involving the right coronary artery (RCA) giving rise to an inferior myocardial infarction (1–2% of cases) or the aortic valve causing acute AR. Severe acute AR is poorly tolerated and the patient rapidly develops severe left ventricular failure. The diastolic murmur of acute AR is short and may be difficult to hear. The murmur is short because the left ventricle has not had time to dilate, the diastolic pressure in the ventricle equalises rapidly with aortic diastolic blood pressure and regurgitant flow ceases early in diastole. Rupture into the pericardial sac causes tamponade characterised by hypotension, pulsus paradoxus and an elevated JVP.

Other complications include:
- Neurological complications (stroke or paraparesis) in up to 20% of patients.
- Acute renal failure due to involvement of the renal vessels.
- Small bowel infarction due to involvement of the superior mesenteric artery.
- Facial swelling due to superior vena caval obstruction.
- Bronchial compression.
- Claudication due to in the involvement of the femoral arteries.

An echocardiogram confirms extension of the aortic dissection to involve the aortic valve associated with severe AR and haemorrhage into the pericardium.

What is the definitive treatment of this condition?

Type A dissections should all be managed surgically. Without surgery, 25% of patients die within the first 24 hours and 75% in the first month. The proximal end of the dissection is repaired to prevent extension into the aortic valve and coronary arteries. Where the aorta is very dilated, an aortic graft may be required. If the aortic valve is involved it can often be repaired but occasionally requires replacement. Type B dissections should be managed medically unless there are complications, e.g. lower limb ischaemia. Selected cases may be suitable for intravascular stenting.

What conditions are associated with aortic dissection?

- Hypertension – found in 70–80% of cases.
- Cystic medial necrosis – Marfan's syndrome (5–9%) and Ehlers-Danlos syndrome.
- Bicuspid aortic valve – found in 7–14% of cases.
- Pregnancy (third trimester and early post-partum).
- Trauma and cardiac surgery.
- Rarities – coarctation, Noonan's syndrome, Turner's syndrome, arteritis.

At operation the aorta is noted to be dilated and a proximal dissection flap identified. A successful aortic repair is performed with preservation of the aortic valve. The patient makes an excellent recovery and is discharged on atenolol 50 mg daily and amlodipine 10 mg daily.

What arrangements should be made for follow-up of this patient?

The entire aorta is frequently abnormal in patients who have had an aortic dissection. In this case, the aorta is dilated indicating that the patient has a pre-existing thoracic aortic aneurysm. The surgical procedure to repair the dissection is usually restricted to the ascending aorta and the disease process may progress elsewhere.

At follow-up, the patient should be asked for symptoms that might indicate further dilatation of the aorta or subacute rupture, e.g. back pain, dysphagia and dyspnoea. One of the most important aspects of follow-up is careful control of blood pressure (systolic blood pressure should be controlled to <120 mmHg). This patient has a dilated aorta that will require follow-up clinically and with imaging. CT and MRI are the gold standard investigations for follow-up of aortic pathology.

Indications for surgical repair of a thoracic aortic aneurysm include:
- Thoracic aortic aneurysm >60 mm.
- Thoracic aneurysm >55 mm in the context of Marfan's syndrome.

- Rapid expansion of the aneurysm or the dissected segment.
- Symptoms related to the aneurysm.
- Severe AR.

The patient is booked for yearly follow-up with contrast CT of the aorta. What are the possible complications arising from this form of imaging?

The complications of contrast CT can be divided into those associated with the radiation dose and those due to the use of contrast agents. The increased risk of **cancer** associated with CT thorax/abdomen is significant and therefore has to be taken into consideration.

The majority of contrast agents contain iodine. An **allergic reaction** to contrast media occurs in approximately 1 in 300 investigations. Most of these are mild reactions (urticaria/skin rash, pyrexia); however, severe anaphylactoid reactions may occur. Allergic reactions are more common in patients with a known allergy to iodine or shellfish. **Renal toxicity** is particularly common in patients with diabetes or pre-existing renal impairment and occurs in approximately 2% of cases. Renal toxicity can be minimised by using non-ionic low osmolar contrast media and with pre-hydration.

Anaphylaxis is treated with i.v. hydrocortisone 200 mg, chlorpheniramine 10 mg, i.v. fluids and adrenaline 0.5–1.0 mg i.m.

CASE REVIEW

This 50-year-old man presents with a history of sudden-onset chest pain that radiates through to the back. The history is suggestive of an aortic dissection, although a myocardial infarction as an alternative diagnosis. He is hypertensive on admission and the presence of ECG changes of left ventricular hypertrophy indicates that his hypertension is long standing. There are no other clinical features to help with the diagnosis and in particular no other warning features in the history or examination. The CXR shows a unilateral pleural effusion, which would be unusual for a myocardial infarction but which can be seen in aortic dissection. Before further investigations can be performed, the patient becomes hypotensive and develops pulmonary oedema. The diastolic pressure falls to 30 mmHg, suggesting volume loss or acute AR; the raised JVP suggests heart failure or pericardial tamponade. The diagnosis is confirmed with echo and contrast CT, which show extension of the aortic dissection into the aortic root (type A dissection) involving the aortic valve and with leakage of blood into the pericardium, causing pericardial tamponade. The patient undergoes emergency surgery with repair of the aortic root and aortic valve. Following surgery he will require regular imaging of the aorta since he is at risk of further enlargement and aneurysm formation of the aorta beyond the repair site.

KEY POINTS

- An aortic dissection is due to a split in the aortic wall between the intima and the media. Important predisposing conditions include Marfan's syndrome and hypertension.
- Aortic dissection is an important differential in the diagnosis of chest pain.
- The mortality from aortic dissection is 1% per hour.
- The diagnosis should be considered in those patients with a family history or clinical features of Marfan's syndrome and in those patients presenting with a sudden onset of very severe chest pain radiating through to the back.
- Warning signs for aortic dissection in a patient presenting with chest pain include the development of neurological features, a blood pressure difference between the arms or clinical AR.
- The CXR is abnormal in 90% of cases.

- A contrast CT of the aorta should be preformed immediately when aortic dissection is suspected. Transthoracic echocardiography may be helpful but can usually only detect dissections involving the aortic root.
- Type A dissections involve the aortic root; they can be complicated by acute AR, pericardial tamponade, inferior myocardial infarction and rupture.
- In type A dissection emergency surgery should be performed. While this is being arranged the blood pressure should be controlled with intravenous beta blockade, nitrates or nitroprusside, aiming for a systolic blood pressure of 100 mmHg.
- Type B dissections do not involve the aortic root and carry a better prognosis. If they are uncomplicated they can be managed medically with rigorous blood pressure control.

Case 6 A 45-year-old man with chest pain and breathlessness

A 45-year-old business executive presents to A&E with a 2-hour history of central crushing chest pain and breathlessness. He is a non-smoker, previously very fit and well and attends a gym four times a week. There is no family history of ischaemic heart disease. His cholesterol measured at an insurance medical was 3.3 mmol/L. His observations on admission are as follows: pulse 105 bpm; blood pressure 80/50 mmHg; O₂ saturations 90% on room air. He is apyrexial. An ECG is performed and is shown in Figure 6.1.

What abnormalities are present on the ECG?

The ECG demonstrates a sinus tachycardia of 94 bpm. There is right-axis deviation and T-wave inversion in lead III and the anterior chest leads.

What are the main differential diagnoses on the basis of the ECG and the history?
ECG findings

The ECG findings do not give a clear diagnosis in this case. T-wave inversion is a non-specific finding that can be seen in a wide variety of conditions. The list is slightly shorter when the changes are limited to the anteroseptal leads (Table 6.1). Any cause of right ventricular strain or dilatation can cause anteroseptal T-wave changes. When the cause of right ventricular strain is long standing, there may be electrocardiographic evidence of right ventricular hypertrophy (tall R waves in the anteroseptal leads). Deep symmetrical T-wave inversion is usually a feature of ischaemia (Wellens' syndrome, see p. 43). T-wave memory characterised by T-wave inversion is seen after a rapid arrhythmia or cardioversion, it is usually short lived.

Cardiology: Clinical Cases Uncovered. By T. Betts, J. Dwight and S. Bull. Published 2010 by Blackwell Publishing.

Right-axis deviation is defined as an axis >90 degrees. The cardiac axis is usually dominated by the left ventricle since this has the greater myocardial mass; the axis can be shifted to the right by right ventricular hypertrophy, Wolff-Parkinson-White syndrome, dextrocardia, left posterior hemiblock or, most commonly, by reversed arm electrodes.

There are a number of ECG abnormalities that can be associated with pulmonary embolism (Table 6.2). The ECG changes are related predominantly to right heart strain and are therefore more common following large or multiple pulmonary emboli. Unfortunately, the ECG is normal in 50% or more of patients with pulmonary emboli.

History

The main differential diagnosis is between an **acute coronary syndrome (ACS)** and **pulmonary embolism**, both of which can give rise to central chest pain. The pain is usually pleuritic in the case of small peripheral pulmonary emboli but with large emboli involving the proximal pulmonary arteries it can be central and mimic myocardial infarction. The breathlessness is characteristically sudden in onset (it can be insidious in patients with chronic thromboembolic disease). Haemoptysis occurs in the context of pulmonary infarction and is uncommon, although helpful diagnostically.

Pericarditis with tamponade due to a pericardial effusion is a possible differential diagnosis but the history is rather acute. Aortic dissection is also in the differential diagnosis but the character of the pain is not typical. It would be unusual for an acute coronary syndrome to present with this degree of hypotension and hypoxia unless the patient had severe coronary disease (left main stem or triple vessel disease) or a large anterior myocardial infarction (in which case there should be ST elevation in the anterior leads). Saturations of 90% in a non-smoker of this age could be due pulmonary embolism or pulmonary oedema secondary to myocardial infarction.

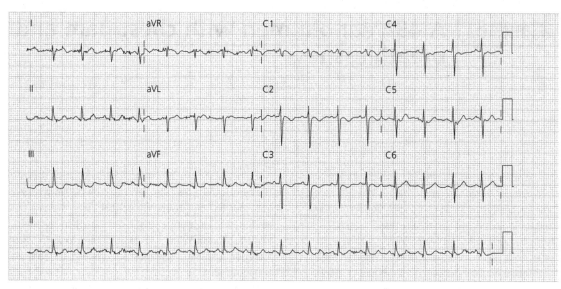

Figure 6.1 The patient's ECG.

Table 6.1 Causes of T-wave inversion in the anteroseptal leads

---

Ischaemic heart disease

Right heart strain:
- Primary pulmonary hypertension
- Secondary pulmonary hypertension (e.g. left-to-right shunt, cor pulmonale)
- Pulmonary embolism
- tricuspid regurgitation (TR)

Conduction abnormalities:
- Right branch bundle block (RBBB)
- Wolf-Parkinson-White syndrome
- Brugada syndrome

Pericardial disease

Right ventricular dysplasia

T-wave memory following:
- Ventricular tachycardia
- Cardioversion
- Paroxysmal rapid atrial dysrhythmias

Table 6.2 ECG findings in pulmonary embolic disease

Tachycardia >100 bpm
S I, Q III, T inversion III
Incomplete right bundle branch block (RBBB)
Right-axis deviation
T-wave inversion V2
ST elevation in V1
RBBB
Atrial fibrillation
Atrial flutter
Qr in V1

What additional aspects of the history and examination would help you to establish diagnosis?

For a diagnosis of thromboembolic disease it is impor-tant to establish whether there has been a recent history of immobility or surgery. As a business executive, the patient may have recently been on a long-haul flight. A history of haemoptysis or calf pain or swelling is helpful. Pulmonary embolism is more likely if there is a past history or family history of thromboembolic disease. The absence of exertional angina, a smoking history and a low cholesterol make the diagnosis of an acute coronary syn-drome less likely.

The important examination findings in pulmonary embolic disease are given in Table 6.3. Unfortunately, the examination features of pulmonary embolism and acute coronary syndrome overlap. Both may be associated with an elevated venous pressure, hypotension, tachycardia and hypoxia. However, in the hypotensive and hypoxic patient with an acute coronary syndrome there is usually

Table 6.3 Examination findings in pulmonary embolism

Cyanosis
Tachycardia
Tachypnoea
Hypotension
Elevated jugular venous pressure (JVP)
Right ventricular heave
Accentuated pulmonary second sound
Right ventricular third heart sound
Pleural effusion/ pleural rub
Hepatomegaly
Deep venous thrombosis (DVT)
Fever

Table 6.4 The Wells scoring system for pulmonary embolism

Clinical finding	Points
Clinical signs and symptoms of DVT (i.e. objectively measured leg swelling or pain with palpation of deep leg veins)	3.0
Alternative diagnosis less likely than pulmonary embolism	3.0
Immobilisation (i.e. bed rest except for bathroom access for at least 3 consecutive days) or surgery in the past 4 weeks	1.5
Previously objectively diagnosed DVT or pulmonary embolism	1.5
Heart rate >100 bpm	1.5
Haemoptysis	1.0
Malignancy (treatment for cancer that is ongoing, within the past 6 months or palliative)	1.0

Total points	Risk of pulmonary embolism	Probability of pulmonary embolism (%)
<2 points	Low	1–28
2–6 points	Moderate	28–40
≥7 points	High	38–91

DVT, deep vein thrombosis.

clear clinical or radiographic evidence of pulmonary oedema; if this is absent then a pulmonary embolism has to be considered. The examination may be entirely normal in patients with small pulmonary emboli.

What scoring system may be used to estimate the probability of pulmonary embolism?

There are a variety of scoring systems used to evaluate the probability of pulmonary embolism. The most commonly used is the modified Wells scoring system given in Table 6.4. The scoring system is heavily weighted by the clinical judgement that there is not a more likely alternative diagnosis. In this case, based on the clinical findings, the score would be 4.5 if we assume that an acute coronary syndrome is unlikely, or 1.5 if an acute coronary syndrome remains a likely diagnosis.

> The patient returned to the UK from a business trip in Australia 2 weeks previously. On clinical examination the patient is cyanosed and cool peripherally with a respiratory rate of 30 breaths/minute. His jugular venous pressure (JVP) is elevated to the angle of the jaw. There is a soft third sound heard over the right sternal border. The troponin I is elevated at 3.5 µg/L (normal range <1 µg/L); the D–dimer is elevated to five times the normal range. Arterial blood gases on 40% O_2 are as follows:
>
> | | | |
> | --- | --- | --- |
> | pH | 7.30 | (7.35–7.45) |
> | pCO_2 | 3.2 kPa | (4.7–6.0) |
> | pO_2 | 7.0 kPa | (11.3–12.6) |
> | HCO_3 | 15 mmol/L | (19–24) |
> | BE | –10 | (+/– 2) |

How would you interpret the arterial blood gases?

Arterial blood gases show **type 1 respiratory failure** ($pO_2 < 8$ kPa) with a low carbon dioxide (**metabolic acidosis**). There is a large alveolar–arterial gradient (Box 1.1). The bicarbonate is low – this can be due to chronic hyperventilation; however, in this case there is an arterial acidosis and a base deficit, indicating that the patient has a metabolic acidosis. In a large pulmonary embolism, hypotension leading to hypoxia and poor tissue perfusion causes a lactic acidosis. Although these findings are useful in assessing the size of the pulmonary embolism, they are not particularly useful in distinguishing a large pulmonary embolism from a myocardial infarction with pulmonary oedema, since both are associated with hypoxia and a lactic acidosis.

> #### Box 1.1 Alveolar–arterial gradient
>
> The alveolar–arterial gradient (A–a gradient) is a measure of the efficiency of gas transfer in the lung. It is measured using the arterial O_2 (PaO_2), the alveolar O_2 (PAO_2) and the arterial CO_2 ($PaCO_2$). The maximum normal alveolar arterial gradient is (room air having 20% O_2 or a PIO_2 of 20 kPa) is given by the equation:
>
> $PAO_2 - PaO_2$
> Where:
>
> $PAO_2 = PIO_2 - PaCO_2/0.8 = 20 - 7.5 = 12.5\,kPa.$
>
> $PAO_2 - PaO_2 = 12.5 - 11.3 = 1.2$
>
> In this case, the PIO_2 is 40 kPA and the $PaCO_2$ is 3.2. The PAO_2 is therefore 36 kPa. The A–a gradient is 36 – 7 = 29.
>
> A shortcut is simply to look at the CO_2 – if this is normal then take the inspired O_2 (% = kPa) and subtract the arterial O_2 in kPa, if the figure is greater than 8 then there is a significant A–a gradient.
>
> A large gradient indicates that there is a ventilation–perfusion inequality. A ventilation perfusion inequality is either due to areas of lung that are well perfused but cannot absorb oxygen due to lung damage, or due to failure to perfuse normal lung tissue, as in the case of a right to left shunt or a pulmonary embolism.

Do the results of the troponin and D-dimer help in establishing the diagnosis?

It is now well recognised that the cardiac troponin can be elevated in pulmonary embolism. The rise in troponin is related to the size of the pulmonary embolism. Very high levels of troponin are unlikely to be due to pulmonary embolic disease. An elevated D-dimer is rather a non-specific finding and can be elevated in inflammation, trauma, infection and myocardial infarction. Therefore, the D-dimer is used in those patients with a low probability score using the Wells criteria to decide whether further investigation is necessary, a positive D-dimer indicating the requirement for further investigation in a low-probability patient. In those patients with an intermediate or high probability of pulmonary embolism the D-dimer does not yield further useful information.

What CXR findings may be helpful?

The characteristic peripheral wedge-shaped shadow or areas of atelectasis in pulmonary infarction are uncommon in central pulmonary emboli and when present are difficult to distinguish from infection. The presence of an apparently clear CXR in the context of severe hypoxia supports the diagnosis of pulmonary embolism. The regions of the lung affected by pulmonary emboli may appear relatively oligaemic; however, this is quite a subtle feature. Unilateral or bilateral pleural effusions may be present but are non-specific.

The CXR is reported as showing clear lung fields and the heart size is normal. A provisional diagnosis of pulmonary embolism and cardiogenic shock due to right heart failure is made.

What is your immediate management?

The usual assessment of airway breathing and circulation is required. More specifically, the patient should be nursed lying flat or with a head-down tilt. A large-bore cannula should be inserted and the patient should be resuscitated with intravenous fluids (500 mL over 10–15 minutes) and given high-flow oxygen. Large volumes of intravenous fluids are contraindicated since they may exacerbate the right heart failure in this condition. Pain relief may present a difficult problem; opiates should be avoided if possible, as they are venodilators and may induce a further fall in blood pressure as a result of reduced right ventricular filling.

The patient responds to intravenous fluid replacement (blood pressure 100/70 mmHg), pulse 100 bpm) but remains hypoxic (O_2 saturation 90%).

What further imaging may be helpful at this point?

If available, a **transthoracic echocardiogram** can be very useful diagnostically. Large pulmonary emboli give rise to pulmonary hypertension and right ventricular dilatation and failure on echocardiography. Myocardial infarction gives rise to a regional wall motion abnormality in the left ventricle and impaired left ventricular function. Pericardial tamponade can be excluded with echocardiography.

A normal **perfusion scan** excludes pulmonary embolic disease and would be a useful investigation provided the CXR is normal and there is no history of asthma. An alternative is the **ventilation perfusion scan**, which can help in identifying areas of poor perfusion due to intrinsic lung disease from those due to pulmonary embolism. However, in most cases where there is a history of lung disease or an abnormal CXR, a **CT pulmonary angiogram** is performed. This investigation has a high sensitivity and specificity for pulmonary

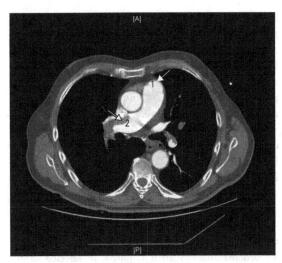

Figure 6.2 CT pulmonary angiogram of a patient with a large pulmonary embolism. 1, pulmonary embolism. 2, pulmonary artery.

embolic disease. The gold standard is a pulmonary angiogram; however, this investigation has largely been superseded by the CT pulmonary angiogram.

> *A CT pulmonary angiogram is performed (Figure 6.2). Bilateral large pulmonary emboli are shown.*

What treatment options are available and how would you choose between them?

The treatment of pulmonary embolism depends on the severity of haemodynamic compromise. All patients are given **oxygen** and **low-molecular-weight heparin**. If the patient is hypotensive then **intravenous fluids** should be administered (usually 500 mL normal saline over 15–30 minutes).

In patients with massive life-threatening pulmonary embolism, a bolus of tissue plasminogen activator (tPA) (50 mg) can be given. In more stable patients with a massive pulmonary embolism then tPA is given as an infusion (100 mg over 90 minutes). In cardiothoracic surgical centres open **pulmonary thrombectomy** remains an option but has been largely superseded by **thrombolysis**. Right-heart catheterisation and local delivery of thrombolysis into the pulmonary artery is an alternative; however, this is not proven to be more effective than systemic administration.

> *This patient went on to have thrombolysis with tPA.*

Table 6.5 Causes of thrombophilic tendency

Primary:
- Antithrombin deficiency
- Protein C deficiency
- Protein S deficiency
- Factor V Leiden
- Prothrombin 20210 mutation
- Disorders of plasmin generation
- Dysfibrinogenaemia
- Hyperhomocysteinaemia

Secondary:
- Pregnancy
- Immobility
- Trauma
- Post-operative status
- Oral contraceptive pill
- Hormone replacement therapy
- Antiphospholipid syndrome
- Hyperhomocysteinaemia
- Malignancy
- Nephrotic syndrome
- Myeloproliferative disorders
- Heparin-induced thrombocytopenia
- Paroxysmal nocturnal haemoglobinaemia
- Behçet's disease
- Increasing age

Thrombolysis is followed by administration of low-molecular-weight heparin and then anticoagulation with **warfarin**. In all cases it is important to continue heparin for 48 hours after the target INR has been achieved with warfarin therapy due to the initial prothrombotic effects of warfarin therapy. The duration of warfarin therapy is usually for at least 3 months. In patients without an obvious precipitating factor and massive pulmonary embolism, or patients with recurrent pulmonary embolism, there is an argument for life-long anticoagulation.

Should this patient have: (1) A thrombophilia screen? (2) Further investigation to rule out an underlying malignancy?

Thrombophilic conditions are divided into primary, which are inherited, and secondary. They are summarised in Table 6.5. There is much debate concerning the value of thrombophilia testing in patients with thromboembolism. Routine testing would be justified if the findings were likely to change the patient's management. Since a patient with a pulmonary embolism is already by definition at higher risk of recurrence, then the question is whether the finding of an abnormality on the thrombophilia screen adds to that risk. The evidence for this is not strong. A pragmatic approach is usually adopted and a thrombophilia screen is advised for:

- Thromboembolism in patients <40 years of age.
- A family history of thromboembolism.
- Thrombosis in an unusual site.
- Recurrent thromboembolism.

Anticoagulation or a recent large pulmonary embolism renders the screening for the inherited disorders of thrombosis unreliable, although there are some DNA-based tests. Where indicated, the thrombophilia screen should be performed 1 month after completion of the course of warfarin.

Routine screening for an underlying malignancy is not recommended, particularly where there is an obvious predisposing risk factor. However, a careful history, examination (including a rectal examination) and routine haematology, liver function tests and prostate specific antigen are appropriate.

Eight months later the patient is re-referred to outpatients. Warfarin therapy was discontinued 2 months previously. His primary complaint is of breathlessness; he has an exercise tolerance of 100 m and complains of swollen ankles and fatigue.

What may account for this presentation?

A **further pulmonary embolism** should be excluded. However, the patient has developed features of chronic right heart failure (swollen ankles and fatigue) the most probable cause for which would be **secondary pulmonary hypertension**. Up to 40% of patients following pulmonary embolism have some right ventricular dysfunction, which may go on to give right heart failure. In up to 0.5% of patients the pulmonary thrombus does not resolve with anticoagulant therapy and there is evidence of residual thrombus in the pulmonary arteries, which becomes organised and unresponsive to further anticoagulant therapy. Treatment for secondary pulmonary hypertension is largely symptomatic: diuretics for leg oedema and oxygen if required. In selected cases, pulmonary thrombo-endarterectomy (surgical removal of the remaining thrombus in the pulmonary vessels) may be appropriate. All patients with chronic pulmonary hypertension should be on long-term warfarin therapy. The use of vasodilator therapy for secondary pulmonary hypertension is currently under investigation and sildenafil and bosentan may be effective in this condition.

An echocardiogram demonstrated a normal left heart. The right ventricle was dilated with moderate tricuspid regurgitation (TR) and an estimated pulmonary artery pressure of 60 mmHg. A further contrast CT scan of the pulmonary arteries demonstrated organised laminated thrombus in the proximal pulmonary arteries and the patient was referred for pulmonary thrombo-endarterectomy.

CASE REVIEW

This 45-year-old business executive presents with chest pain and breathlessness to A&E. Although a myocardial infarction is the major differential diagnosis, in the history a recent long-haul flight and the absence of risk factors for coronary disease point to a diagnosis of pulmonary embolism. The examination features of hypoxia, hypotension and right heart failure indicate a massive pulmonary embolism. The ECG findings of right heart strain, the absence of pulmonary oedema on the CXR and an elevated D-dimer and troponin are consistent with this diagnosis. CT pulmonary angiography confirms the presence of central large pulmonary emboli. The patient is treated with fluid resuscitation and thrombolysis. He later presents with a rare but important long-term complication of pulmonary embolism: right heart failure secondary to pulmonary hypertension. This is treated with pulmonary thrombo-endarterectomy.

KEY POINTS

- Pulmonary embolism is a common differential diagnosis for patients presenting with chest pain or breathlessness. The diagnosis is often made having excluded other likely causes, rather than on the clinical presentation alone.
- The probability of pulmonary embolism is estimated from the clinical scoring system (Wells score or Revised Geneva score).
- Important common examination findings in order of frequency are tachypnoea, tachycardia, signs of deep vein thrombosis (DVT), cyanosis and fever. Features of right heart failure are uncommon and only occur in large or recurrent pulmonary emboli.
- The ECG changes of pulmonary embolism are rather non-specific and tend to occur only with a large or recurrent pulmonary emboli giving rise to pulmonary hypertension. They are characteristically those of right heart strain (S1, q3, T3 pattern, anterior T-wave inversion, right bundle branch block (RBBB) and right axis).
- A negative D-dimer is only useful as a rule-out test in patients with low probability of pulmonary embolism.
- Troponins may be elevated and are indicative of myocardial damage due to a large pulmonary embolism.

- In the A&E department an echocardiogram is useful in distinguishing a massive pulmonary embolism from myocardial infarction in patients presenting in cardiogenic shock. The findings of normal left ventricular function, an elevated pulmonary artery pressure and a dilated right ventricle strongly support the diagnosis of a large pulmonary embolism. In the case of small pulmonary emboli, the echocardiogram is usually entirely normal.
- A definitive diagnosis is made using a ventilation perfusion scan or CT pulmonary angiogram.
- Treatment depends on the haemodynamic status of the patient. All patients are given oxygen and low-molecular-weight heparin. In the shocked patient with evidence of right ventricular failure clinically or on echocardiography, the initial treatment is with cautious intravenous fluid supplementation followed by thrombolysis. Stable patients are anticoagulated with low-molecular-weight heparin followed by warfarin (usually for at least 3 months).
- The long-term complication of pulmonary hypertension should be considered in all patients with a history of pulmonary embolism presenting late with right heart failure, breathlessness and fatigue.

A 34-year-old man with chest pain following a viral illness

A 34-year-old man presents to his GP with a history of central chest pain. He is otherwise fit and well with no past medical history. On examination he is well; pulse 80 bpm; blood pressure 130/80 mmHg; there are no abnormalities on cardiovascular or respiratory examination. His ECG is shown in Figure 7.1.

What abnormalities are present on this ECG and what features help to distinguish these abnormalities from those seen in acute myocardial infarction?

The ECG shows widespread ST elevation in leads I, II, aVF and V2–V6; these changes are characteristic of acute pericarditis. Unlike the ST-segment elevation of myocardial infarction, the ST segments elevation is concave. Whereas the ST elevation in myocardial infarction usually conforms to one vascular territory (anterior or inferior), ST elevation in acute pericarditis frequently involves more than one vascular territory, as in this case. Serial ECGs in ST-elevation myocardial infarction (STEMI) usually demonstrate a loss of R-wave amplitude as a result of myocardial loss. In acute pericarditis the R-wave height is preserved, unless the patient develops a pericardial effusion or myocarditis. A subtle feature present in some cases of acute pericarditis, but not in myocardial infarction, is PR-segment depression. There is no reciprocal ST-segment depression (seen in myocardial infarction but not pericarditis) and the T waves are not inverted (T-wave inversion can be a feature of both myocardial ischaemia and pericarditis).

What causes are there of this condition?

The causes of pericarditis are listed in Table 7.1. The most

common presentations are with idiopathic or viral pericarditis. Pericarditis may complicate myocardial infarction, either in the first 48–72 hours or 4–6 weeks later (Dressler's syndrome).

What other clinical features in the history and examination may be present in this condition?

Patients with pericarditis frequently have a prodromal illness with malaise fever and chest pain, particularly with viral and idiopathic causes. The pain of pericarditis is central and may radiate to the shoulder or to the upper border of the trapezoid muscles. The pain may be exacerbated by inspiration and is relieved by sitting forwards. In uncomplicated pericarditis, there is frequently nothing to find on examination. A pericardial friction rub may be heard through systole and diastole but may be transient and positional. The patient may have additional clinical features of the underlying cause, e.g. a history of viral infection or sore throat, recent chest infection, etc.

On arrival in the A&E department the patient looks well but is complaining of central chest pain on inspiration. A friction rub is heard over the precordium. He gives a history of a viral illness 10 days previously. Routine investigations are normal apart from a D-dimer, which is elevated, and an elevated troponin I (1.2 μg/L).

How would you interpret these findings?

A pericardial friction rub is often confused with a murmur. The characteristic description is that of the sound generated by walking in fresh snow or a 'scratchy' sound. Unlike most murmurs, the sound of a friction rub is not related to diastole or systole but appears to run though the heart sounds. A D-dimer may be sent in patients with pleuritic-sounding chest pain because the

Cardiology: Clinical Cases Uncovered. By T. Betts, J. Dwight and S. Bull. Published 2010 by Blackwell Publishing.

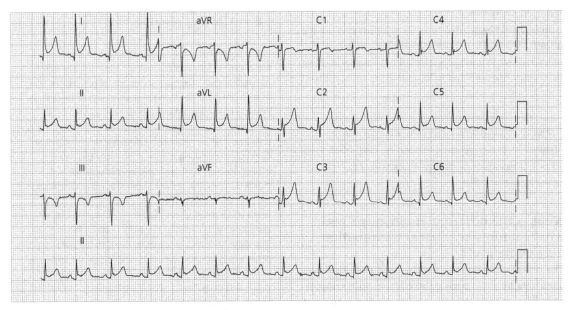

Figure 7.1 The patient's ECG.

Table 7.1 Causes of pericarditis

Idiopathic (non-specific, probably viral in most cases)

Infectious:
- Viral, e.g. coxsackie A and B, human immunodeficiency virus (HIV), hepatitis viruses
- Bacterial, e.g. Gram-positive and Gram-negative organisms, rarely mycobacterium
- Fungi (immunocompromised patients), e.g. *Histoplasma* or *Candida*

Non-infectious:
- Acute myocardial infarction
- Renal failure
- Malignancy
- Radiation therapy
- Autoimmune disorders, e.g. rheumatoid arthritis, systemic lupus erythematosis, hypothyroidism
- Trauma
- Drugs, e.g. hydrallazine, procainamide, doxorubicin

diagnosis of pulmonary embolism has been considered. Unfortunately the D-dimer may be elevated simply as a result of the pericardial inflammatory process. For a similar reason, the C-reactive protein and erythrocyte sedimentation rate are often elevated and there may be a raised white cell count. Troponins I or T are commonly mildly elevated in pericarditis, presumably due to a mild underlying myocarditis. However, a large troponin rise is uncommon and points towards a diagnosis of myocardial infarction or primary myocarditis.

What further investigations may be helpful?

A **chest X-ray (CXR)** may reveal an associated pneumonia or cardiomegaly, which may indicate the development of a pericardial effusion (a flask-shaped heart). An **echocardiogram** may show a pericardial effusion but, more importantly, the presence of normal left ventricular function on echocardiography helps to exclude myocardial infarction or myocarditis. **Viral serology** may be sent but is not usually helpful in the acute management of the patient. In recurrent acute pericarditis, or where there is a clinical suspicion of a non-viral or idiopathic cause, an **autoimmune profile** may be helpful in identifying an underlying connective tissue disease.

What treatment would you offer and what advice would you give to the patient?

Most patients with pericarditis will respond to anti-inflammatory drugs. For those cases that do not respond, a short course of corticosteroids may be helpful. Patients intolerant of non-steroidal agents or with recurrent pericarditis may respond to colchicine. Patients with pericarditis should be advised to avoid vigorous exercise for at least 2 weeks. There is an increased risk of ventricular and atrial dysrhythmias, particularly in those who have an elevated troponin and mild underlying myocarditis.

The patient was treated with aspirin and made a good recovery. Six weeks later he presents to his GP with breathlessness and fatigue. A CXR is performed, which shows cardiomegaly. Routine bloods including FBC and electrolytes are normal.

What is the differential diagnosis and what features on clinical examination may be helpful?

The differential diagnosis is between a **post-viral cardiomyopathy** and a **pericardial effusion with tamponade**. The clinical features of tamponade are not dependent upon the size of the pericardial effusion. If a pericardial effusion develops rapidly then the features of tamponade may be present with relatively little fluid in the pericardium. The clinical features of tamponade are shown in Table 7.2. With a large pericardial effusion

Table 7.2 Features of cardiac tamponade

Clinical:
- Tachycardia
- Hypotension
- Pulsus paradoxus
- Elevated jugular venous pressure (JVP)
- Quiet heart sounds (with large effusion)
- Oliguria

ECG:
- Diminished QRS voltages
- Electrical alternans

Table 7.3 Echocardiographic features of tamponade

Right atrial and left atrial collapse
Right ventricular diastolic collapse
Increased inspiratory tricuspid flow velocities
Decreased inspiratory transmitral flow velocities
Loss of inspiratory collapse of the inferior vena cava
Reversal of pulmonary venous flow in inspiration.

Box 7.1 Pulsus paradoxus

Pulsus paradoxus is the fall in systolic blood pressure associated with inspiration during normal breathing. It is usually less than 10 mmHg and is due to preferential filling of the right ventricle during inspiration and of the left ventricle during expiration. The pressure exerted by a pericardial collection of fluid exaggerates this effect. Pulsus paradoxus can be measure by manually recording systolic blood pressure during normal respiration. The cuff is inflated to above the measured systolic pressure and deflated slowly. The degree of paradox is the difference in the pressure reading when the Korotkoff sound is first heard and is intermittent (present in inspiration but not expiration) and when the Korotkoff sound is heard throughout the respiratory cycle. Exaggerated pulsus paradoxus is not a feature of a cardiomyopathy and should not be confused with pulsus alternans (alternating strong and weak beats), which is a features of severe left ventricular dysfunction.

---

the heart sounds may be quiet and the apex beat impalpable. The ECG voltages may be low due to the effusion or may demonstrate electrical alternans where the QRS amplitude varies as the heart swings in the enlarged pericardial sac. The clinical features of tamponade are due to raised pressure within the pericardial sac and its effects on filling of the left and right ventricles. The patient is usually tachycardic and hypotensive (however a normal blood pressure does not exclude tamponade). The peripheries are cold and the venous pressure is elevated. All these features however may be present in a cardiomyopathy. In tamponade the X descent of the JVP waveform is preserved and the Y descent lost, however this is often difficult to identify clinically. Kussmaul's sign – a rise or failure to fall of the venous pressure during inspiration is a feature of pericardial constriction and *not* tamponade. A pericardial friction rub may be present despite the accumulation of pericardial fluid in tamponade. Exaggerated pulsus paradoxus may be present (Box 7.1).

What is the definitive investigation in this condition and what does it show?

An **echocardiogram** will distinguish between a cardiomyopathy and pericardial effusion. A diagnosis of tamponade is made on the basis of a number of echocardiographic criteria (Table 7.3).

On examination, the patient is cool peripherally. Pulse 110 bpm; blood pressure 120/50 mmHg with 20 mmHg of paradox. His jugular venous pressure (JVP) is elevated to the earlobes. Heart sounds are quiet and he has clinical evidence of bilateral pleural effusions. An ECG shows small QRS complexes. His echocardiogram shows a global 3-cm pericardial effusion with evidence of right ventricular collapse. Routine investigations are normal, with the exception of an elevated urea (12 mmol/L) and creatinine (160 μmol/L).

How should this patient be managed?

Pericardial drainage (Box 7.2). In the absence of haemodynamic compromise pericardial effusions may be treated conservatively and monitored. A diagnostic pericardial tap may need to be performed if the cause is unknown. Fluid is sent to microbiology, biochemistry and for cytology; in the case of a malignant pericardial effusion the diagnostic yield is usually high. However, where there is haemodynamic compromise (cool peripheries, right ventricular collapse on echo or deteriorating renal function) and evidence of tamponade, the effusion needs to be formally drained.

| *A decision is made to insert a pericardial drain.*

Box 7.2 Pericardial drainage

Pericardial drainage is performed under local anaesthetic. The procedure is performed under echocardiographic guidance to demonstrate the location of the fluid. The fluid may be loculated or more prominent over the anterior or inferior surfaces of the heart and this determines the approach (subxiphisternal, apical or anterior). The procedure is more difficult and liable to give rise to complications if the pericardial effusion is small (<1 cm). If a pericardial drain is required it is inserted over a guide wire placed in the pericardial sac through a hollow needle (Seldinger method). The major complications arise as a result of trauma to the right atrium, right ventricle or coronary artery, which may give rise to a haemopericardium and (rarely) may require surgical intervention. If a drain is inserted it is usually removed within 24 hours after a further echocardiogram has been performed to establish that the fluid has been adequately drained and that that there is no persistent evidence of tamponade.

Of what potential complications of this procedure should the patient be informed ?

- Direct laceration of a coronary artery.
- Right or left atrial or ventricular perforation.
- Cardiac arrhythmias.
- Vagal mediated hypotension.
- Pneumothorax.
- Laceration of the liver (rare).

A pericardial drain is inserted and 1 litre of straw-coloured fluid is removed. The patient improves clinically and the pericardial drain is remover the following morning at which point an echocardiogram show a thin rim of residual fluid. The cytology report confirms the presence of occasional neutrophils; microbiology of the fluid is negative. The biochemistry results are as follows: protein 20 g/L; lactate dehydrogenase (LDH) 220 IU/L.

How would you interpret these findings?

These findings are consistent with a post-viral pericarditic effusion. In a similar manner to the analysis of a pleural effusion, pericardial effusions are classified into exudates and transudates. In an exudate, the LDH is greater than 200 IU/L and the protein content is greater than 50% of the serum protein content. Most pericardial effusions are exudates. In practice, the distinction is not that helpful since pericarditis due to viral disease often gives rise to a mixed picture due to dilution as a result of coexistent heart failure, while a transudate due to heart failure may be concentrated as a result of diuretic therapy. However, a very high protein content suggests bacterial or malignant disease. A blood-stained effusion may indicate malignancy; however, the significance of this is lost if the patient has been anticoagulated.

What important long-term complication may arise from pericarditis and what are the clinical features?

Constrictive pericarditis is a rare condition that can follow most causes of acute pericarditis. TB is no longer the most common cause in the western world, and most cases are seen following acute viral or bacterial pericarditis, cardiac surgery and radiotherapy. Patients present with fatigue, and features of right heart failure (**hepatomegaly, ascites, peripheral oedema**). **Kussmaul's sign** (a rise in JVP on inspiration) is present in constriction. The

JVP demonstrates a pronounced Y descent. A third sound may be present, often referred to as a **pericardial knock**. Unlike tamponade, *pulsus paradoxus is not present*.

The main differential diagnosis of constrictive pericarditis is a **restrictive cardiomyopathy**. The clinical features are so similar in these conditions that the diagnosis can usually only be established with imaging and Doppler echocardiography. Echocardiography demonstrates normal systolic function in both conditions and because of impaired ventricular filling there is usually bi-atrial enlargement. Pericardial thickening (>3.5 mm in thickness) on CT or MRI and calcification of the pericardium point to a diagnosis of constrictive pericarditis. There are subtle differences on Doppler echocardiography between constriction and restriction. The diagnosis may require additional confirmation with right and left heart catheterisation.

Pericardial biopsy will yield a tissue diagnosis where the cause is unknown; however, in practical terms the diagnosis is usually confirmed at operation for constrictive pericarditis where the pericardium is stripped (pericardectomy). Pericardectomy for constrictive pericarditis carries a significant mortality (10–15%).

CASE REVIEW

This 34-year-old man presents with a history of pleuritic central chest pain shortly after the onset of a viral illness. This history is characteristic for viral pericarditis. Examination demonstrates a pericardial friction rub. Inflammatory markers are elevated, consistent with infection or inflammation, and the troponin is elevated, indicative of a mild myocarditis. The ECG demonstrates widespread concave ST elevation and helps to confirm the diagnosis. As the patient is well he is discharged with a non-steroidal anti-inflammatory agent.

He re-presents 6 weeks later with fatigue, breathlessness and features of right heart failure. On examination he is tachypnoeic and tachycardic, his JVP is elevated and his blood pressure is 120/50 mmHg with 20 mmHg of paradox. Heart sounds are quiet and there are bilateral pleural effusions. These features are all consistent with a pericardial effusion causing cardiac tamponade. The alternative diagnosis of a post-viral cardiomyopathy is ruled out by the finding of a large pericardial effusion on echocardiography that is causing haemodynamic compromise, restricting filling to the right ventricle. This is treated with pericardial drainage and the patient makes an excellent recovery.

Pericarditis is a common presentation to the A&E department. Most cases are benign and viral in origin and treated with non-steroidal anti-inflammatory agents. It is important to be aware that pericarditis may be a manifestation of malignancy and where this is expected a chest CT and diagnostic pericardial tap (when there is pericardial fluid) may be required. The development of cardiac tamponade is a rare, but life-threatening, complication of pericarditis of all causes.

KEY POINTS

- Acute pericarditis usually presents with central chest pain. The main differential diagnosis is between pericarditis, a pulmonary embolism and an acute coronary syndrome. Clues to a diagnosis of pericarditis are that the patient looks well, the pain is positional and often pleuritic and there may be a preceding viral illness.
- Most cases are viral or idiopathic but in recurrent cases autoimmune pathology or malignancy needs to be considered. Patients with bacterial pericarditis are usually very unwell.
- Clinical examination may be normal but the diagnosis is confirmed when a pericardial friction rub (sound of footsteps crunching snow) is demonstrated.
- The ECG may be normal but the characteristic changes are of concave or saddle-shaped ST elevation occurring in multiple ECG leads. Unlike an STEMI the ECG changes often do not conform to a single coronary artery territory, there is no reciprocal ST-segment depression and there may be evidence of depression of the PR segment.
- The CXR is usually normal unless there is a pericardial effusion, underlying malignancy or pulmonary infection.
- If the patient is well then no further intervention is required and the patient is treated with non-steroidal anti-inflammatory agents. The patient should be advised to avoid vigorous exercise for 2 weeks after an attack.
- The most serious short-term complication of pericarditis is cardiac tamponade. This presents with fatigue, breathlessness, tachycardia, hypotension, an elevated JVP and poor peripheral perfusion. The diagnosis is confirmed by echocardiography. Cardiac tamponade is treated with pericardial drainage.
- Pericardial constriction is a rare complication of pericarditis and usually presents with evidence of chronic right-sided heart failure in the absence of left ventricular dysfunction on echocardiography. It is a very difficult condition to diagnose and has to be distinguished from a constrictive cardiomyopathy. A combination of investigations including MRI, echocardiography and right- and left-heart catheterisation may be helpful.

Case 8 An 80-year-old woman with acute severe breathlessness

An 80-year-old woman is admitted via ambulance in extremis to A&E. She is very dyspnoeic and unable to give a history. Medications found with her are as follows: frusemide 80 mg po od; atenolol 50 mg po od; warfarin; digoxin 0.125 mg po od

Routine observations are as follows: temperature 37°C; pulse 130 bpm, irregularly irregular; blood pressure 190/100 mmHg; respiratory rate 40 breaths/min, O₂ saturations are 88% on 10 L/min O₂ through a rebreath mask. Examination reveals central cyanosis and cool peripheries. Auscultation of the chest reveals widespread inspiratory crepitations; pulses are absent below the femoral arteries in both legs. The following investigations are available:

Arterial blood gases: pH 7.12; pO₂ 5.8 kPa; pCO₂ 3.2 kPa; bicarbonate 16 mmol/L. Routine electrolytes: sodium 130 mmol/L; potassium 5.5 mmol/L; creatinine 300 μmol/L. Glucose 6.0 mmol/L. Her chest X-ray (CXR) is shown in Figure 8.1.

What is the probable diagnosis?

The clinical features strongly point to a diagnosis of pulmonary oedema. Pulmonary emboli and severe pneumonia would be alternative causes for an acutely ill woman of this age with hypoxia and acidosis. Beta-blocker overdose may give rise to pulmonary oedema and acidosis; however, the patient has a marked tachycardia. The degree of hypertension virtually rules out pulmonary emboli as the cause of her presentation. The absence of clinical features of sepsis (peripheral vasodilatation and fever) would make a diagnosis of pneumonia less likely.

What are the findings on the arterial blood gases and what is cause for each abnormality?

Type 1 respiratory failure

The pO₂ is low with a low CO₂. There is a large A–a gradient, indicating a ventilation perfusion mismatch.

Metabolic acidosis

The patient is likely to have a profound lactic acidosis owing to poor tissue perfusion. This will be exacerbated by a metabolic acidosis related to her renal failure. The acidosis should correct with treatment of the underlying cause, there is no indication for the use of bicarbonate.

What abnormalities are seen on the CXR and what is the differential diagnosis of the radiographic findings?

The CXR shows cardiomegaly and airspace shadowing. Airspace shadowing can be caused by consolidation, due to infection, pulmonary haemorrhage or infection. Consolidation due to infection is characterised by the presence of air bronchograms. Fluid can represent cardiogenic or non-cardiogenic pulmonary oedema (Table 8.1).

The features suggesting cardiogenic pulmonary oedema on a CXR are; cardiomegaly, Kerley B lines (fine horizontal lines adjacent to the pleura due to fluid in the interlobular septa), upper lobe blood diversion and bilateral pleural effusions.

What features on examination would point specifically to a cardiogenic cause for pulmonary oedema in this woman?

The clinical features of heart failure causing pulmonary oedema are summarised in Table 8.2. However the features that are particularly helpful when present are:

- An abnormal apical impulse.
- Elevated jugular venous pressure (JVP).
- Third heart sound.
- Peripheral oedema.

Cardiology: Clinical Cases Uncovered. By T. Betts, J. Dwight and S. Bull. Published 2010 by Blackwell Publishing.

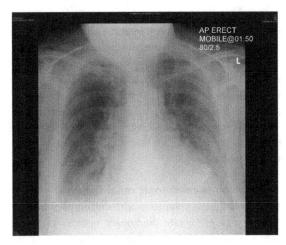

Figure 8.1 CXR of patient on arrival in A&E.

Table 8.1 Causes of non-cardiogenic pulmonary oedema

Imbalance of Starling's forces:
- Decreased plasma oncotic pressure (hypoalbuminaemia)
- Decreased interstitial pressure (decompression of pneumothorax, severe asthma)

Increased alveolar–capillary permeability:
- Infection
- Drugs
- Toxins
- Acute pancreatitis
- Aspiration of gastric contents
- Disseminated intravascular coagulation
- Shock lung

Other:
- Lymphatic insufficiency
- High altitude
- Pulmonary embolism
- Neurogenic
- Eclampsia
- Post-coronary artery bypass graft/cardioversion
- Post-anaesthesia

Table 8.2 Clinical features of heart failure

Fluid overload/congestion:
- Orthopnoea/paroxysmal nocturnal dyspnoea
- Raised jugular venous pressure (JVP)*
- Gallop rhythm
- Pulmonary inspiratory crackles
- Peripheral oedema*
- Ascites*
- Hepatic distension*

Low output:
- Tachycardia
- Low blood pressure/narrow pulse pressure*
- Cool extremities
- Poor capillary refill
- Confusion/drowsiness
- Oligouria
- Pulsus alternans (terminal)

*May be absent in acute heart failure.

The most useful finding on examination of the cardiac apex is a displaced apical impulse. Radiographic evidence of cardiomegaly has a sensitivity of 50% and a specificity of 80% for systolic dysfunction. However, up to 50% of patients develop heart failure as a result of diastolic dys-function and in these patients the heart size is often normal. Peripheral oedema is a common finding in the elderly due to immobility and venous insufficiency and therefore a non-specific finding. A third heart sound is created by the early diastolic filling phase of the left ventricle when the ventricular compliance is poor. It may be confused with a split second sound; however, a third sound occurs approximately 150 ms into diastole, i.e. much later. A fourth heart sound may occur in heart failure but is less specific; it occurs in conjunction with the atrial filling phase of diastole, again in the context of a ventricle with poor compliance. The presence of a third and fourth heart sound produces a gallop rhythm; with a tachycardia these sounds fuse, producing a summation gallop.

An ECG showing Q-wave formation, suggesting previous infarction, left bundle branch block (LBBB) or left ventricular hypertrophy and strain, is helpful. A completely normal ECG helps to rule out a diagnosis of cardiogenic pulmonary oedema. The presence of atrial fibrillation is not particularly helpful since it is present in over 10% of the population at this age.

Additional findings on cardiovascular examination are of a prominent apex beat, which is displaced to the mid-axillary line. There is a soft systolic murmur present throughout the precordium and a gallop rhythm.

What are the possible causes of pulmonary oedema in this woman and how may they be distinguished by further investigation?

Acute myocardial infarction

The drug history points to a history of either angina or hypertension. There is clinical evidence of vascular disease with absence of femoral pulses. She is unable to give a history of pain, which may be absent in this age group. The diagnosis may be obvious with the presence of ST elevation on the ECG. However, in the context of a history of hypertension and in this age group, either LBBB or left ventricular hypertrophy and strain may be found. ST changes will not be helpful as the patient is on digoxin and may well be digoxin toxic in the context of her renal failure. A small troponin rise is common in patients presenting with cardiogenic pulmonary oedema and does not prove that the cause is a plaque event causing acute myocardial infarction; however, a large rise in troponin does suggests acute myocardial infarction. Echocardiography usually shows a regional wall motion abnormality consistent with the site of infarction.

Hypertensive crisis

Hypertension is not uncommon in acute pulmonary oedema due to catecholamine release and peripheral vasoconstriction. Therefore, the finding of hypertension in patients with heart failure does not reflect a good cardiac output. The blood pressure tends to fall with the treatment of pulmonary oedema and the patient may then becomes relatively hypotensive. The features pointing to hypertension as a primary cause would be the presence of left ventricular hypertrophy clinically, on ECG, and echocardiographic evidence of left ventricular hypertrophy, particularly in the context of normal systolic function. The presence of papilloedema or haemorrhages on fundoscopy, blood and protein in the urine, or disseminated intravascular coagulation on the blood film point to a diagnosis of malignant hypertension. Phaeochromocytoma is a rare but important cause of presentation with hypertension and pulmonary oedema, a profound tachycardia is usually present.

Flash pulmonary oedema associated with renal artery stenosis

The presence of renal failure and peripheral vascular disease indicate the possibility of renal artery stenosis. The diagnosis is often made having excluded other causes. The patient presents with recurrent episodes of pulmonary oedema; between these episodes the patient may be relatively asymptomatic. Echocardiography reveals normal left ventricular function. Renal asymmetry on ultrasound is suggestive but its absence does not exclude renal artery stenosis, further investigation (see Case 24) may be required. As the cause of renal artery stenosis in this age group is atherosclerosis, the patients often have coexisting ischaemic heart disease and it is often difficult to be certain that this is the cause of pulmonary oedema.

Acute or acute-on-chronic renal failure

Fluid overload in combination with uncontrolled hypertension may precipitate pulmonary oedema in renal failure. The diagnosis is suggested by a significantly elevated creatinine on blood chemistry. Chronic renal disease is suggested by the presence of a normochromic normocytic anaemia and the demonstration of small kidneys on ultrasound examination.

A rise in creatinine is common in patients presenting with acute pulmonary oedema and usually reflects pre-renal failure or an element of acute tubular necrosis. Where renal failure is secondary to cardiogenic pulmonary oedema, renal function usually recovers with restoration of an adequate cardiac output.

Fast atrial fibrillation

Paroxysmal atrial fibrillation can present with acute pulmonary oedema, especially in conjunction with pre-existing ischaemic, hypertensive or valvular heart disease. In a patient with new-onset fast atrial fibrillation who is critically unwell with pulmonary oedema, electrical cardioversion may be necessary. However, it is a mistake to assume that fast atrial fibrillation is the cause of pulmonary oedema in a patient with a history of chronic atrial fibrillation. The catecholamine drive associated with acute pulmonary oedema will inevitably result in a marked increase in heart rate in patients with chronic atrial fibrillation. Although digoxin is usually given to patients with atrial fibrillation and heart failure, the rate will slow when the pulmonary oedema is treated with diuretics and vasodilators. This patient is already on digoxin and warfarin and therefore can be assumed to have chronic atrial fibrillation; attempted electrical or chemical cardioversion will not be successful and may be harmful. Since the patient is already on digoxin and has renal failure, digoxin levels are likely to be high and further digoxin therapy should be avoided.

Critical myocardial ischaemia

Left main stem or severe triple vessel coronary disease may present as acute pulmonary oedema in the absence of major left ventricular systolic dysfunction on echocardiography. The usual scenario is the patient who presents with acute pulmonary oedema and has a history of angina. The presentation with heart failure is often out of proportion to the troponin rise and the ECG demonstrates widespread ST depression. By the time an echocardiogram is performed the left ventricular dysfunction associated with ischaemia has reversed with treatment of the pulmonary oedema. These patients require further investigation with coronary angiography.

Valvular heart disease

It is important to remember that in the context of a patient with acute pulmonary oedema that the heart sounds may be obscured by noisy breath sounds. When the cardiac output is low, the murmur of critical aortic stenosis may be quiet or inaudible. Papillary muscle rupture in the context of ischaemic heart disease or chordal rupture in the context of mitral valve prolapse may present with acute pulmonary oedema. Acute aortic or mitral valve damage due to endocarditis may also present in this way. It is important to re-examine the patient following treatment to establish whether a murmur is present. Therefore, all patients presenting with pulmonary oedema should have echocardiography as soon as possible after admission. It would be unusual for the patient to be hypertensive in the context of pulmonary oedema due to valvular heart disease, except in the case of acute aortic regurgitation (AR) in the context of an ascending aortic arch (type A) dissection and occasionally with severe mitral stenosis (MS).

Acute myocarditis

This is a rare cause of cardiogenic oedema and is highly unlikely in this woman. The diagnosis is made on the basis of the history, echocardiographic and angiographic findings. Acute myocarditis may give rise to ST elevation on the ECG; however, the ECG changes are frequently non-specific. There is usually no history of coronary disease, hypertension or valvular diseases. There is a relatively short illness followed by presentation with hypotension, left ventricular failure. The echocardiogram shows a dilated left ventricle with global dysfunction and coronary angiography is normal. The troponin is

elevated if the patient presents early in the course of the illness. The patient is usually hypotensive at the time of presentation.

Thyrotoxicosis

Thyrotoxicosis should always be excluded as a cause of heart failure. In the elderly there are often no other clinical features of thyrotoxicosis. Thyrotoxicosis does not account for all the clinical features in this patient but may exacerbate the features of otherwise stable cardiac disease.

Dilated cardiomyopathy

Patients with a dilated cardiomyopathy usually have a less acute presentation and are normotensive or hypotensive at the time of presentation with left ventricular failure. The exception is where the dilated cardiomyopathy is secondary to hypertension or a phaeochromocytoma.

The patient has a troponin I rise of 4.6. The ECG is shown in Figure 8.2. An echocardiogram performed shows global severe left ventricular dysfunction, moderate left ventricular dilatation and hypertrophy. A diagnosis of pulmonary oedema due to left ventricular systolic dysfunction is made.

Patients with acute heart failure are often classified according to their fluid status and perfusion. Patients with acute-on-chronic heart failure are often oedematous, the blood pressure is normal or low and the peripheries are relatively warm. In cardiogenic shock due to myocardial infarction presenting in acute heart failure, the patient is often not fluid overloaded and the features are predominantly of pulmonary oedema and a low-output state with cold peripheries. In acute heart failure secondary to a hypertensive crisis there may be little evidence of chronic fluid retention and the picture is similar in that the patient is cool peripherally and the predominant feature is pulmonary oedema.

What does the ECG demonstrate and what is the underlying pathology?

Widespread ST depression and **ST elevation in lead aVR** are findings consistent with severe ischaemia. The presence of ST elevation in aVR is strongly associated with left main stem coronary artery stenosis and triple vessel coronary artery disease. ST elevation of >1 mm in aVR is associated with an in-hospital mortality of up to 20% in non-STEMI.

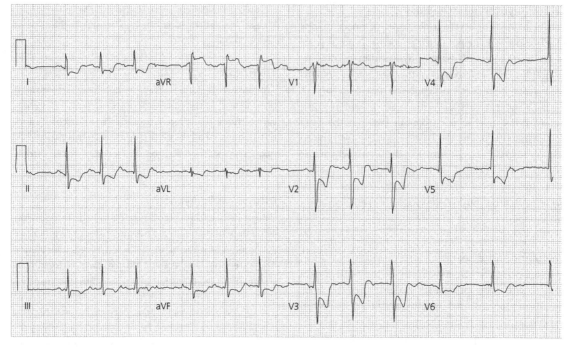

Figure 8.2 The patient's ECG.

How would you manage this patient?

There are two aspects to the treatment of this patient. First is the treatment of acute heart failure. An algorithm for the management of acute heart failure is given in Figure 8.3. In this case the management will be predominantly with oxygen, intravenous diuretics and nitrates. The dose of loop diuretic in those patients not on oral diuretics is usually frusemide 40 mg; if the patient is already on frusemide then the usual oral dose can be given intravenously. A urinary catheter is not required in most patients with left ventricular failure; however, it is recommended in hypotensive patients and those with pre-existing severe renal disease. The standard treatment for an acute coronary syndrome should be commenced (see p. 42). The question of whether to continue beta blockade is important. In the context of acute pulmonary oedema, beta blockade has to be withdrawn initially despite evidence of an acute coronary syndrome.

She is given 40 mg of frusemide intravenously and commenced on intravenous nitrates. One hour after commencing therapy she remains acutely unwell. O₂ saturations are 86% on 10 L O₂ via a rebreath mask, blood pressure is now 140/70 mmHg and the respiratory rate is 35 breaths/min; there has been no urine output.

What other interventions would you consider?

Continuous positive airways pressure (CPAP)

Patients who remain in type 1 respiratory failure despite therapy may respond to CPAP. There is little evidence that CPAP improves mortality in acute heart failure but it may avoid the requirement for ventilation or is helpful as a bridge to definitive treatment of the underlying cause.

High-dose intravenous diuretics

Patients with renal failure are resistant to diuretic therapy. Doses of 120–240 mg frusemide as a short infusion (1–2 hours) may be required to generate a diuresis.

Haemofiltration

Haemofiltration will rapidly remove fluid and treat the pulmonary oedema. However, this is usually undertaken if the cause is reversible and there is a reasonable prospect of recovery from the underlying cause of the pulmonary oedema.

Balloon pump

A balloon pump may be used to augment coronary flow in diastole and offload the left ventricle in patients in

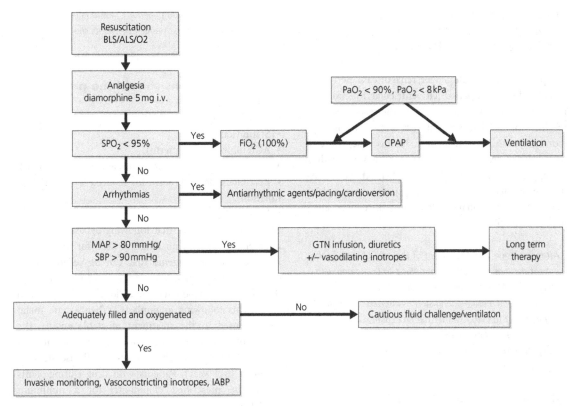

Figure 8.3 Algorithm for management of acute heart failure. ALS, advanced lift support; BLS, basic life support; CPAP, continuous positive airways pressure; GTN, glyceryl trinitrate; IABP, intra-aortic balloon pump; MAP, mean arterial pressure; SBP, systolic blood pressure; SPO₂, arterial oxygen saturation.

cardiogenic shock (see Case 26, p. 202). Again, this is only a bridge to definitive treatment, e.g. revascularisation.

What factors would influence your decision regarding resuscitation status?

A decision has to be made whether to ventilate this patient if the respiratory failure does not respond to the above measures. Malignant ventricular dysrhythmias are also common in this situation and a decision has to be made regarding the resuscitation status. The major factors are:

- The patient's pre-morbid state.
- The prospects for recovery of left ventricular function.
- The prospects for recovery of renal function.
- The age of the patient.
- The patient's wishes.

It is important to contact the patient's relatives or GP to obtain an idea of the pre-morbid state of the patient.

If there has been extensive or multiple myocardial infarction in the past, then the prognosis for recovery of left ventricular function is poor. Patients with pre-existing renal disease have a poor prognosis and therefore it is important to establish whether the renal failure is chronic, or acute and therefore potentially reversible. It is frequently impossible and often inappropriate in critically ill patients to obtain their own views; however, where available, a living will should be taken into account even though these documents are not legally binding.

The patient responds to high-dose frusemide and CPAP. Five days later her creatinine is 210 μmol/L. A repeat echocardiogram shows moderate, globally impaired left ventricular function. An angiogram is performed and demonstrates a 90% distal left main stem stenosis. Her case is discussed with the cardiac surgeons.

What factors contribute to the perioperative risk for coronary bypass surgery and what alternatives are available?

The patient's age, female gender, renal disease, peripheral vascular disease, impaired left ventricular function and recent non-STEMI all contribute to the risks of surgery in this woman. The surgical risk is assessed using a scoring system (the Euroscore). In this case, the estimated risk of death during surgery is 33%. With medical therapy the 1-year mortality is higher. An alternative used in selected high-risk elderly patients is angioplasty to the left main coronary artery, a procedure increasingly used in a number of centres.

After discussion with the patient of the risks of surgery, the patient declines an operation but elects to be treated with angioplasty. An angioplasty to the distal left main stem is performed and a drug-eluting stent is inserted. The patient is transferred to the CCU after the procedure with a balloon pump in situ; 24 hours later the balloon pump is removed. The patient makes an uncomplicated recovery and is discharged 5 days later.

What are the long-term risks of this procedure?

• Restenosis.
• Stent thrombosis.

The patient returns to outpatients 1 month later. She is well but complains about the number of tablets she has been prescribed.

What medications should the patient be taking?

• Aspirin (long term).
• Statin (long term).
• ACE inhibitor (long term).
• Clopidogrel (at least 1 year with a drug-eluting stent).
• Beta blockade (long term for reduced left ventricular function).*
• Diuretic.*

Many patients believe that following bypass surgery or intervention there is no longer a need for medication. However, the only agents that can be reliably withdrawn are the patient's antianginal agents (provided that the patient is angina free). Clopidogrel is given to all patients following angioplasty. When a bare metal stent is used in the treatment of stable angina, the course of clopidogrel need only be for 1 month (in the context of unstable coronary disease this is extended to 1 year). Patients with drug-eluting stents should be prescribed clopidogrel for a minimum period of 1 year.

---

*In some instances left ventricular function returns to normal following bypass surgery and beta blockade and diuretic therapy can be withdrawn.

CASE REVIEW

This 80-year-old woman presents to A&E with acute dyspnoea. The diagnosis of acute heart failure is suggested by the examination findings of a raised JVP, displaced apex beat, gallop rhythm and basal crepitations. The diagnosis is confirmed by the findings of an abnormal ECG, radiological features of pulmonary oedema on the CXR and an echocardiogram demonstrating left ventricular systolic dysfunction. The additional findings of hypertension and renal failure raise the possibility of renal artery stenosis as a cause of her pulmonary oedema. The ECG findings of severe ischaemia and a troponin rise suggest that coronary artery disease is the cause of her left ventricular failure. Although the patient is in fast atrial fibrillation, this is chronic and not felt to be the cause of her sudden deterioration. Conventional treatment with diuretics, oxygen and vasodilators fails to produce an adequate response and the patient requires treatment with CPAP ventilation. On recovery, coronary angiography is performed and demonstrates a left main stem coronary stenosis. Although coronary bypass grafting is considered, she is felt to be a high-risk case for surgery due to her age, renal failure and impaired left ventricular function. The patient is successfully treated with angioplasty to the left main coronary artery.

The mortality in the first year following presentation with acute left ventricular failure is approximately 30%. It is very important to establish and treat specific causes. Coronary artery disease, hypertension and valvular heart disease are the most common causes of left ventricular dysfunction in this age group. In patients with severe left ventricular dysfunction and patients with angina, a significant proportion of viable myocardium should be considered for revascularisation.

KEY POINTS

- In patients presenting with acute breathlessness, the most common differential diagnoses are acute left ventricular failure, asthma, pulmonary embolism, an exacerbation of chronic obstructive airways disease (COPD) and pneumonia.
- Nearly all cases of pulmonary oedema are due to cardiac disease; however; this is not a diagnosis in itself. Careful evaluation is required to establish the cause of the heart failure.
- Useful clinical signs include an elevated JVP, basal crepitations, a third and/or fourth heart sound; however, these are not always present.
- Diagnostic features of pulmonary oedema due to left ventricular failure on the CXR are cardiomegaly, upper lobe blood diversion, Kerley B lines, 'bats wing' perihilar shadowing and bilateral pleural effusions.

- An ECG is helpful; in acute pulmonary oedema the ECG is nearly always abnormal
- Acute management is with oxygen, vasodilators and intravenous diuretics. Patients not responding to these treatments may require CPAP.
- If there is no pre-existing diagnosis, an echocardiogram should be performed as soon as possible.
- In patients presenting with acute heart failure without a prior history of orthopnoea, paroxysmal nocturnal dyspnoea, ankle oedema or myocardial infarction, so-called flash pulmonary oedema, reversible ischaemia, dysrhythmias and renal artery stenosis should be considered.
- The decision to escalate treatment, including ventilation, balloon-pump support or intravenous inotropes, depends upon the likelihood of a reversible cause and the patient's pre-morbid state.

Case 9 A 50-year-old man with exertional breathlessness

A 50-year-old man is referred to medical outpatients with breathlessness on exertion and an irregular pulse. At best, his exercise tolerance is 100 m on the flat and he cannot manage a flight of stairs without stopping; 6 months previously he was attending the gym three times weekly and regarded himself as very fit. He is a non-smoker. When last measured, his total cholesterol was 7.5 mmol/L. He takes simvastatin 40 mg po od. There is no past history of note; in particular there is no history of diabetes or hypertension or ischaemic heart disease.

What is the differential diagnosis for the cause of his breathlessness?

The common differential diagnoses in a 50-year-old man with exertional breathlessness are:

- Heart failure.
- Atrial fibrillation or flutter.
- Silent myocardial ischaemia.
- Asthma.
- Chronic obstructive airways disease (COPD).
- Lung cancer or pulmonary metastases.
- Anaemia.
- Chronic pulmonary thromboembolic disease.
- Obesity.
- Interstitial fibrotic lung disease.

The onset of symptoms and the exercise tolerance prior to the illness are key in establishing the cause of the breathlessness. The history suggests a relatively recent onset in a man who has had an excellent exercise tolerance previously and is a non-smoker. The diagnosis of chronic lung disease is therefore unlikely. Chest pain is not reported; however, it is important to question the patient further about chest tightness or discomfort on exertion. In a relatively young, non-diabetic man, ischaemic heart disease is unlikely to be the cause for breathlessness in

the absence of symptoms of angina. Although asthma is a possibility, the exercise tolerance is very poor in this man and there is no evidence of reversibility of the symptoms. Fast atrial fibrillation may trigger symptoms of heart failure and, when prolonged, may cause a cardiomyopathy. Chronic pulmonary embolic disease, interstitial fibrotic lung disease, anaemia and lung cancer cannot be excluded on the basis of the above history.

What other features in the history may help to establish the diagnosis?
Cough

A history of cough may be present in COPD, asthma, interstitial lung disease, lung cancer and heart failure. The cough is usually non-productive in asthma, heart failure and fibrosing alveolitis. In heart failure, as with asthma, the cough may be predominantly nocturnal. A chronic productive cough (especially if daily for more than 3 months of the year for 2 years in succession) would point to a diagnosis of COPD. Copious amounts of sputum are a feature of bronchiectasis.

Haemoptysis

Haemoptysis is a red-flag symptom for lung carcinoma but may also be present in COPD, bronchiectasis, pulmonary embolism and heart failure. Haemoptysis is a feature of pulmonary infarction due to pulmonary embolism and this is a feature of the acute presentation of pulmonary embolic disease. Haemoptysis due to heart failure is usually a feature of pulmonary oedema (pink frothy sputum) and is unlikely as an outpatient presentation (the exception is in some cases of heart failure due to severe mitral stenosis).

Wheeze

Wheeze can be a feature of asthma, COPD and heart failure. It is not uncommon for patients with heart failure to present with wheeze in addition to breathlessness and to have received a trial of bronchodilators. In these cases, the history may be of a presumed viral upper

Cardiology: Clinical Cases Uncovered. By T. Betts, J. Dwight and S. Bull. Published 2010 by Blackwell Publishing.

respiratory illness that appears prolonged and unresponsive to antibiotics. There may be some symptomatic response to bronchodilators; however, the breathlessness remains and the exercise tolerance is poor. The wheeze of asthma and heart failure may be predominantly nocturnal.

Orthopnoea

This is a feature of heart failure and COPD. Orthopnoea in heart failure is due to the development of pulmonary oedema associated with the increased venous return when lying flat. The patient is more comfortable when propped up on two or more pillows and reports that they become more breathless if they slip down from the pillows.

Orthopnoea in COPD is due to the mechanical advantages of supporting the accessory muscles of respiration by sitting with the arms fixed on the side of the bed or chair. These patients are usually breathless at rest and have characteristic examination findings of COPD (barrel chest, use of accessory muscles, etc.). It is not difficult therefore to distinguish between the orthopnoea of heart failure and COPD (except when the patient has both).

Paroxysmal nocturnal dyspnoea

This is a classic symptom of heart failure that is fairly specific for the diagnosis; however, it is present only in a minority of patients. Characteristically, the patient wakes at night with breathlessness that is relieved by standing or sitting.

Ankle oedema

Although common in the elderly, the presence of ankle oedema in a man of this age would strongly support the diagnosis of heart failure. Ankle oedema may also be a feature of COPD; contrary to common belief this is due to cor pulmonale only in minority of cases. The mechanism is unclear but fluid retention as a result of the effects of renal hypoxia and activation of the renin angiotensin system is one possibility. Fluid retention in COPD usually only occurs when resting oxygen saturations fall to less than 93%.

Prolonged immobility, recent surgery, history of thromboembolic disease

Chronic pulmonary thromboembolic disease is a relatively rare cause of chronic breathlessness and the diagnosis is usually made when other causes have been excluded.

Occupational history

This is particularly important in identifying patients with fibrotic lung disease, e.g. pneumoconiosis and asbestosis, and extrinsic allergic alveolitis (e.g. farmer's lung).

Hobbies/pets

Patients with extrinsic allergic alveolitis may have birds as pets (bird fancier's lung).

Family history

Patients with dilated or hypertrophic cardiomyopathy may report a family history of cardiac disease or sudden death.

Alcohol intake

Patients with heart failure due to an alcoholic cardiomyopathy usually develop atrial fibrillation early in the course of the illness. The alcohol intake required is approximately 10 units per day for a period of more than 2 years but is highly variable. Heavy alcohol consumption should not be assumed to be the cause until other causes have been excluded.

The patient reports mild ankle oedema for the last 2 months and two-pillow orthopnoea. He describes upper abdominal pain and loss of appetite over the past 2 months. There is no history of cough, wheeze or paroxysmal nocturnal dyspnoea. He has been a heavy drinker in the past but is now only drinking 10 units of alcohol per week. There is no family history of cardiac disease.

What is the differential diagnosis for the patient's upper abdominal pain and loss of appetite and what further questions would you ask?

Peptic ulcer disease

A history of dyspepsia would help to confirm this diagnosis. Loss of appetite would be unusual in peptic ulcer disease.

Gastric carcinoma

A history of weight loss would point to a diagnosis of malignancy. However, weight loss can also be seen in the advances stages of COPD and in heart failure (cardiac cachexia). There may be a history of vomiting or haematemesis. The patient may have become anaemic due to gastrointestinal bleeding and may have a history of melaena.

Liver metastases

A history of weight loss would be expected. A lung primary with liver secondaries would account for both the breathlessness and upper abdominal pain.

Hepatic congestion

This is a fairly common symptom in patients with heart failure. An elevated JVP gives rise to hepatic congestion, which accounts for the epigastric discomfort and a sense of fullness that gives rise to a loss of appetite.

Mesenteric ischaemia

Patients with mesenteric ischaemia usually have evidence of vascular disease elsewhere. The pain is usually after eating and may be relieved by GTN. Ischaemia of the large bowel gives rise to bleeding per rectum.

The patient has gained weight over the past month, despite the loss of appetite. There are no other upper GI symptoms and he does not report rectal bleeding or melaena. On examination: O_2 saturations 98% on room air; pulse 120 bpm, irregular; blood pressure 120/70 mmHg; JVP – elevated to the angle of the jaw. Apex beat – impalpable. Auscultation – soft apical systolic murmur, 3rd heart sound. Chest examination – bibasal inspiratory crackles. Abdominal examination – 3 cm tender hepatomegaly. Pitting oedema both ankles.

What is the most probable diagnosis?
Cardiac failure and atrial fibrillation

The absence of a smoking history, examination features of COPD and normal oxygen saturation virtually exclude COPD or respiratory disease. Atrial fibrillation may be present in heart failure, COPD or pulmonary embolic disease and is a relatively non-specific finding. The apex beat is often impalpable in patients with heart failure and the heart size may be normal in diastolic heart failure, so this does not exclude the diagnosis. A third sound strongly supports the diagnosis of heart failure (note a fourth sound will not be present as the patient is in atrial fibrillation).

The tender hepatomegaly is consistent with hepatic venous congestion due to heart failure. Inspiratory crackles are a feature of fibrotic lung disease, COPD and heart failure. Extensive fine crackles throughout the lung fields in a patient who is not particularly breathless at rest and who has no other signs of heart failure suggest a diagnosis of fibrosing alveolitis. Pitting oedema may be a feature of right or left heart failure, hypoalbuminaemia, venous/

Table 9.1 New York Heart Association (NYHA) classification of breathlessness

Class I – no limitation: ordinary physical activity does not cause undue fatigue, dyspnoea or palpitation.
Class II – slight limitation of physical activity: comfortable at rest. Ordinary physical activity results in fatigue, dyspnoea or palpitation.
Class III – marked limitation of physical activity: comfortable at rest but less than normal activity produce symptoms.
Class IV – inability to carry out any physical activity without discomfort.

lymphatic obstruction or immobility and does not help greatly in confirming diagnosis.

How would you classify the severity of his symptoms?

This patient is New York Heart Association (NYHA) class III. The NYHA classification of breathlessness is given in Table 9.1.

An ECG is performed and demonstrates atrial fibrillation and left bundle branch block (LBBB). A CXR demonstrates mild cardiomegaly; the lung fields are clear. His echocardiogram is reported as follows:

Left ventricular dilatation: left ventricular diastolic dimension 6 cm, Left ventricular systolic dimension 5.5 cm.
Ejection fraction 25% with global hypokinesis.
Aortic and mitral valves structurally normal.
Moderate central jet of mitral regurgitation (MR).
Dilated left atrium 5.5 cm.
Right heart moderately dilated with impaired function.
Tricuspid valve normal. Mild tricuspid regurgitation (TR) with an estimated pulmonary artery pressure of 20 mmHg.

How does the measured ejection fraction in this patient compare to that of a normal heart?

The ejection fraction is half the normal value and indicates severe left ventricular dysfunction (Box 9.1).

What is the clinical significance of the finding of global hypokinesia and right heart dilatation?

Characteristically, ischaemic heart disease primarily

Box 9.1 Measurement of left ventricular function

The ejection fraction on echocardiography is an estimate of left ventricular function. It is calculated from the left ventricular volume derived from images of the left ventricle (Figure 9.1). The difference in left ventricular volume in systole and diastole is used to calculate the proportion of blood ejected during each cardiac cycle. Since the heart does not empty completely during normal systole, the normal left ventricular ejection fraction is 55–60% rather than 100%. Many patients will not understand this concept and become concerned that their heart is working at only 55% efficiency. The accuracy of the measurement is highly dependent on the quality of the images and therefore the skill of the operator. Where adequate images cannot be obtained with standard echocardiography, bubble contrast echocardiography may provide better image definition. Alternative non-invasive methods for measuring left ventricular function include myocardial scintigraphy (multi-gated acquisition [MUGA] scan) and MRI. The left ventricular function on echo is usually reported as being normal, mild, moderate or severely impaired according to the estimated ejection fraction (Table 9.2).

Table 9.2 Left ventricular function and ejection fraction

Normal: >55%
Mild impairment: 46–55%
Moderate impairment: 35–45%
Severe impairment: <35%

causes impairment of left ventricular function; the presence of right ventricular dilatation indicates that the patient has either had long-standing left ventricular dysfunction with pulmonary hypertension and right heart failure or that the patient has a dilated cardiomyopathy. Since there is no evidence of pulmonary hypertension on echocardiography, the right ventricular involvement is likely to be due to a primary cardiomyopathic process. The diagnosis of a dilated cardiomyopathy rather than an ischaemic cardiomyopathy is also suggested by the absence of regional wall motion abnormalities, which are more common in ischaemic heart disease due to localised myocardial damage related to coronary artery occlusion.

What is the significance of the finding of mitral regurgitation?

The finding of mitral regurgitation (MR) on echocardiography in patients with left ventricular failure is not uncommon. However, this does not indicate that MR is the cause of the heart failure. In a dilated cardiomyopathy the mitral valve annulus is stretched as the ventricle dilates. As a result, the leaflets no longer coapt in systole giving rise to a central jet of 'functional' MR. In heart failure due to mitral valve disease the ventricle will also be dilated; however; the mitral valve is usually structurally abnormal and the jet of MR is eccentric due to prolapse of one of the mitral valve leaflets. Patients with heart failure and significant functional MR have a poorer prognosis.

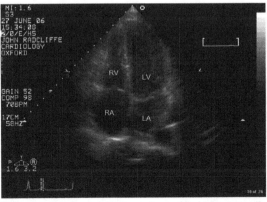

(a)

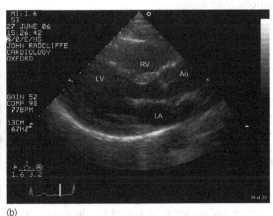

(b)

Figure 9.1 Examples of echocardiographic views. (a) Four chamber apical view. (b) Parasternal long axis view. Ao, aorta; LA, left atrium; LV, Left ventricle; RA, right atrium; RV, right ventricle.

What further investigations may be required to establish the diagnosis in this patient?

Heart failure is a syndrome and not a diagnosis. It is important to investigate for reversible causes. The causes of left ventricular failure are given in Table 9.3. The classification can be confusing. Hypertension ischaemic heart disease, diabetes, tachycardias and high output states can all give rise to the appearances of a dilated cardiomyopathy but are usually classified separately. Routine investigations for a dilated cardiomyopathy would include:

- FBC (anaemia).
- Liver function tests (alcoholic liver disease, haemochromatosis).
- Creatine kinase (muscular dystrophies).
- Thyroid function tests.
- Glucose.
- Lipid profile.
- Ferritin (haemochromatosis).
- Urinary catecholamines (phaeochromocytoma).

The above investigations are all normal, with the exception of the cholesterol which remains elevated at 7.5 mmol/L and the liver function tests are as follows:
Bilirubin – 30 μmol/l (normal 3–17).
Alanine aminotransferase (ALT) – 70 IU/L (normal 10–45).
Alkaline phosphatase – 450 IU/L (normal 95–320).
Albumin – 39 g/L (normal 35–50).

What are the possible causes of the abnormal liver function tests and what further investigations should be considered?

Alcoholic liver disease

Despite the fact that the patient has reduced his alcohol intake alcoholic liver disease remains a possibility. The presence of a raised mean corpuscle volume (MCV) would tend to support the diagnosis.

Simvastatin

Simvastatin can cause a rise in liver enzymes, in particular the ALT. The simple way of establishing whether this is the case is to discontinue the drug, since the abnormalities are reversible.

Hepatic congestion

These abnormalities are quite typical for those seen in hepatic congestion due to heart failure. With severe hepatic congestion the patient may become jaundiced

Table 9.3 Aetiology of left ventricular failure

Ischaemic heart disease

Hypertension

Valvular heart disease

Myocarditis

Dilated cardiomyopathy:
- Idiopathic
- Alcohol
- Post-viral
- Genetic, e.g. Becker muscular dystrophy
- Haemochromatosis
- Phaeochromocytoma
- Sarcoid

Hypertrophic cardiomyopathy

Restrictive cardiomyopathy:
- Radiotherapy
- Amyloid
- Eosinophilia related

Pericardial disease

High-output heart failure:
- Anaemia
- Thyrotoxicosis
- A–V malformations

Diabetic cardiomyopathy

Tachycardia mediated:
- Atrial flutter
- Atrial fibrillation

and develop ascites. Some patients first present to a gastroenterologist, particularly when the features of right heart failure predominate.

Chronic hepatitis

In the absence of another cause, chronic active hepatitis, hepatitis B or C and other causes of chronic liver disease would need to be considered.

An abdominal ultrasound and gamma-glutamyl transpeptidase (GGT) would be helpful.

The abdominal ultrasound confirms a large liver. There is evidence of marked hepatic venous congestion; however, the scan is otherwise normal. The GGT is normal.

What further investigations would you consider?

Although these investigations suggest an idiopathic dilated cardiomyopathy, ischaemic heart disease should be excluded in a man of this age with hypercholesterolaemia. Coronary angiography, myocardial perfusion scanning, stress echocardiography and MRI may be helpful and their use varies between centres.

What drug therapy would you introduce?

ACE inhibitors

All patients with heart failure are started on ACE inhibitors, which substantially reduce mortality and improve symptoms. This is a class effect and a variety of ACE inhibitors have been shown to be effective in clinical trials. The agent used should be titrated up to full dose. Where patients are intolerant of ACE inhibitors (usually due to cough) an angiotensin II blocker may be substituted.

Loop diuretics

The vast majority of patients with symptomatic left ventricular function will require treatment with a loop diuretic (e.g. furosemide or bumetanide). The dose is titrated according to response and the degree of fluid overload.

Beta blockade

Beta blockers have been shown to reduce mortality and improve symptoms in patients with left ventricular systolic dysfunction. They are titrated gradually to the maximum tolerated doses. Not all beta blockers have been shown to be beneficial. Those with proven benefit

Table 9.4 Beta blockers used in heart failure

Bisoprolol
Carvedilol
Metoprolol
Nebivolol

Table 9.5 Contraindications to beta blockade in heart failure

Asthma
Chronic obstructive airways disease (COPD) with significant variability
Heart rate <60 bpm
Severe conduction disease (not bundle branch block)
Systolic blood pressure <100 mmHg

are shown in Table 9.4. Contraindications to beta blockade in heart failure are given in Table 9.5.

How would you manage the atrial fibrillation in this patient?

- **Beta blockade.** The conventional therapy for heart failure and atrial fibrillation has, until recently, been digoxin. There is little doubt that digoxin is effective at improving symptoms in patients with heart failure and atrial fibrillation. However, digoxin has not been shown to have a mortality benefit in heart failure. Beta blockers are the preferred agents to control rate. The exception is in those patients with pulmonary oedema where digoxin is often used initially until the pulmonary oedema has resolved and then a beta blocker is introduced.
- **Anticoagulation.** The presence of congestive cardiac failure and atrial fibrillation puts this man at high risk of thromboembolic events (see CHAD2 score, Box 19.1, p. 163). Anticoagulation should be started with a low loading dose of warfarin (e. g. 5 mg daily) and should be monitored carefully in view of the abnormal liver function.
- **Cardioversion.** The decision whether to cardiovert this patient is based on:
  - The probability of restoring sinus rhythm
  - The probability of maintaining sinus rhythm
  - The probability that the cardiomyopathy is rate related.

The probability of restoring sinus rhythm is reduced with:

- Increasing age.
- Duration of atrial fibrillation >1 year.
- Increased left atrial size (>5 cm).
- Associated valvular or left ventricular disease

In this man the duration of the atrial fibrillation is probably less than 1 year; however, the patient has a dilated left atrium and left ventricle. Similar factors influence the likelihood of maintaining sinus rhythm and even if sinus rhythm is restored the patient is likely to require life-long antiarrythmic therapy or atrial fibrillation ablation therapy.

Cardioversion is usually attempted where the cardiomyopathy is felt to be rate related. In these patients the resting heart rate is usually >120 bpm and the rate responds poorly to the treatment of the heart failure. Often the diagnosis of a rate-related cardiomyopathy is only confirmed retrospectively when the echocardiogram returns to normal and the patient remains stable off heart failure therapy following cardioversion.

The patient is seen 3 months later, by which time he on the following medication: bisoprolol 10mg od; ramipril 10mg od; furosemide 80mg od; warfarin 4mg od.

He reports that his breathlessness is improved; however, his exercise tolerance is only 150m and he remains short of breath on exertion. On examination: pulse 70bpm in atrial fibrillation; blood pressure 110/70mmHg; JVP +10cm, heart sounds normal; bibasal crepitations.

What further therapeutic options are available?

Figure 9.2 illustrates the stepwise approach to therapy in patients with heart failure.

Spironolactone

This potassium-sparing diuretic is an aldosterone antagonist. In clinical trials it has been shown to be beneficial in reducing morbidity and mortality in heart failure. The serious side-effect of the drug is hyperkalaemia and renal failure and it is contraindicated where the baseline potassium is >5mmol/L or the serum creatinine >220μmol/L.

Angiotensin II blockade

The angiotensin II receptor blockers, valsartan and candesartan, have been used in conjunction with ACE inhibitors with further benefit.

Digoxin

Although the atrial fibrillation rate has been adequately controlled there is still a role for digoxin in patient with uncontrolled symptoms of heart failure on first-line medication.

Cardiac resynchronisation therapy

In some patients with a broad QRS complex and LBBB, cardiac output can be improved by pacing the left and right ventricles. The improvement in the stroke volume of the heart is achieved by ensuring that the septum and the lateral wall of the heart contract simultaneously. The procedure involves insertion of a pacemaker with an additional lead that paces the left ventricle via the coronary sinus. The National Institute for Health and Clinical Excellence (NICE) guidelines for indications for cardiac

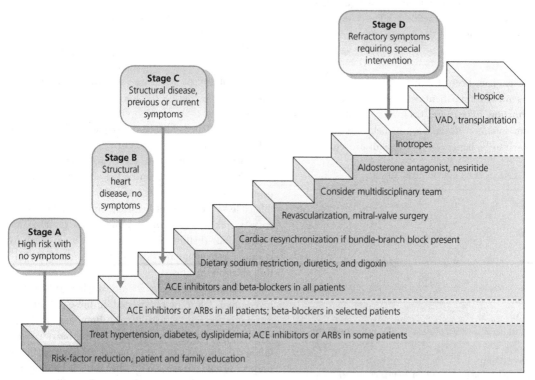

Figure 9.2 Stepwise progression of drug therapy in heart failure. ACE, angiotensin-converting enzyme; ARBs, angiotensin receptor blocks; VAD, ventricular assist device. From Jessup M, Brozena S. Medical progress – heart failure. *N Eng J Med* 2003; 348: 2007–2018. Copyright 2002 Massachusetts Medical Society.

Table 9.6 National Institute for Health and Clinical Excellence (NICE) criteria for cardiac resynchronisation therapy (all criteria need to be met)

Patient experiencing or have recently experienced New York Heart Association (NYHA) class III of IV symptoms

They are in sinus rhythm:
- Either with a QRS duration of 150 ms or longer, estimated by the ECG
- Or with a QRS duration of 120–149 ms and with evidence of mechanical dysynchrony that is confirmed by echocardiography

Patient has an ejection fraction of 35% or less

Patient receiving optimal pharmacological therapy

resynchronisation therapy are given in Table 9.6. This patient fails to qualify as he is in atrial fibrillation.

Cardiac transplantation and left ventricular assist devices

Where all standard therapeutic options have been tried, heart transplantation or the use of a mechanical heart has to be considered.

The patient improves with the introduction of digoxin and spironolactone and is discharged to the care of his GP.

What advice and what further measures should be taken to reduce the risk of decompensation in this patient?

Heart failure is one of the most common causes of admission to hospital. Most of these admissions are patients with an established diagnosis of heart failure who deteriorate in the community. The following advice should be given:

- **Regular weight** – patients should be advised to weigh themselves each day or on alternate days. A rapid rise in weight (>1 kg) over a few days is due to fluid retention and is an indication that heart failure is worsening and should prompt a visit to their GP.
- **Salt** – patients should be advised to avoid added salt.
- **Drugs** – the purpose of each drug therapy should be explained to the patient to improve compliance. The patient should be advised not to take non-steroidal drugs (e.g. ibuprofen).
- **Exercise** – most patients should be advised to take regular gentle aerobic exercise, this improves long-term outcome and symptoms.
- **Warning symptoms** – the patient should be informed of the warning symptoms of orthopnoea, paroxysmal nocturnal dyspnoea and ankle swelling, which indicate decompensation and syncope, and postural hypotension, which may indicate the need to reduce diuretic or vasodilator therapies.

The introduction of community heart failure specialist nurses has been shown to reduce hospital readmissions with heart failure and improve drug compliance.

What is the long-term prognosis in this patient and what is the usual mode of death?

The mortality rate from heart failure is 30% in the first year and 10% each year subsequently. The mode of death is split evenly between sudden death due to ventricular dysrhythmias and death due to progressive heart failure. The high incidence of sudden death in these patients has prompted the use of AICD devices in these patients, particularly if there is a history of syncope or documented ventricular arrhythmias (see Case 22, p. 181).

CASE REVIEW

This previously fit 50-year-old man presents with a history of breathlessness, ankle oedema and orthopnoea. The diagnosis of heart failure is supported by the findings of an elevated JVP, a third heart sound on auscultation and the presence of hepatomegaly and pitting oedema. An echocardiogram confirms that has a dilated cardiomyopathy with biventricular failure. The history of heavy alcohol consumption in the past would support a diagnosis of heart failure secondary to an alcohol-related cardiomyopathy. Atrial fibrillation occurs early in the course of this form of cardiomyopathy. There is no history of coronary disease and his routine investigations are normal, with the exception of abnormal liver function tests that are probably related to hepatic congestion. The patient makes a partial response to standard therapy with ACE-inhibition diuretics and beta blockade. His risk of systemic embolism is high and he therefore requires anticoagulation with warfarin. Spironolactone and digoxin are added and his symptoms improve further.

KEY POINTS

- Heart failure is a common condition with an incidence of 1% per annum of the population and a prevalence of 2–3% of the population. The incidence increases with age.
- Heart failure still caries a very poor prognosis; 30% of patients will die within 1 year of the diagnosis being made and approximately 10% per annum, subsequently.
- Heart failure is broadly classified into patients with systolic dysfunction on echocardiography and those with the clinical features of heart failure but normal systolic function on echocardiography (heart failure normal ejection fraction [HFNEF]).
- The important features in the history that suggest a heart failure include orthopnoea, paroxysmal nocturnal dyspnoea, ankle oedema and fatigue.
- The important clinical examination findings that are relatively specific include an elevated JVP, a displaced apex beat, basal crepitations and leg oedema.
- The diagnosis is supported by the finding of an abnormal ECG and cardiomegaly or evidence of pulmonary venous congestion on the CXR.
- Echocardiography should be performed in all patients with suspected heart failure. The cause of heart failure may be obvious on echocardiography, e.g. if there is evidence of severe aortic or mitral valve disease or where there is a regional wall motion abnormality from a prior myocardial infarction. However, in the majority of cases the echocardiogram confirms systolic dysfunction but does not reveal the cause.

- Further investigation is required to exclude, ischaemic heart disease, thyroid disease and rarer conditions that may present with heart failure.
- Atrial dysrhythmias commonly accompany heart failure and approximately a fifth of patients have atrial fibrillation. Patients with fast atrial arrhythmias may develop a tachycardia-mediated cardiomyopathy that will resolve with restoration of sinus rhythm.
- Where no specific cause for the findings of left ventricular dilatation and systolic dysfunction can be identified, the patient is usually classified as having an idiopathic dilated cardiomyopathy.
- Treatment of heart failure involves a stepwise approach, initially with the introduction of a loop diuretic, ACE inhibition and beta blockade to which spironolactone, digoxin and angiotensin II blocker may be added. In selected cases, cardiac resynchronisation therapy and the implantation of an AICD should be considered.
- Patient education is important in the management of patients with heart failure. The patient should be informed of the importance of the multiple medications that they have to take and the importance of monitoring their weight and fluid intake. They should also be aware of the warning features that may indicate that their heart failure is decompensating, such as ankle oedema, increasing breathlessness and weight gain, and should know when to seek medical advice.

Case 10 — A 72-year-old woman with breathlessness on exertion

A 72-year-old woman is referred by her GP with a 6-month history of breathlessness on exertion – she is now limited to 200 m on the flat. She is usually fit and well with a good exercise tolerance. There is no history of hypertension or diabetes. She does not report angina or a history of coronary disease; however, she remembers being told that she had a heart murmur as a child. A year ago she had a small, left-sided cerebrovascular accident from which she has made a complete recovery. She has a history of recurrent urinary tract infections and has suffered from rheumatoid arthritis since the age of 50 years. She is a life-long non-smoker and does not drink alcohol.

Examination findings in the GP's letter are as follows: pulse 80 bpm, regular; blood pressure 140/80 mmHg; JVP not elevated. Heart sounds normal; apex not felt. Chest auscultation: bibasal inspiratory crepitations. ECG normal.

An echocardiogram has been obtained and is reported as follows:

Left ventricle: non-dilated with normal contractility.
Left atrium non-dilated.
Normal aortic valve.
Normal mitral valve with trivial mitral regurgitation (MR).
Reversed E:A ratio, suggestive of left ventricular diastolic dysfunction.
Atrial septal aneurysm with small left-to-right shunt on colour Doppler.
Normal right heart.
Pulmonary artery pressure not elevated.

The GP has commenced an angiotensin-converter enzyme (ACE) inhibitor and diuretic on the basis that the patient may have heart failure but there has been no improvement in the patient's symptoms. She also takes naproxen 500 mg po tds and methotrexate weekly for her rheumatoid arthritis.

Cardiology: Clinical Cases Uncovered. By T. Betts, J. Dwight and S. Bull. Published 2010 by Blackwell Publishing.

What are the causes of chronic heart failure in the presence of normal left ventricular function?

- Restrictive cardiomyopathy (e.g. amyloid).
- High output failure (e.g. anaemia).
- Pericardial constriction.
- Diastolic heart failure.
- Renal failure.
- Uncontrolled hypertension.
- Arrhythmias (e.g. heart block, fast atrial fibrillation or flutter).

The above causes should be considered in patients with obvious clinical features of heart failure and normal systolic function on echocardiography. If the history and clinical signs are not convincing for heart failure, then an alternative diagnosis should be considered.

What is the significance of the atrial septal defect (ASD) on the echocardiogram in the context of the clinical presentation and how do you explain the absence of any abnormality on auscultation of the heart?

Patients often report murmurs in childhood, which subsequently disappear. Most of these are flow murmurs. Occasionally, the murmur is due to rheumatic heart disease or an atrial or ventricular septal defect. A small ventricular septal defect in childhood produces a loud pansystolic murmur that is know as the *maladie de Roger*; the septal defect usually closes during adolescence and the murmur disappears.

The auscultatory findings for an ASD are dependent upon the size of the defect and the size of the left-to-right shunt. With a large left-to-right shunt, the right ventricular stroke volume increases. There is increased flow through the pulmonary valve producing a pulmonary ejection systolic murmur. The right ventricle takes longer to empty and is no longer affected by changes in filling due to respiration giving rise to a wide fixed splitting of the second heart sound. As a consequence, the right ventricle dilates and the pulmonary artery pressure rises giving rise to pulmonary hypertension. Patients can therefore present with breathlessness and fatigue in their late 60s and 70s.

In this case the ASD is small and there is no evidence of pulmonary hypertension or right ventricular overload on the echocardiogram. The ASD does not therefore account for the breathlessness in this patient. There is an association between ASDs and paradoxical emboli giving rise to stroke (venous thromboembolism passing through the ASD giving rise to stroke). This association is stronger in those patients with an atrial septal aneurysm in combination with the ASD. In a patient of this age, the previous stroke is much more likely to be related to carotid artery disease, cerebrovascular disease or atrial arrhythmias.

What is meant by diastolic dysfunction on the echocardiogram? What evidence is there for diastolic heart failure in this case?

The echocardiogram has reported a reversal of the E:A ratio, suggestive of diastolic left ventricular dysfunction. This indicates that a greater proportion of left ventricular filling is dependent upon atrial contraction. This occurs when the left ventricle is non-compliant or stiff. Up to 50% of cases of heart failure are said to be related to diastolic heart failure, perhaps more correctly referred to as heart failure with normal systolic function. However, there is evidence of diastolic dysfunction on echo in up to 50% of the population over 70 years and this finding alone does not mean that diastolic heart failure is the cause of the patient's breathlessness.

The risk factors for diastolic heart failure are given in Table 10.1. This patient does not give a history of hypertension or coronary disease and there is no evidence of left ventricular hypertrophy on the echo. The incidence

Table 10.1 Risk factors for diastolic dysfunction

Age
Female > male
Reduced ejection fraction
Hypertension
Diabetes
Coronary disease
Myocardial infarction

of diastolic heart failure in the absence of these three factors is <2%. The ECG is normal making a diagnosis of heart failure very unlikely. Significant diastolic dysfunction is usually associated with a dilated left atrium which is not a feature of this case. The diagnosis of diastolic heart failure is therefore not proven in this case.

What further investigations would be appropriate?

- Full blood count (FBC).
- Electrolytes.
- Renal function.
- Thyroid function tests.
- Oximetry.
- Chest X-ray (CXR).
- Brain natriuretic peptide (BNP).

These are routine tests for patients presenting with suspected heart failure. Where there is doubt about the diagnosis and a respiratory cause is suspected, spirometry is useful and available in most GP surgeries and outpatient departments.

The following investigations become available:

FBC: Hb 8.6 g/dL; white cell count (WCC) 11.0 × 10⁹; platelet count 222; MCV: 110 fL; iron, B12 and folate normal; erythrocyte sedimentation rate (ESR) 60; Na 130 nmol/L; K 5.8 mmol/L; Ur 18.0 mmol/L; creatinine 260 μmol/L; albumin 40 g/L. Thyroid function normal. O₂ saturations 93% on room air. BNP 400 pg/mL.

What is the significance of the raised BNP in this patient?

BNP is released in heart failure in response to wall stress on the left ventricle. Its normal function is to promote a salt and water diuresis by the kidney. It has been promoted as a screening test to identify patients with heart failure. Levels of BNP <100 pg/mL effectively rule out the diagnosis, whereas levels >500 pg/mL make the diagnosis very likely. Unfortunately, there are a number of confounders which make the interpretation of BNP results difficult (Table 10.2). In this case the BNP level is not diagnostic and may be elevated as a result of renal impairment.

What are the possible causes of the anaemia in this patient, which is most likely and what further investigations would you perform?

The patient has the picture of the anaemia of chronic disease (the raised MCV is secondary to methotrexate

Table 10.2 Confounders that may increase brain natriuretic peptide (BNP) levels

---

Age
Female sex
Pulmonary disease
Systemic hypertension
Hyperthyroidism
Cushing's syndrome
Glucocorticoid usage
Conn's syndrome
Hepatic cirrhosis with ascites
Renal failure
Paraneoplastic syndrome
Subarachnoid haemorrhage

---

therapy). In the context of this presentation the causes include:

- **Chronic renal disease.**
- **Rheumatoid arthritis.**
- **Heart failure.** The anaemia of heart failure is usually in patients with severe left ventricular dysfunction. The cause is thought to be due to the effects of tumour necrosis factor on the bone marrow. The presence of anaemia due to heart failure is associated with a poor prognosis. Treatment with erythropoietin may be helpful for symptoms and may improve prognosis.
- **ACE inhibition.** ACE inhibition is rarely the sole cause of anaemia in a patient but may exacerbate an anaemia due to other causes. The mechanism is via inhibition of erythropoietin production by the kidney.
- **Haematological malignancy/myelodysplasia.** The raised ESR may indicate a haematological malignancy, e.g. myeloma.

The following further investigations may be appropriate.

- **Plasma protein and urinary electrophoresis.**
- **Erythropoetin** level (depressed in renal disease).
- **Bone marrow** if the erythropoietin level is normal.
- **MSU/urine analysis.**
- **Renal ultrasound.**

The following investigations are performed:
- *Plasma electrophoresis:*
  - ○ *IgG 12.0 g/L (normal 6.0–13.0).*
  - ○ *IgA 2.5 g/L (normal 0.9–3.0).*
  - ○ *IgM 1.0 g/L (normal 0.4–2.5).*
  - ○ *Kappa band.*
- *Bone marrow – normal.*

- *MSU – profuse growth of E. coli.*
  - ○ *Trace of protein and blood.*
  - ○ *Bence Jones protein absent.*
- *Renal ultrasound: bilateral small kidneys with cortical scarring.*

What is the significance of the Kappa paraprotein band in this patient?

This is likely to be a monoclonal gammopathy of unknown significance (MUGA). Even though the patient is anaemic and myeloma can cause renal disease, the diagnosis of myeloma is less likely in the presence of a normal bone marrow and in the absence of suppression of immunoglobulin production and significant proteinuria. The raised erythrocyte sedimentation rate (ESR) is likely to be due to the urinary tract infection. The cause of the renal disease is likely to be recurrent pyelonephritis.

The finding of a paraprotein raises the possibility of amyloid affecting the heart. Amyloid heart disease is one of the causes of a restrictive cardiomyopathy; the characteristic clinical features are as follows:

- Preserved systolic function.
- Severe left ventricular hypertrophy on the echocardiogram with small complexes on the ECG and in the absence of a history of hypertension.
- Dilatation of the left atrium.
- Diastolic left ventricular dysfunction.
- Myocardial speckling or bright echoes, particularly in the septum on echocardiography.

There are no features on ECG or echocardiography to suggest amyloid heart disease in this patient.

The CXR is reported to show diffuse airspace shadowing; there are no pleural effusions and there is no evidence of peribronchial cuffing or upper lobe blood diversion; the heart size is normal.

How would you interpret the CXR findings and what further investigations would you perform?

The major differentials are the causes of interstitial lung disease. The airspace shadowing of fibrosing alveolitis can look similar to pulmonary oedema. The absence of upper lobe blood diversion, pleural effusions and peribronchial cuffing make a diagnosis of pulmonary oedema unlikely. This patient has rheumatoid arthritis and is on methotrexate, both of which can give rise to pulmonary fibrosis.

Other investigations that should be considered include:
- Lung function tests.

- Exercise testing with oximetry.
- High-resolution CT scan of the chest.
- Autoimmune profile.

It is important to remember that lung-function tests are not normal in left ventricular failure; typical findings are of a mild restrictive defect, decreased gas transfer and occasionally an obstructive defect. Exercise testing with oximetry may unmask hypoxia in fibrosing lung disease that may account for the breathlessness in this patient. Antinuclear antibodies (ANA) and IgG are elevated in usual interstitial pneumonitis (UIP).

> *The high-resolution CT is reported as showing diffuse ground-glass shadowing, the distribution of which is unchanged with images taken supine and prone. Lung-function tests report a forced expiratory volume in 1 s (FEV$_1$) of 1.07 L and a forced vital capacity (FVC) of 1.3 L. The carbon monoxide transfer factor corrected for lung volumes is 50% of normal.*

What is the most likely diagnosis?
Rheumatoid lung disease
The lung-function tests demonstrate a restrictive pattern with an FEV$_1$:FVC ratio of 0.85. The reduced carbon monoxide transfer factor is a measure of alveolar diffusion capacity and is markedly reduced (particularly for a non-smoker), consistent with alveolar fibrosis rather than pulmonary oedema. Ground-glass shadowing can be seen in pulmonary oedema but the shadowing redistributes with the patient imaged in the prone position. The diagnosis is therefore fibrosing alveolitis, probably secondary to rheumatoid lung disease.

What changes would you make to the patients medication and why?
Stop ACE inhibitors, non-steroidal anti-inflammatory drugs and diuretics
The combination of these agents is particularly nephrotoxic. There is no longer an indication for diuretic therapy, which has in any case made no difference to the patient's symptoms. Consideration should be given to using an alternative agent to methotrexate, in case the pulmonary fibrosis is related to this agent. If the renal function improves, an ACE inhibitor may be introduced again at a later date for control of hypertension and to preserve the remaining renal function if required.

Should any action be taken regarding the ASD?
Most centres would recommend percutaneous closure of an ASD, particularly if there is a history of stroke where no other aetiology (e.g. carotid disease, atrial fibrillation or hypertension) has been identified. In the young patient, percutaneous closure of the ASD would be recommended. In the elderly, a decision to close an ASD will depend upon the haemodynamic importance of the shunt and the probability that paradoxical embolism (the risk of a clot from the venous circulation embolising through the ASD) is the cause of the stroke. The risk of stroke is higher if the ASD is associated with a septal aneurysm. In view of the patients comorbidities and the risk of the procedure (stroke, dislodgement of the device), an ASD closure may not be appropriate.

CASE REVIEW

This is an increasingly typical case of an elderly patient with multiple comorbidities presenting with breathlessness. This is therefore a rather 'grey case'. Where there are a number of comorbidities, identifying heart failure as the cause can be difficult. Although the presence of normal left ventricular function on the echocardiogram is reassuring, up to 50% of patients with heart failure have normal systolic function. These patients are assumed to have diastolic heart failure. However, the diagnosis of diastolic heart failure is largely by exclusion of other causes. Even where there is evidence of abnormal left ventricular filling indicating diastolic dysfunction on echocardiogram, this does not mean that diastolic heart failure is the cause of the patient's symptoms. The normal ECG and absence of risk factors for diastolic heart failure, such as hypertension or ischaemic heart disease, makes the diagnosis of diastolic heart failure unlikely. The diagnosis may therefore rely largely on excluding alternative causes of breathlessness. In this patient anaemia and rheumatoid lung disease are possible alternative diagnoses. Further investigations reveal that the patient has evidence of pulmonary disease with a restrictive defect on lung-function tests. High-resolution CT confirms the presence of pulmonary fibrosis. The cause of the breathlessness in this patient is therefore not the diastolic dysfunction reported on echocardiography. Treatment with ACE inhibition and high-dose diuretics could have had serious consequences in this patient with renal impairment.

KEY POINTS

- In elderly patients with multiple comorbidities, identifying heart failure as a cause of breathlessness may be difficult.
- An abnormal ECG, left ventricular systolic dysfunction on echocardiography, evidence of heart failure on CXR and a raised BNP may help to confirm the diagnosis.
- Heart failure with normal systolic function on echocardiography may be due to anaemia, diastolic heart failure, arrhythmias, a restrictive cardiomyopathy, pericardial constriction or other causes of fluid overload (e.g. renal failure).
- Diastolic heart failure accounts for 50% of cases of heart failure. The prognosis in diastolic heart failure is the same as for systolic heart failure. Treatment is usually with ACE-inhibition beta blockers and diuretics.
- Amyloid heart disease presents with diastolic heart failure, with evidence of left ventricular hypertrophy on echocardiography in the absence of a history of hypertension, and small voltage complexes on the ECG.
- In the absence of an abnormal ECG, a history of hypertension, diabetes or ischaemic heart disease, diastolic heart failure is unlikely, even where there may be echocardiographic evidence of abnormalities of left ventricular filling.
- Poor cardiac output should not be assumed to be the cause of renal dysfunction in patients with heart disease and should be investigated appropriately.
- Heart failure is one of the causes of a normochromic normocytic anaemia. It is associated with a poor prognosis and may be treated with erythropoietin.
- Pulmonary fibrosis may present with similar clinical features to heart failure (breathlessness, widespread pulmonary crackles, features of right heart failure and a restrictive defect on lung-function testing). The diagnosis of pulmonary fibrosis can be made with high-resolution CT scanning.
- ASDs can be an incidental finding on echocardiography. Patients with a documented ASD should be considered for percutaneous closure if they are haemodynamically significant or if they are felt to be the cause of a stroke due to paradoxical embolism.

Case 11 A 50-year-old man with a murmur

A 50-year-old plumber is referred by his GP following an insurance medical during which a systolic murmur was identified. He was noticed to have a heart murmur when examined for an inguinal hernia repair 10 years previously but has not had any recent follow-up.

What is the differential diagnosis of the systolic murmur?

Systolic murmurs are a very common finding on examination; many are innocent or flow murmurs. Causes are listed in Table 11.1.

What examination findings may be used to characterise the murmur and identify its cause?

- Site – the location of the murmur in relation to the surface anatomy. Usually the point of maximal intensity, some murmurs are heard throughout the precordium.
- Character:
  - Ejection.
  - Pan.
  - Late.
  - Mid.
- Intensity.
- Radiation, e.g. carotids in aortic stenosis and axilla for mitral regurgitation (MR).
- Heart sounds:
  - second heart sound – soft in aortic stenosis (AS).
  - third heart sound – present in MR due to increased ventricular filling in early diastole.
  - fourth heart sound – in AS due to atrial filling of a hypertrophied non-compliant left ventricle.

Cardiology: Clinical Cases Uncovered. By T. Betts, J. Dwight and S. Bull. Published 2010 by Blackwell Publishing.

What other features on clinical examination may help to identify the cause?

- **General inspection** – for features of endocarditis.
- **Pulse**, e.g. slow rising in AS, equality of pulses and strength of femoral pulses in aortic coarctation.
- **Blood pressure**, e.g. reduced pulse pressure in AS, or hypertension with coarctation of the aorta.
- **JVP** – large 'V' waves associated with tricuspid regurgitation (TR).
- **Apex beat** – displaced or hypertrophied.
- **Hepatomegaly** – pulsatile in TR.

The patient does not report any symptoms and is fit and well. Cardiovascular examination: pulse 60 bpm, regular with a normal character; blood pressure 160/70 mmHg. JVP is not elevated. Heart sounds are normal. There is a 4/6 pansystolic murmur heard in all areas and radiating to the axilla. The apex beat is displaced 2 cm laterally. There are no other abnormal findings.

Why is this unlikely to be an innocent murmur?

- The murmur has a wide radiation.
- The apex beat is displaced.

The clinical features that suggest an innocent systolic murmur are shown in Table 11.2. Flow murmurs are usually ejection in character. They are associated with high-output states. Flow murmurs are characterised by the fact that the murmur is localised, does not radiate and is not associated with other abnormalities on the cardiovascular examination. They are not necessarily innocent and can be associated with:

- Anaemia.
- Pregnancy.
- Thyrotoxicosis.
- Sepsis.
- Paget's disease.
- Arteriovenous malformations or fistulae.

Table 11.1 Causes of a systolic murmur

Innocent murmur
Flow murmur
Aortic stenosis (AS)
Mitral regurgitation (MR), including mitral valve prolapse
Tricuspid regurgitation (TR)
Ventricular septal defect (VSD)
Prosthetic aortic valve
Coarctation of the aorta
Hypertrophic obstructive cardiomyopathy
Pulmonary stenosis

Table 11.2 Features of an innocent systolic murmur

Absence of cardiovascular symptoms
Character – usually ejection or mid-systolic
Site – usually left sternal edge or pulmonary area
Radiation – no significant radiation.
Intensity – usually soft
Positional – often
Heart sounds – normal
Added sounds – none
Apex – normal

What is the most likely diagnosis and why?
Mitral regurgitation

The most likely diagnosis is MR. The murmur is pan-systolic, heard throughout the precordium and is associated with cardiomegaly. A ventricular septal defect (VSD) remains a possibility; however, while the murmur of a loud VSD may be heard in all areas it would not radiate to the axilla. Cardiomegaly in the context of a VSD would suggest a large shunt that causes right ventricular enlargement and would be associated with a right ventricular heave.

The most common valvular pathologies associated with a systolic murmur are AS and MR. The features that suggest MR as opposed to AS in this case are:

- A normal character pulse.
- Normal pulse pressure.
- Normal second sound.
- Pan systolic vs ejection systolic.
- Left ventricular dilatation.
- Radiation of the murmur to the axilla.

It is often surprisingly difficult to distinguish between AS and MR. The pulse in severe AS is slow rising; however, it can be normal, particularly in the elderly. The

pulse in MR is usually of good volume and may even have a slight collapsing quality in severe MR.

The murmur of AS is characteristically ejection systolic; however, in severe AS the aortic second sound is quiet and the murmur may be interpreted as pansystolic. The murmur of MR is characteristically pansystolic; however, in mitral valve prolapse the murmur can be limited to late systole and appear more ejection in character. The classical pansystolic murmur starts at the first sound and runs up to, and just beyond, the second sound. Because there is a large pressure gradient between the ventricle and atrium throughout systole the murmur is of constant intensity. The murmur may obscure the second sound at the apex (when the aortic valve shuts there is still a significant pressure in the left ventricle forcing blood though the incompetent valve into the low-pressure left atrium). Confusion is often created by the statement that the second sound cannot be heard in MR since it is obscured by the murmur. The second sound is not lost in MR and while it may be difficult to hear at the apex, it is usually quite distinct over the aortic and pulmonary areas. MR is rarely heard in the carotids; however, a loud murmur of AS can often be heard at the apex and axilla.

In MR the left ventricle is volume overloaded and the apex beat displaced. In AS the ventricle is pressure over-loaded, giving rise to left ventricular hypertrophy. In cases of severe AS the left ventricle may dilate with the onset of left ventricular failure; however, by this time the patient is usually severely symptomatic. Significant left ventricular dilatation in an asymptomatic patient with a systolic murmur therefore points to MR rather than AS.

What further investigations should be performed and what would you expect them to show?
ECG

The ECG in MR is often normal. As the left ventricle dilates, the ECG may demonstrate tall voltages consistent with left ventricular hypertrophy.

CXR

The CXR has largely been superseded by echocardiography but may demonstrate left ventricular and left atrial dilatation. A normal CXR does not exclude haemodynamically significant MR.

Echocardiography (Figure 11.1)

The echocardiographic features that may be seen in MR depend on the aetiology (see Table 11.3) and include:

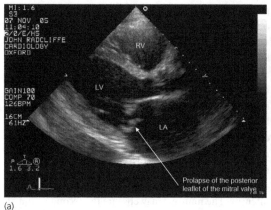
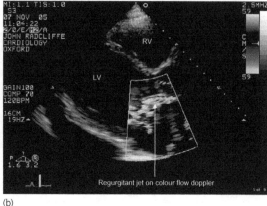

(a)   (b)

Figure 11.1 Echocardiographic findings in mitral regurgitation (MR). (a) Long axis view of mitral valve prolapse. (b) Colour Doppler showing regurgitant jet.

Table 11.3 Aetiology of mitral regurgitation (MR)

Leaflet abnormalities:
- Rheumatic heart disease (usually in conjunction with mitral stenosis)
- Mitral valve prolapse
- Connective tissue disease (Marfan's syndrome, Ehlers–Danlos syndrome, pseudoxanthoma)
- Endocarditis
- Congenital (cleft or parachute valve)

Annulus abnormalities:
- Dilatation (functional MR due to left ventricular dilatation)
- Annular calcification

Abnormalities of the chordae tendinae:
- Endocarditis
- Rheumatic heart disease
- Mitral valve prolapse
- Marfan's syndrome
- Osteogenesis imperfecta

Papillary muscle dysfunction:
- Ischaemia or infarction
- Left ventricle dilatation
- Rheumatic heart disease
- Hypertrophic cardiomyopathy
- Infiltration (sarcoid)
- Myocarditis

- Left ventricular dilatation.
- Left atrial dilatation.
- Structural abnormality of the mitral valve (mitral valve prolapse or rheumatic mitral valve disease, chordal rupture).
- Colour or pulse-wave Doppler evidence of MR.

The ECG is normal.

Echocardiography demonstrates a mildly dilated left ventricle with normal function and normal left atrial dimensions. There is prolapse of the posterior leaflet of the mitral valve with moderate MR.

What is the mechanism of mitral valve prolapse and how should this patient be managed?

In **mitral valve prolapse** the pathology is usually due to redundancy of the valve leaflets and stretching of the chordae. The valve remains competent in the first part systole but the valve leaflets cannot be kept competent when the ventricle reduces in size, since the increased slack on the valve leaflets and chordae cannot be compensated for by papillary muscle contraction. As a result one leaflet bows back into the left atrium and the leaflet tips separate, giving rise to regurgitation and a late systolic murmur. With time, the chordae and valve leaflets stretch further and the valve becomes incompetent throughout systole.

Trivial MR is often reported on an echocardiogram and is not clinically significant in the presence of a structurally normal valve. This level of MR is significant and is associated with a structural abnormality of the valve.

No intervention or drug therapy is required. MR can be tolerated for many years but requires regular follow-up. Antibiotic prophylaxis is currently recommended; however, it is not required in the recently published American Heart Association (AHA) and NICE guidelines. The patient can undertake all levels of exercise but should be advised to report any deterioration in exercise tolerance or symptoms of heart failure. Patients with MR of moderate severity are usually followed up yearly with echocardiography.

Three years later the patient is referred urgently by his GP and reports deterioration in his exercise tolerance over the past 3 months. He now has an exercise tolerance of 300 m on the flat and has noticed mild ankle oedema.

What features on clinical examination would you look for that might indicate an increase in the severity of MR?

- Onset of atrial fibrillation.
- Evidence of heart failure (raised JVP, basal crepitations, ankle oedema).
- Third heart sound.
- Loud pulmonary second sound.
- Left ventricular dilatation.
- Right ventricular heave.

The left atrium dilates early in MR in response to regurgitation of blood in systole. The probability of **atrial fibrillation** increases as the left atrial size increases. The ventricle dilates progressively in response to volume overload. In order to maintain a satisfactory cardiac output the left ventricular stroke volume increases to accommodate the volume of blood regurgitating into the left atrium. A **third sound** is generated as a result of a combination of reduced ventricular compliance in response to dilatation and the increased diastolic left ventricular filling. A persistently high left atrial pressure gives rise to pulmonary hypertension, which is manifest clinically as a loud pulmonary second sound and right ventricular hypertrophy and dilatation.

In acute MR due to ischaemic rupture of a papillary muscle or rupture of the chordae tendinae, these features are not reliable. The left ventricle may not have had time to dilate and may be of normal dimensions on echocardiography. Acute MR is not well tolerated and pulmonary oedema is the predominant feature.

On clinical examination he is in atrial fibrillation at a rate of 100 bpm; blood pressure 140/70 mmHg. JVP is elevated to 10 cm above the sternal angle. The pulmonary second sound is loud. His murmur is unchanged. Auscultation of the chest reveals bibasal crepitations.

His echocardiogram is reported as follows:

Left ventricle dilated – end systolic dimension 4.5 cm, end diastolic dimension 6.6 cm.

Left atrial dilatation – 5.2 cm diameter.
Severe MR on colour Doppler.
Flow reversal in the pulmonary veins.
Ejection fraction – 50%.
Right ventricular function normal.
Elevated peak pulmonary artery pressure – 40 mmHg + JVP.

Why is the patient in heart failure despite a near normal ejection fraction and what is the significance of the elevated pulmonary artery pressure?

In severe MR the ejection fraction is usually greater than normal. This is because the left ventricle is offloading into the left atrium, which is at low pressure (14–16 mmHg), rather than into the aorta, which is at diastolic pressure. The ejection fraction therefore gives a false impression of the left ventricular function. When MR is severe, the pressure rises in the left atrium to the extent that the normal flow of blood into the pulmonary veins is reversed. Chronically elevated left atrial pressures give rise to pulmonary hypertension. (The pulmonary artery pressure is estimated by continuous-wave Doppler using the velocity of the regurgitant jet across the tricuspid valve; the height of the JVP has to be added to the value to give the estimated pulmonary artery pressure.) The presence of an elevated pulmonary artery pressure, dilatation of the left ventricle and onset of atrial fibrillation all support the diagnosis of severe MR with decompensation. The intensity of the murmur is often unhelpful. In acute severe MR, e.g. due to chordal rupture, the murmur may be quiet since the left atrium has not had time to dilate and the regurgitant volume is small.

How would you manage this patient?

The clinical features suggest that the MR is no longer well compensated. The patient therefore requires surgery (Box 11.1). The functional and long-term outcome for surgery in MR is better with valve repair than replacement. A transoesophageal echocardiogram is therefore performed to establish whether the valve is suitable for repair. Prolapse of the posterior leaflet of the mitral valve is easier to repair than prolapse of the anterior leaflet. Rheumatic MR is seldom suitable for mitral valve repair. In all surgery for valvular heart disease the patient will need formal assessment of their dentition and, where necessary, extractions prior to surgery to minimise the risk of subsequent endocarditis.

In the period before surgery the patient should be anticoagulated in view of the risk of thromboembolism, started on digoxin and given diuretics and an ACE inhibitor.

The results of mitral valve repair are excellent. However, once there is echocardiographic evidence of significant left ventricular impairment the long-term prognosis is poor and once the ejection fraction falls below 30%, or there is severe pulmonary hypertension with impaired right ventricular function, the risks of surgery are much higher, emphasising the importance of regular follow-up of these patients.

> *The patient undergoes transoesophageal echocardiography which confirms prolapse of the P2 segment of the posterior segment of the mitral valve that is suitable for surgical mitral valve repair. Following surgery, he is asymptomatic and a repeat echocardiogram demonstrates trivial MR; left ventricular volumes and function have returned to normal.*

> **Box 11.1 Indications for surgery in MR**
>
> - Symptoms (breathlessness, fluid overload).
> - Any deterioration in left ventricular function (ejection fraction <55%).
> - Progressive left ventricular dilatation in the presence of severe MR.
> - Acute MR secondary to ischaemic papillary muscle rupture.

What outcome can be expected?

If MR is treated surgically before there has been a significant deterioration in left ventricular function or severe pulmonary hypertension there is usually an excellent outcome. Left ventricular volumes return to normal and the pulmonary hypertension is completely reversed.

CASE REVIEW

This 50-year-old plumber is referred with a systolic murmur. He is asymptomatic. A clinical diagnosis of MR is made on the basis of the character of the murmur (pan-systolic) and its radiation (axilla). Echocardiography confirms the diagnosis. There is prolapse of the posterior leaflet of the mitral valve with moderate MR. This condition is well tolerated. As his left ventricular function is normal, and he is not symptomatic, he simply requires regular follow-up with echocardiography. Three years later he presents with breathlessness, a reduction in his exercise tolerance and ankle oedema. These features suggest that his MR has become more severe and is now associated with left ventricular failure. Clinical examination reveals an elevated JVP and basal crepitations, confirming the suspected diagnosis from the history. In addition, he has developed atrial fibrillation and features of pulmonary hypertension. These features are confirmed on echocardiography and it is evident that his left ventricular function is now reduced. Surgical intervention is indicated on the basis of symptoms and the development of features of left ventricular impairment and pulmonary hypertension. The echocardiographic features indicate that the valve is suitable for repair; he undergoes successful surgery.

KEY POINTS

- Systolic murmurs are present in 4–5% of patients in the general population. Most are flow murmurs and are not associated with structural heart disease.
- The major differential diagnosis in adults with a systolic murmur is between AS and MR. In MR the murmur extends into the second sound and is of a similar intensity throughout systole (pansystolic). In mitral valve prolapse with mild (late) regurgitation the murmur is late systolic.
- Where it is difficult to distinguish between MR and AS on the auscultatory findings, additional findings on clinical examination such as a displaced apex beat due to ventricular dilatation, the absence of a slow rising pulse and relatively early presence features of pulmonary hypertension in the course of the disease may be helpful in pointing to a diagnosis of MR.
- Causes of MR include mitral valve prolapse, rheumatic heart disease (where there is usually evidence of coexistent MS), ischaemic rupture of a papillary muscle,

and endocarditis. Patients with a severe dilated cardiomyopathy also develop MR as a result of functional regurgitation due to stretching of the mitral valve annulus.
- It is important to monitor all patients with significant MR with regular echocardiography, even if the patient is asymptomatic.
- In MR the ejection fraction may remain normal until late stages of the disease. The valve should be repaired or replaced before significant left ventricular impairment occurs.
- In severe MR the valve should be replaced if the patient is symptomatic (breathlessness, fatigue, right heart failure), if the left ventricular function is below normal (ejection fraction <55%) or if there is significant pulmonary hypertension.
- Mitral valve repair is superior to replacement with a mechanical valve; suitability for mitral valve repair can be assessed with transoesophageal echocardiography.

Case 12 A 30-year-old man with high blood pressure and a heart murmur

A 30-year-old bank executive is referred to outpatients for assessment by his GP. He is known to be hypertensive. On routine follow-up he has been found to have a systolic and diastolic murmur. He is usually very fit and well and on the advice of his GP has recently taken up swimming, which he finds helpful for a long-standing complaint of back pain. He is now swimming up to 30 lengths of the swimming pool twice a week and feels well. The GP has performed some routine bloods including FBC, electrolytes; these are normal. Current medication comprises: amlodipine 5 mg daily; lisinopril 20 mg daily.

What is the differential diagnosis for the auscultatory findings?

The differential diagnosis includes:

- Mixed mitral valve disease.
- Valvular aortic regurgitation (AR).
- Mixed aortic valve disease.
- Patent ductus arteriosus (PDA).
- Ruptured sinus of Valsalva.
- Pericardial friction rub.

In contrast to systolic murmurs, diastolic murmurs are less common and are always pathological. The differential includes a PDA, since the continuous 'machinery' murmur may be mistaken for a systolic and diastolic murmur. A pericardial friction rub may also be interpreted as murmurs in systole and diastole but tends to be more positional and had a scratchy quality that sounds extracardiac.

On auscultation in outpatients an ejection systolic murmur radiating to the carotids is heard. There is an early diastolic murmur heard at the left sternal edge.

What is the differential diagnosis based on these findings and what other clinical signs may help to confirm the diagnosis?

Aortic regurgitation, mixed **aortic valve disease** and a **ruptured sinus of Valsalva** remain on the differential diagnosis.

When listening for the murmur of AR, it is important to lean the patient forward in expiration and listen over the aortic area and left and right sternal edge. The murmur is often localised and quite variable in location; it is a soft-blowing decrescendo murmur heard immediately after the second sound. Since AR is associated with a systolic flow murmur and may accompany aortic stenosis (AS), it is important to listen carefully for an early diastolic murmur in patients with a systolic ejection murmur. Unlike the systolic murmurs of mitral regurgitation (MR) and AS, which are easy to hear but difficult to distinguish, the murmurs of mitral stenosis (MS) and AR are very different but difficult to hear. The murmur of AR is early diastolic and heard best at the left sternal edge with the patient leaning forward in expiration. The murmur of MS is a mid-to-late low-pitched murmur heard at the apex with the patient leaning on the left side.

The sinuses of Valsalva are just above the aortic valve. They can become aneurismal and may rupture into the left ventricle or into the right side of the heart. Rupture into the right side of the heart causes a continuous murmur while rupture into the left ventricle produces clinical features that are identical to AR. The rupture is acute and often associated with pain and the acute onset of shortness of breath.

Aortic regurgitation is often associated with a systolic murmur and need not indicate the presence of AS. In severe AR this is a flow murmur created by the increased stroke volume necessitated by regurgitation of blood through the aortic valve during diastole, which needs to be ejected during the subsequent systole. The clinical

Cardiology: Clinical Cases Uncovered. By T. Betts, J. Dwight and S. Bull. Published 2010 by Blackwell Publishing.

Table 12.1 Eponymous clinical features of aortic regurgitation (AR).

de Musset's sign – head bobbing
Corrigan's pulse – collapsing/waterhammer
Traube's sign – pistol shot femorals
Muller's sign – systolic pulsation of the uvula
Duroziez's sign – systolic murmur over the femoral artery
Quincke's sign – capillary pulsation

signs of AR are associated with a large number of eponyms and are given in Table 12.1.

The following clinical features are helpful in confirming the presence of significant AR:

• Pulse – the pulse in AR is collapsing and large volume.
• Blood pressure – the diastolic pressure is low and there is a large pulse pressure.
• Apex – the ventricle is volume overloaded and dilated, the apex beat is therefore displaced laterally.
• Heart sounds – the second sound is soft in AR there may be a third heart sound due to a volume-overloaded left ventricle.

The following features are present on examination: pulse 70 bpm; blood pressure 200/100 bpm; JVP not elevated; normal aortic second sound; added fourth heart sound; clinically hypertrophied non-dilated left ventricle.

How would you assess clinically the severity of AR in this patient?

The following features indicate severe disease in the context of chronic AR:

• Collapsing pulse.
• Low diastolic blood pressure.
• Length of the diastolic murmur.
• Degree of left ventricular dilatation.
• Clinical features of heart failure, e.g. third heart sound.

With increasing severity the left ventricle dilates to accommodate the blood returning through the aortic valve during diastole. The increased ventricular volume allows for a greater regurgitant volume and therefore the murmur becomes more prolonged. This is not the case in acute regurgitation due to endocarditis or aortic dissection, where the left ventricle has not had time to dilate and therefore the duration of the murmur is purely dependent upon the time taken

to equalise the pressure in the aorta and left ventricle in diastole. If the AR is severe this occurs rapidly and therefore the murmur is short. The fourth sound in this patient is likely to be due to the presence of left ventricular hypertrophy and hypertension. A fourth heart sound is the sound of late ventricular filling associated with atrial contraction; it occurs when the ventricular compliance is reduced either due to hypertrophy or scarring and is therefore always an abnormal finding.

What findings on echocardiography would support the diagnosis of severe AR?

• Left ventricular dilatation
• Premature opening of the aortic valve because of raised left ventricular end diastolic pressure and premature closure of the mitral valve.
• Colour flow Doppler (Box 12.1). The width of the AR jet immediately below the aortic valve and the length of the jet (the extent to which the colour fills the left ventricle) indicate severity (Figure 12.1)
• Diastolic flow reversal in the aortic arch.

Box 12.1 Echo Doppler

Doppler is a technique used to measure the velocity of flow of blood within the cardiac chambers. Doppler uses the reflection of ultrasound by moving red blood cells; the frequency of the reflected ultrasound from the red cells is related to their velocity.

Continuous-wave Doppler is used to measure high velocities but cannot localise the signal. It is particularly useful for assessing the severity of AS. The pressure gradient across the aortic valve can be estimated from the velocity of the jet across the aortic valve using the Bernoulli equation (Pressure gradient = $4V^2$). **Pulsed-wave Doppler** is designed to allow a sample volume to estimate the velocity at a particular location (e.g. at the orifice of the mitral valve) and is useful for detecting low velocity jets. **Colour flow mapping** is a technique whereby the direction and velocity are colour coded. A sample area is placed over the two-dimensional image on echocardiography and the flow can be visualised. Flow away from the transducer is in blue and that towards the transducer is in red (BART convention – Blue Away Red Towards). This is useful for looking at valve regurgitation (see Figure 11.1, p. 114).

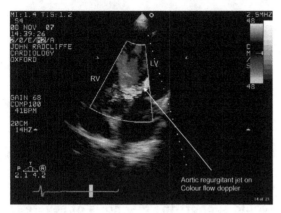

Aortic regurgitant jet on Colour flow doppler

Figure 12.1 Colour flow mapping of aortic valve apical five-chamber view.

An echocardiogram is performed and reported as follows: Suboptimal views:

Left ventricle: non-dilated, severe left ventricular hypertrophy, normal left ventricular systolic function.
Left atrium: mildly dilated at 4.2 cm.
Aortic root: 4.0 cm.
Aortic valve thickened (bicuspid?), aortic peak gradient 20 mmHg, moderate AR.
Normal mitral valve.
Normal right heart.

What are the possible aetiologies for the aortic valve disease in this patient and what other clinical features would you ask for in the history and look for on examination?

Table 12.2 lists the possible aetiologies of AR. Rheumatic aortic valve disease is uncommon in the western world and would be unusual with a normal mitral valve, which is usually also affected. There is no history to suggest

Table 12.2 Aetiology of aortic regurgitation (AR)

Bicuspid/degenerative
Rheumatic fever
Endocarditis
Hypertension
Marfan's syndrome
Aortic dissection
Ankylosing spondylitis
Large vessel vasculitis
Syphilis

aortic dissection. There is no history of malaise or fever to suggest endocarditis. Inflammatory aortic valve disease is a possibility and the history of back pain may suggest ankylosing spondylitis; however, the patient is relatively young for this diagnosis. A history of sexually transmitted disease would point to a diagnosis of syphilitic aortitis and regurgitation but this is now very rare. Marfan's syndrome is an important diagnosis not to miss in the patient with AR, since these patients are at risk of aortic dissection. The patient should be asked about a family history of aortic dissection or Marfan's syndrome and examined for the associated physical findings (see p. 72).

Aortic root dilatation is often seen in AR and is not particularly helpful in identifying the cause. However, the aortic root in Marfan's syndrome is characteristically flask-shaped with the maximal dilatation at the sinuses of Valsalva (i.e. close to the aortic valve).

A high systolic pressure is very common in AR and is due to the increased stroke volume. However, in this case the left ventricle is not dilated and therefore the systolic hypertension cannot be accounted for in this way. The aetiology may simply be a bicuspid aortic valve or hypertension. The combination of a bicuspid aortic valve and hypertension in a young patient should raise the suspicion of a coarctation of the aorta. The patient should be examined for a blood pressure difference between the arms or reduced femoral pulses (brachial to femoral pressure difference >10 mmHg). In coarctation there may be an interscapular murmur from the site of the dissection or a widespread crescendo decrescendo murmur throughout the chest wall from intercostals collaterals.

What further investigations would you perform?

The views in this case are suboptimal and insufficient to exclude a bicuspid aortic valve or coarctation of the aorta. **Transoesophageal echocardiography** will help to identify both lesions. A **CXR** may reveal rib notching or other features consistent with aortic coarctation. MRI is now the investigation of choice to identify the anatomy of aortic coarctation.

The aortic valve is reported as bicuspid on transoesophageal echocardiography and a coarctation of the aorta is reported with a gradient of 50 mmHg. A CXR demonstrates rib notching. A coarctation of the aorta is confirmed on MRI.

What is the usual site of a coarctation and what treatment should be considered?

The CXR in aortic coarctation may demonstrate rib notching due to intercostals, collaterals and dilatation of the ascending aorta with a kink in the descending aorta (reversed 3 sign). The anatomy is best demonstrated with MRI although multislice or spiral CT may be used. In the adult, aortic coarctation is almost always located at the junction of the distal aortic arch and the descending aorta, just below the origin of the left subclavian artery. The gradient across the coarctation is an indication of the severity and a gradient of 20 mmHg is an indication of a significant coarctation. Untreated coarctation leads to death from ischaemic heart disease, heart failure or stroke, usually before the age of 50 years. A total of 85% of patients with coarctation have a bicuspid aortic valve. Coarctation of the aorta is also associated with aneurysms of the circle of Willis and premature coronary artery disease. Treatment can be with intravascular stenting or, more commonly, surgery. The aortic disease is mild there are no indications for aortic valve replacement at this stage.

The patient is treated surgically and makes an excellent recovery. He is started on an angiotensin-converting enzyme (ACE) inhibitor.

What is the purpose of the ACE inhibitor?

There is some evidence that ACE inhibition may slow progression of left ventricular dilatation and heart failure in patients with AR. The evidence for calcium antagonists is more controversial.

The patient is lost to follow-up and is referred 15 years later with breathlessness, ankle swelling and orthopnoea, which have developed over the past month. He is no longer taking an ACE inhibitor.

What complications related to his aortic coarctation may account for his breathlessness?

Patients with aortic coarctation require long-term follow-up. They are susceptible to a number of long-term complications including:
- Persistent hypertension.
- Dilatation and aneurysm formation of the aorta.

- Re-coarctation or residual stenosis at the site of surgery.
- Coronary artery disease.
- AS.
- AR.
- Bacterial endocarditis.
- Rupture of aortic or cerebral aneurysm.

The causes of breathless in this patient could include hypertensive left ventricular disease, the onset of coronary disease or progression of his aortic valve disease, the cause of which may be endocarditis.

What further questions would you ask him?

It is important to exclude endocarditis as a cause of his deterioration. You would ask about:
- Recent dental abscess or dental treatment.
- Fever or night sweats.
- Weight loss, malaise or anorexia.
- Skin rashes.
- Transient neurological events.
- Haematuria.

The patient does not report any clinical symptoms to suggest endocarditis. On examination he looks well. There are no stigmata of endocarditis and he is afebrile.

Pulse is 100 bpm; blood pressure 140/40 mmHg; JVP elevated +5 cm; apex beat displaced 5 cm laterally. There is an aortic systolic murmur, early diastolic murmur at the left sternal edge, and mid- to late-diastolic murmur at the apex.

What is the cause of the mid- to late-diastolic murmur at the apex?

This is an Austin Flint murmur. This murmur is similar to that present in MS. The cause is uncertain but is thought to be due to the vibration of the anterior leaflet of the mitral valve between the regurgitant jet of blood through the aortic valve and blood entering in diastole through the mitral valve.

What further investigations would you perform?
- FBC.
- Electrolytes and liver-function tests.
- C-reactive protein.
- Blood cultures.
- Urine analysis.
- Transoesophageal echocardiogram.

Table 12.3 Indications for surgery in pure aortic regurgitation (AR)

Symptomatic AR
Progressive left ventricular dilatation (>1 cm over 12 months)
Falling ejection fraction
Left ventricular end diastolic dimension >7 cm
Left ventricular systolic dimension >5.5 cm

Even in the absence of other clinical features, endocarditis should be excluded in patients with known valvular disease and recent haemodynamic deterioration. A transoesophageal echocardiogram will help to exclude endocarditis (the views on transthoracic echocardiography will be inadequate) and will also enable the site of the coarctation repair to be assessed.

The results of his blood tests and urine analysis are normal. His echocardiogram is reported as showing severe left ventricular dilatation with severe AR. The ejection fraction is 40%. There is flow reversal in the aortic arch. The ascending aortic arch is dilated at 6.0 cm. At the site of the coarctation repair there is no gradient. There are no vegetations on the aortic valve.

What are the indications for surgical intervention in this patient and what operation should be performed?

The indications for surgery in AR are given in Table 12.3. In this case the presence of symptoms and a severely dilated left ventricle with impaired function are an indication for surgical replacement of the aortic valve. In addition, the aorta has dilated to over 5.5 cm in diameter and should therefore be repaired in its own right. Aortic dilatation is associated with aortic coarctation and also with a bicuspid aortic valve and may present late after surgical correction of either of these lesions. The patient requires a composite aortic valve and root replacement.

CASE REVIEW

This 30-year-old man is referred with hypertension and a diastolic murmur; he is otherwise well. Clinical examination reveals both an ejection systolic and an early diastolic murmur. A transthoracic echocardiogram reveals severe left ventricular hypertrophy, moderate AR and a thickened aortic valve with mild AS. The presence of resistant hypertension in a young patient with coexistent AR raises the possibility of the combination of a coarctation of the aorta and bicuspid aortic valve. This is confirmed on transoesophageal echocardiography. The coarctation is haemodynamically significant, with a gradient across the coarctation of 50 mmHg. The coarctation is repaired surgically. He is lost to follow-up and presents 15 years later with the clinical features of heart failure. The AR is now judged clinically severe on the basis of a collapsing pulse, low diastolic pressure and dilated left ventricle. He has additional features of left ventricular failure. An echocardiogram now reveals severe AR and evidence of decompensation. In addition, the aortic arch is now dilated to 6.0 cm, indicating a significant risk of spontaneous rupture or dissection. The patient requires aortic valve surgery on the basis of symptoms and the echocardiographic findings. The presence of aortic root dilatation means that the surgery should include an aortic root replacement (a composite graft).

KEY POINTS

- Aortic coarctation is a rare but important cause of hypertension in young people. The clinical features include radiofemoral delay and absent foot pulses.
- Aortic coarctation may be associated with a bicuspid aortic valve and AR.
- Untreated, aortic coarctation usually results in death before the age of 50 years.
- Diastolic murmurs are less common than systolic murmurs and are usually due to AR or MS. They are usually quiet and difficult to hear.
- AR produces an early diastolic decrescendo murmur best heard at the left sternal edge with the patient leaning forward.
- The severity of AR can be assessed clinically by the presence of a collapsing pulse, a low diastolic pressure, displacement of the apex beat and the presence of heart failure and a third heart sound.
- Most causes of proximal aortic dilatation may give rise to a functionally regurgitant valve. The majority of cases of AR are secondary to hypertension or are associated with degenerative AS or bicuspid aortic valve disease. In the young hypertensive patient it is important to exclude associated aortic coarctation.
- Acute AR may be due to endocarditis, aortic dissection or a ruptured sinus of Valsalva.
- AR is well tolerated and most patients remain asymptomatic for many years. The exception to this rule is in patients with AR that accompanies AS. This lesion is often poorly tolerated and the patient develops symptoms earlier than those with isolated valve abnormalities.
- The progression of left ventricular dilatation and symptoms may be delayed in patients with pure AR by the introduction of ACE inhibitors and calcium-channel blockers, together with blood pressure control.
- All patients with moderate or severe aortic valve disease should receive follow-up with regular echocardiography. As with all cases of valvular heart disease, the primary indication for replacement of the aortic valve is the presence of symptoms that can be attributable to the valvular disease. Echocardiographic indications for surgery include severe left ventricular dilatation, impairment of left ventricular function or associated severe AS.

Case 13   A 64-year-old man with collapse and a murmur

A 64-year-old man is brought to A&E after collapsing in the street. On arrival he looks well, is alert and orientated with a blood pressure of 105/85 mmHg and a regular pulse of 72 bpm.

What key questions should be asked about the collapse?

- Was there a loss of consciousness?
- Was there any warning or a prodrome?
- What was he doing immediately prior to the collapse?
- Was there incontinence or tongue biting?
- Were there any other associated symptoms (palpitations, chest pain)?
- Did he recover quickly or feel groggy and disorientated?
- Were there any witnesses?
- Has this happened before?

The patient tells you that he had been out shopping and had just started running to catch a bus. He felt breathless and light-headed for a second before collapsing. He lost consciousness for 5–10 seconds before making a very quick recovery. This is the only time he had collapsed, although he has felt dizzy on exertion on a few recent occasions. There was no incontinence or tongue biting and no witnesses have accompanied him.

What are the main differential diagnoses?
Cardiac cause
- Bradyarrhythmias, such as sinus pauses or transient complete heart block. Often called 'Stokes-Adams' attacks, these typically produce sudden, short-lived collapses with no warning and quick recovery, although it is unusual to occur with exertion.

- Tachyarrhythmias, such as atrial fibrillation, supraventricular tachycardia and ventricular tachycardia, may cause collapse at the onset of the tachycardia due to the sudden fall in cardiac output before compensatory peripheral vasoconstriction can occur. Palpitations and additional symptoms are present if the tachycardia persists after consciousness has been regained.
- Low cardiac output due to outflow tract obstruction resulting from aortic valve stenosis or asymmetrical septal hypertrophy (HOCM). This typically occurs during exertion as the obstruction results in a fixed, low cardiac output that cannot increase with exercise. Peripheral resistance falls during exercise due to skeletal muscle vasodilatation and the amount of blood delivered to the brain decreases proportionally.

Neurological cause
- Epileptic seizures are often (but not always) accompanied by tongue biting or incontinence and are usually followed by a post-ictal phase when the patient is groggy and disorientated. An eye-witness account can be particularly useful. They are sometimes preceded by an aura.

Neurocardiogenic cause
- Vasovagal syncope is typically preceded by a prodrome of nausea and sweating and a feeling of faintness that may precede the actual collapse by a few minutes. It is more likely to occur if patients have been standing still for a while and if they are dehydrated, or if they are exposed to noxious stimuli. Typical patients are young women with recurrent events. Patients may feel groggy and be hypotensive for a while afterwards.

What other questions should be asked?
- Are there any cardiac symptoms?
  ○ Any palpitations, chest pains or breathlessness might indicate cardiac disease.

Cardiology: Clinical Cases Uncovered. By T. Betts, J. Dwight and S. Bull. Published 2010 by Blackwell Publishing.

- Are there any neurological symptoms?
  - Headaches, limb weakness, loss of sensations might indicate a neurological space occupying lesion.
- What medication is he on?
  - Antihypertensive treatments may lower blood pressure. Antiarrhythmics may cause bradycardia. Antidepressants and antipsychotics may cause arrhythmias. Diabetic medication may cause hypoglycaemia.
- Is there any family history of collapses, fits or sudden cardiac death?
  - In younger patients, syncope may be a consequence of inherited channelopathies such as long QT syndrome (LQTS).

He tells you that for the last year he has noticed a gradual deterioration in exercise capacity. He now gets quite breathless after walking 50 m and over the last few weeks this has been accompanied by heaviness across his chest. He has no neurological symptoms. He is taking ibuprofen for hip pain. There is no family history of note.

Can you narrow down your differential diagnosis?

The associated symptoms sound cardiac. The exertional breathlessness may be a manifestation of heart failure due to left ventricular dysfunction, valvular heart disease, hypertrophic cardiomyopathy or ischaemia. The chest tightness sounds typical for exertional angina.

What features in the physical examination are important?

In this setting following a collapse, a quick assessment of basic vital signs is always important. As there is likely to be a cardiac cause of his syncope, a detailed cardiac exam is required as well as a basic neurological assessment.

His blood pressure is 105/85 mmHg; radial pulse weak but regular at 78 bpm; O₂ saturations 98% on room air. He is fully alert and orientated. Conjunctiva look pale. Apex beat is not displaced but it is prominent and sustained.

The second heart sound is quiet. There is a loud, rasping ejection systolic murmur, heard best at the right upper sternal edge. The murmur radiates to the carotids.

The lung fields are clear. Abdominal examination is unremarkable. A basic neurological examination is unremarkable

What is the likely diagnosis (or diagnoses) and the mechanism of his syncope?
Aortic stenosis (AS)

His physical examination is consistent with AS. His blood pressure demonstrates a narrow pulse pressure. His radial pulse is low volume. Severe AS typically has a low volume or 'slow-rising' pulse; however, this may not be as obvious in the radial artery, particularly in older individuals. The character of the pulse is best assessed by palpating the carotid pulse. The ejection systolic murmur, loudest in the aortic area that radiates to the carotids, is consistent with the diagnosis.

AS may present with one or more of the triad of exertional breathlessness, exertional chest pain and/or dizzy spells or syncope on exertion.

Angina

The exertional chest heaviness may be entirely the result of AS, or may indicate coexisting coronary artery disease.

The mechanism of his exertional syncope could result from a sudden fall in cerebral perfusion, resulting either from a low cardiac output in the setting of sudden physical activity, or a ventricular arrhythmia resulting from a sudden fall in coronary artery perfusion at the onset of physical activity.

Based on the history and physical examination, is he likely to have mild, moderate or severe AS?

He is likely to have severe AS. He has symptoms (breathlessness, angina and now syncope), a low-volume pulse and narrow pulse pressure. He has a prominent, sustained apex beat, which would suggest there is significant left ventricular hypertrophy (LVH).

Left ventricular hypertrophy causes the ventricular muscle to thicken, which in turn makes the left ventricular cavity smaller. This results in a sustained, strong, heaving apex beat. The apex beat does not move laterally unless left ventricular dilatation occurs. This is not seen until left ventricular function deteriorates, the ventricle thins, weakens and dilates, or it may occur if there is coexisting severe aortic regurgitation.

The loudness of the murmur is not related to the severity of the stenosis.

What simple tests should be requested in A&E?

• ECG – to assess rhythm and look for evidence of conduction disease, previous myocardial infarction, LVH and rare conditions that predispose to arrhythmias and syncope such as LQTS and Wolff-Parkinson-White syndrome.

• Blood tests:

  ○ FBC – anaemia may also cause or exacerbate breathlessness and angina.

  ○ Renal function – abnormal potassium may contribute to arrhythmias.

  ○ Blood glucose – hypoglycaemia may cause collapse. Hyperglycaemia is a risk factor for coronary artery disease.

  ○ Cholesterol – hypercholesterolaemia is a risk factor for ischaemic heart disease.

• CXR – CXR can assess cardiac size (looking for cardiomegaly) and may show calcification on a heavily stenosed aortic valve.

The ECG is shown in Figure 13.1.

The FBC shows Hb 6.9 g/dL; MCV 69 fL; WCC 7.2 × 10⁹/L; platelets 344 × 10⁹/L. Electrolytes and renal function are all within the normal range. CXR shows a cardiothoracic ratio of 0.5, no obvious calcification within the cardiac silhouette, mild upper lobe blood diversion but no interstitial oedema.

How should these results be interpreted?

• ECG findings are consistent with severe AS (LVH and left-axis deviation).

• The FBC shows a microcytic anaemia.

• CXR findings are also consistent with severe AS with LVH but not left ventricle dilatation.

What is the likely cause of his anaemia?

The anaemia is most likely due to chronic blood loss. This is usually from the GI tract. He is on long-standing non-steroidal anti-inflammatory drugs for chronic hip pain and may have duodenal ulceration. Alternatively,

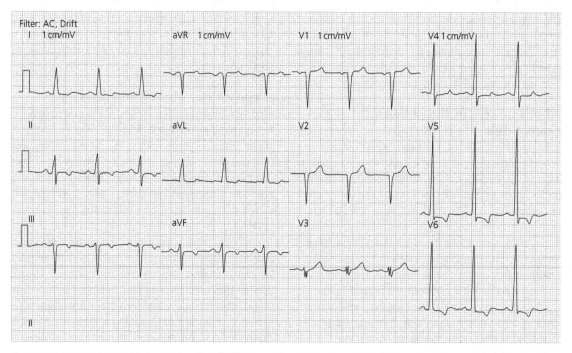

Figure 13.1 A 12-lead ECG with sinus rhythm, left-axis deviation, left ventricular hypertrophy (LVH) and strain pattern. The predominantly positive QRS deflection in lead II and negative deflection in lead aVF indicate that the axis is between 0 and −30°. The sum of the deep S wave in lead V1 and tall R wave in V5 is 53 mm (a total >35 mm indicates LVH). The ST segment depression and inverted T waves in leads V5 and V6 represent a left ventricular strain pattern.

there is an association between AS and angiodysplasia of the lower GI tract that can also lead to chronic blood loss.

The patient is admitted to the medical wards for further assessment. While on bed rest he remains well and symptom free.

What specialist non-invasive test should be performed next?

Echocardiography is the gold-standard test to confirm the diagnosis of valve disease and assess the severity of the lesion (Figure 13.2). Echocardiography will also assess left ventricular function (an important prognostic indicator) and guide subsequent treatment strategies.

The following morning a transthoracic echocardiogram is performed. The report is as follows: there is concentric LVH (left ventricle wall thickness 1.8 cm). Left ventricular systolic function is mildly impaired (estimated ejection fraction 49%).

The aortic valve is bicuspid and calcified with restricted opening. Peak aortic valve gradient is 92 mmHg. Estimated aortic valve area (AVA) is 0.6 cm². There is mild AR. The mitral valve appears structurally normal with trivial mitral regurgitation (MR). The right ventricle is a normal size with normal systolic function. The tricuspid and pulmonary valves function normally.

How would you interpret this report?

The findings are consistent with severe AS (peak valve gradient >64 mmHg, AVA <0.6 cm²) and having already

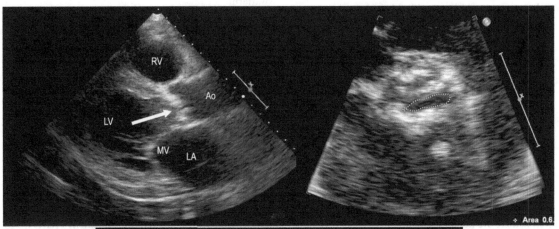

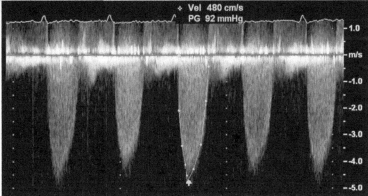

Figure 13.2 Transthoracic echocardiogram images demonstrating severe aortic stenosis (AS). The top left panel is a parasternal long axis view. A bright, thickened, calcified aortic valve with restricted opening is indicated by the arrow. The top right panel is a parasternal short axis view with the aortic valve, appearing as a white, echo-bright circle, shown 'en face'. The image is frozen in systole showing the maximum size of the valve orifice, the area of which has been traced around (dotted lines) and measured as 0.6 cm². The lower panel shows a continuous wave Doppler tracing aimed across the aortic valve which measures the velocity of blood flow. From this the valve gradient (VG) is estimated to be 92 mmHg. Ao, aorta; MV, mitral valve; LV, left ventricle, RV, right ventricle.

resulted in LVH is now beginning to cause left ventricular dysfunction.

A congenitally bicuspid aortic valve often predisposes to AS.

What treatment should be considered?

Drug treatment with diuretics may improve exertional breathlessness. Angiotensin-converting enzyme (ACE) inhibitors and other vasodilators are contraindicated in severe AS but may potentially be prescribed safely for coexisting conditions such as hypertension in patients with mild to moderate AS.

There is no medication that relieves the mechanical obstruction caused by a stenosed aortic valve. Once aortic valve stenosis is severe, affects left ventricular function or causes limiting symptoms, surgical valve replacement should be considered as the treatment of choice.

His anaemia should be treated with a cautious blood transfusion (sudden fluid overload may provoke pulmonary oedema in the setting of AS) and oral iron supplementation.

Should any additional investigations be performed?
Coronary angiography

Prior to considering surgical valve replacement, a coronary angiogram should be performed to look for coexisting coronary artery disease. This should be considered even if there are no angina symptoms as it is preferable to perform coronary artery bypassing for significant coronary artery disease at the same time as the valve replacement if appropriate. If necessary, aortography can be performed to assess aortic regurgitation and the valve may be crossed to measure the 'pull-back' pressure gradient (difference between left ventricular and aortic systolic pressures) although echocardiography has effectively made this redundant.

Upper GI endoscopy and colonoscopy

It is important to identify the cause of anaemia. If there is a GI malignancy, this may affect the prognosis and alter the decision for surgery. If there is a source of bleeding, this needs to be addressed as the aortic valve surgery requires cardiopulmonary bypass, which involves aggressive anticoagulation. A metallic aortic valve prosthesis would require life-long anticoagulation with warfarin.

Should the patient be allowed home for outpatient referral to cardiology or should this be undertaken on this admission?

The onset of symptoms carries a poor prognosis, with there being particular concern if there is syncope, pulmonary oedema or signs of congestive cardiac failure. Once these symptoms have developed, 3-year survival is 30–50%. It is particularly important to act soon if there are signs of left ventricular impairment. As this man has exertional symptoms and now has had syncope, his surgery should ideally be performed within the next 30 days, which would require inpatient referral to cardiology.

CASE REVIEW

This 64-year-old man presented with the typical triad of symptoms resulting from severe AS. He has a congenitally bicuspid aortic valve which predisposes to AS, often presenting in the seventh or eighth decade of life. There is often a long latent period as the calcification and stenosis progresses, leading to left ventricular pressure load and hypertrophy. By the time he developed symptoms he had many of the features of severe AS, including physical, ECG and echo markers of LVH, a low volume, slow rising pulse and a narrow pulse pressure.

Exertional chest pain may be the result of coexisting coronary artery disease, which should always be looked for before contemplating surgery as it is common in this age group. AS is also associated with angiodysplasia and lower GI blood loss. His anaemia may have exacerbated his symptoms and allowed the AS to manifest earlier than it may have done otherwise.

The development of symptoms heralds a poor prognosis. Sometimes asymptomatic patients are discovered (by detection of a heart murmur) and are found to have severe AS. There is some debate over the role of surgical valve replacement for asymptomatic individuals, however the rate of progression of valve disease may be rapid and it is important to operate before left ventricular dysfunction occurs. Further assessment of aortic valve and left ventricular function may be undertaken by looking at ST-segment depression and the blood pressure response to exercise testing.

Surgical valve replacement is the treatment of choice, even in octogenarians. Mortality from aortic valve replacement is <2% in otherwise fit individuals, but rises to 10% or more in the very old or in patients who have developed congestive cardiac failure and impairment of left ventricular function, emphasising the need for early surgery. As he is in his 60s a metallic valve prosthesis would be selected, meaning life-long anticoagulation with warfarin. Patients in their late 70s or early 80s may elect to have a bioprosthetic heart valve that has an expected life span of 10 years but does not require anticoagulation.

KEY POINTS

- Aortic stenosis may be asymptomatic, or cause dyspnoea, chest tightness, dizzy spells or syncope.
- Aortic stenosis typically has a crescendo–decrescendo ejection systolic murmur that is loudest at the upper right sternal edge and radiates to the carotids.
- The loudness of the murmur does not correlate with severity. Physical signs such as a low-volume, slow rising pulse, narrow pulse pressure, heaving, sustained apex beat, and ECG markers of LVH and strain all indicate severe disease.

- The diagnosis is confirmed with echocardiography, which can also determine the aetiology, grade the severity and comment on LVH and systolic function.
- The development of symptoms, deteriorating left ventricular function and/or critical stenosis are all indicators for aortic valve replacement surgery.
- Coronary angiography should be performed prior to surgery.

Case 14   A 34-year-old man with malaise, chest pains and breathlessness

A 34-year-old man brings himself to A&E with chest pains and breathlessness that developed 6 hours earlier. On closer questioning he says he has felt unwell for 3–4 weeks with general lethargy and fatigue and intermittently feeling hot and sweaty. Two weeks ago he had seen an out-of-hours duty doctor who had prescribed him 5 days of antibiotics as he was febrile at the time but he does not think they had much effect.

What are the key questions in the initial history?

- What is the nature of the pain? Where is it, does it radiate, what makes it better or worse?
- Does he have a cough? Is he producing sputum?
- Is he able to lie flat? Does he describe orthopnoea or paroxysmal nocturnal dyspnoea? Has he had ankle swelling?
- Does he have a history of cardiac or respiratory problems? Has he had any recent immobility or foreign travel?
- Has his appetite decreased? Has he lost weight?

It is important to establish whether his principle complaints have a cardiac or respiratory origin and whether there are any other symptoms that it is important to uncover.

He says that the pain is sharp and localised to the left lateral chest wall. It is worse with deep inspiration. He is a heavy smoker and coughs most days – this has not changed recently. He can lie flat without difficulty. His appetite has disappeared recently and he may well have lost weight over the last few weeks. He is unemployed and does not travel. He has no known cardiac or respiratory disease.

Cardiology: Clinical Cases Uncovered. By T. Betts, J. Dwight and S. Bull. Published 2010 by Blackwell Publishing.

On physical examination he is unkempt. There are scratches and marks on both arms. He looks malnourished. His temperature is 37.8 °C; blood pressure 130/50 mmHg; pulse 88 bpm, regular; O_2 saturations on air 95%. His JVP is prominent with a large impulse. Auscultation reveals a pansystolic murmur and an early diastolic murmur at the lower left sternal edge. There is a scratchy 'squeal' that coincides with respiration over the left lateral lung field. His liver edge is palpable and pulsatile and the tip of his spleen is also just palpable. There is no ankle oedema.

What are the most likely differential diagnoses?

- Pneumonia/chest infection.
- Pulmonary embolism.
- Bacterial endocarditis.

His fever is likely to be the result of infection, although rarely it may be the consequence of thromboembolic disease (such as deep vein thrombosis or pulmonary embolism) or autoimmune disease. His respiratory signs are consistent with a pleural rub, which could be the result of infection, inflammation or infarction. The raised JVP with large 'V' wave and pulsatile liver suggest right heart failure or tricuspid regurgitation (TR). The most important finding are the systolic and diastolic heart murmurs – the systolic murmur could be consistent with TR, the early diastolic murmur with aortic regurgitation (AR). It is impossible to know if the murmurs are new; however, they are unusual for a man of this age.

The presence of fever and heart murmurs, particularly with a history of malaise, weight loss and other non-specific symptoms, should always raise the suspicion of bacterial endocarditis, which in this instance is the most likely diagnosis. However, whereas 99% of endocarditis patients have a murmur, 3–15% of patients do not manifest a fever.

Considering the likely diagnosis, what specific questions need to be asked? What features on physical examination should be looked for?

He has already denied any previous known heart disease, although he should be asked if he has ever been diagnosed as having rheumatic fever. He should be asked if he has had any recent dental work or other invasive procedures that may have caused a bacteraemia. It is very important to ask about intravenous drug abuse, as this is becoming a relatively common cause of endocarditis, particularly in young adults.

Peripheral stigmata of infective endocarditis are present in 20% of cases (Table 14.1). Underlying valve aetiology in bacterial endocarditis is shown in Table 14.2.

He admits to being an intravenous drug abuser for at least 4 years. He reuses and shares needles with other drug users. On close examination, there are splinter haemorrhages in his fingernails and toe nails (Figure 14.1). There are petechiae on his anterior chest and abdominal wall and his oral mucosa.

Table 14.1 Peripheral stigmata of endocarditis

Petechiae
Splinter haemorrhages
Osler nodes
Clubbing
Arthritis
Splenomegaly
Roth spots
Janeway lesions

Table 14.2 Underlying valve aetiology in bacterial endocarditis

10–20% of cases are on prosthetic valves
Rheumatic heart disease now underlies only 20% of endocarditis cases

Mitral valve prolapse is present in 30% of young adults with endocarditis

Calcific aortic stenosis is present in 50% of elderly with endocarditis

75% of i.v. drug users with endocarditis have no underlying valve abnormality. In 70% cases the tricuspid valve is infected. In 5–10%, left- and right-sided valves may be simultaneously affected.

What immediate investigations would you request?

- Full blood count (FBC), erythrocyte sedimentation rate (ESR).
- Biochemistry, including C-reactive protein and liver function.
- Blood cultures.
- Urinalysis.
- Chest X-ray (CXR).
- ECG.
- Transthoracic echocardiogram.

The FBC may show a raised white cell count and anaemia of chronic disease. The ESR and C-reactive protein will be raised in >90% cases of endocarditis, although they are not specific. It is important to assess renal function as a glomerulonephritis may be present and subsequent antibiotics (aminoglycosides) may be nephrotoxic. Proteinuria and microscopic haematuria are present in approximately 50% of cases.

Blood cultures are vital to confirm the diagnosis and guide treatment through identification of the organism. Good technique is required and ideally three separate sets should be taken from different sites, a minimum of 1 hour apart, before initiating antibiotic therapy. The cultures can be taken at any time; there is no need to wait until there is a spike in the temperature.

A CXR should be taken due to the presenting symptoms of breathlessness and chest pain.

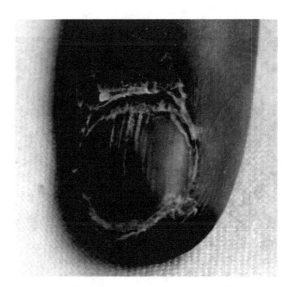

Figure 14.1 Splinter haemorrhages in the nail bed and finger tip.

A 12-lead ECG should be performed to look for evidence of conduction delay.

A transthoracic echocardiogram should be performed to assess cardiac valve structure and function and look for evidence of infection. A vegetation is an oscillating mass attached to a valve and can be seen on transthoracic echocardiography in 60% of native valve endocarditis patients (but only 20% of prosthetic valve patients). A normal transthoracic echo appearance does not exclude endocarditis, in which case a transoesophageal echo should be performed (which has a >90% sensitivity). A transoesophageal echocardiogram may also identify complications such as abscess formation.

The results are: Hb 9.7g/dL; MCV 84 fL; WCC 13.5 10 × 9/L; platelets 146 10 × 9/L; ESR 89mm/hr; C-reactive protein 140mg/L; urea 7.8mmol/L, creatinine 93μmol/L. Microscopic haematuria present on urinalysis.

The ECG shows sinus rhythm at 98bpm, normal axis, PR interval 200ms, QRS 110ms.

CXR shows mild cardiomegaly and a small area of atelectasis in the left lateral lung field with a small left pleural effusion A transthoracic echocardiogram (Figure 14.2) shows a dilated left ventricle with dynamic left ventricular systolic function. There is moderate AR with a thickening of the non-coronary cusp and small (0.3cm) vegetation. The right ventricle is dilated. There is moderate to severe TR and a large tricuspid valve vegetation is seen.

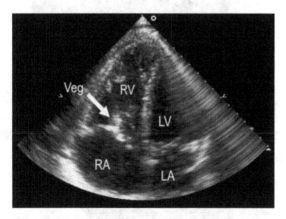

Figure 14.2 Transthoracic echocardiogram showing a large white echolucent tricuspid valve vegetation (arrow). LA, left atrium; LV, left ventricle; RA, right atrium; RV, right ventricle; Veg, vegetation.

What has caused the symptoms of chest pain and breathlessness that led to his presentation? How could this be confirmed?

The most likely cause of sharp 'pleuritic' pain accompanied by breathlessness in someone with tricuspid valve endocarditis is septic pulmonary embolism. The differential diagnosis could be breathlessness due to pulmonary oedema resulting from severe AR; however, this does not fit with the chest symptoms and signs nor the echo assessment of the severity of AR. Left flank pain may result from a splenic abscess rather than pulmonary pathology. Septic pulmonary embolism could be confirmed with a chest CT.

What is the immediate management? What are the likely organisms?

When endocarditis is suspected but the patient is relatively stable and well, initiation of antibiotics may be delayed for 24–48 hours while waiting for the infective organism to be identified from repeated sets of blood cultures. This is particularly important if the patient has been subjected to intermittent antibiotic therapy over the last week. In this way the most appropriate antibiotics can be prescribed. If the patient is very unwell (sepsis, severe valve dysfunction, conduction disturbances, embolic events, etc.), empiric antibiotic therapy may be initiated once a full set of blood cultures has been drawn. Patients should be managed in centres with readily available microbiology expertise, transoesophageal echocardiography and access to cardiovascular surgery; therefore urgent transfer may be indicated. Patients with possible prosthetic valve endocarditis should also be assessed and treated in experienced tertiary referral centres.

The likely organisms are shown in Box 14.1.

In this patient, as he is unwell and has suffered a probable embolic event, antibiotic therapy should be initiated after the three sets of blood cultures are taken. Empiric therapy of native valve endocarditis, before organisms have been identified, is usually recommended as vancomycin 15mg/kg i.v. every 12 hours and gentamicin 1.0mg/kg i.v. every 8 hours. Treatment may be required for 4–6 weeks. Once an organism and its sensitivities have been discovered, antibiotic therapy should be guided by expert microbiology advice.

The patient is started on i.v. vancomycin and gentamicin. A CT, chest and transoesophageal echocardiogram are scheduled for the following day.

Box 14.1 Common infective organisms

- Streptococci are the most common infective organisms, usually the viridians group, *S. pneumoniae, S. pyogenes,* Lancefield group B, C and G and *S. bovis.* Mortality should be around 10%.
- Staphylococci account for 30% of all endocarditis infection, of which 90% are *S. aureus* and 10% are coagulase-negative staphylococci. Infection is particularly severe and often life-threatening. Early appropriate antibiotic treatment is vital. *S. aureus* is the most common infective organism seen in intravenous drug users.
- Enterococci, or which 90% are *E. faecalis*. Antibiotic resistance is common in this group
- Gram-negative organisms account for 10% of infections. They include Enterobacteriaceae, *Pseudomonas* spp. and organisms from the HACEK group (*Haemophilus* spp., *Actinobacillus actinomycetemcomitans, Cardiobacterium hominis, Eikenella corrodens,* and *Kingella kingae*).
- Fungal infection may be seen in the immunocompromised, intravenous drug abusers and patients with indwelling venous lines; 75% are due to *Candida* spp.

In this situation, what are the particular challenges that may need to be overcome during treatment? How should treatment be monitored?

- Intravenous access for administering antibiotics and taking blood samples is notoriously challenging in i.v. drug users. He is likely to require a double-lumen tunnelled ventral venous line (Hickman line) for this purpose.
- Prolonged hospital admission – he may require i.v. vancomycin for 6 weeks if allergic or resistant to penicillin. Sometimes long-term antibiotics may be administered in the community.
- Withdrawal from opiates – as an addict he may start to suffer withdrawal symptoms and need appropriate support. It is vital that he stops injecting drugs to avoid a relapse and repeat infection.
- Risk of blood-borne infection – he is an intravenous drug abuser who has admitted to sharing needles. Any invasive procedure, in particular heart valve replacement surgery, carries potential risk of the operator contracting infections such as HIV or hepatitis C. He should be screened for these as a matter of course.

Treatment may be monitored by assessing his clinical response and laboratory parameters. Simple physical examination of the temperature and severity of the valvular destruction are important. Fever should settle within 5–10 days. Clinical signs of potential complications should be sought (see below). C-reactive protein values usually decrease over the first 7–14 days but may be slightly elevated for 4–6 weeks. Failure of the temperature or C-reactive protein to decrease usually indicates inadequate control of the infection. The ESR is less useful, as it may remain high despite a good therapeutic response. Renal function should be monitored and an ECG performed every few days. If there is a failure to respond to treatment or complications are suspected, echocardiography should be repeated.

What are the potential complications of infective endocarditis? When should surgery be considered?

Complications include:

- **Embolic events.** These occur in 22–43% of patients, the majority being cerebral. They may be more frequent with staphylococcal and enterococcal infections. Emboli usually don not occur until vegetations have reached a certain size and are detectable by echocardiography. Large (>15 mm) and very mobile vegetations may present a greater risk. The high incidence of pulmonary embolism in tricuspid valve endocarditis may be a result of the larger vegetations seen in this setting. The treatment of emboli is antibiotics or surgery, not anticoagulation with warfarin or heparin. There may be a role for aspirin to prevent platelet aggregation on vegetations and subsequent embolisation. Recurrence after embolisation is high. The prognosis of right-sided embolisation is good. If surgery is indicated after cerebral embolism, it is best to perform it within 72 hours of the event and only once cerebral haemorrhage has been excluded.
- **Mitral kissing vegetations.** Large aortic valve vegetations may affect the anterior leaflet of the mitral valve. Early surgery may prevent major damage to the mitral valve.
- **Severe acute MR or AR.** If there is significant destruction of the valve and haemodynamic compromise, urgent surgery is required. Temporary support with inotropes or intra-aortic balloon pumps may be required.
- **Acute renal failure.** This is associated with a poor prognosis, especially in patients with non-staphylococcal endocarditis. Renal failure may result from an immune-complex glomerulonephritis, haemodynamic collapse

Table 14.3 Indications for surgery in infective endocarditis

Acute heart failure

Persistent fever and bacteraemia despite 7–10 days of appropriate antibiotics

Evidence of extension of infection beyond the valve, i.e. abscess formation, complete heart block, etc.

Recurrent emboli despite antibiotic treatment

Obstructive vegetations

Mobile vegetations >10 mm in size

Infection due to organisms with poor response to antibiotic therapy (fungi, *Brucella*, *Coxiella*, etc.)

and shock, antibiotic toxicity, renal infarcts or acquired after cardiac surgery.

- **Conduction damage.** Extension of infection beyond the valve (particularly the aortic valve) into the septum can damage the His bundle, resulting in heart block. Compete heart block may be preceded by gradual PR-interval prolongation, hence the need for regular ECGs. If heart block develops, urgent transoesophageal echocardiography to look for an aortic root abscess is required as immediate surgery is usually warranted.
- **Relapse.** Insufficient length of treatment or suboptimal antibiotics are the usual cause of relapses; however, surgical treatment may be indicated as an alternative to life-long antibiotic treatment.

Prognosis is better if surgery, when indicated (Table 14.3), is performed before major cardiac pathology or haemodynamic deterioration develops.

What is his prognosis?

Prognosis in native valve endocarditis is dependent upon the organism and the time taken to reach a diagnosis. Streptococcal endocarditis, if diagnosed early, is frequently cured by antibiotic treatment. Infection with staphylococci or any organism with a delayed diagnosis has a higher chance of requiring eventual valve surgery and the prognosis will be worse due to the more aggressive or advanced nature of the disease. Overall, approximately 30% of native valve endocarditis patients end up with surgery. Patients with prosthetic valve endocarditis have a worse prognosis than those with native valve

endocarditis. This patient's prognosis will be heavily influenced by his ability to stop injecting intravenous drugs.

What measures are employed to prevent bacterial endocarditis and who should receive them?

All patients who survive the initial infection are at risk of future infections. Good dental hygiene is important and there should be a full dental assessment and appropriate extraction of teeth prior to any valve replacement surgery should be arranged. The use of single-dose antibiotic prophylaxis in all patients with audible murmurs, minor native valve disease and prosthetic valves undergoing dental, upper respiratory and urinary tract procedures has recently been revised by a number of international organisations.

In the UK, NICE guidelines issued in 2008 are that healthcare workers should regard people with the following cardiac conditions as being at risk of developing infective endocarditis:

- Acquired valvular heart disease with stenosis or regurgitation.
- Valve replacement.
- Structural congenital heart disease, including surgically corrected or palliated structural conditions, but excluding isolated atrial septal defect, fully repaired ventricular septal defect or fully repaired patent ductus arteriosus, and closure devices that are judged to be endothelialised.
- Hypertrophic obstructive cardiomyopathy (HOCM).
- Previous infective endocarditis.

These guidelines do not indicate when at-risk patients should receive antibiotic prophylaxis but do state that it should no longer be offered to patients undergoing dental procedures or procedures in the upper and lower GI, genitourinary tract, obstetric procedures, the upper and lower respiratory tract (including ear, nose and throat procedures and bronchoscopy) or childbirth. If a person at risk of infective endocarditis is receiving antimicrobial therapy because they are undergoing a GI or genitourinary procedure at a site where there is a suspected infection, the person should receive an antibiotic that covers organisms that cause infective endocarditis. The North American and European guidelines differ in that they still recommend antibiotic prophylaxis for dental procedures in high-risk patients.

CASE REVIEW

This 34-year-old male intravenous drug user presents with a typical history for endocarditis with weeks of malaise, fatigue and fever. The presence of a murmur, fever and peripheral stigmata of endocarditis facilitated a prompt diagnosis. His blood results were consistent with bacterial endocarditis and the diagnosis was confirmed using echocardiography by the presence of vegetations on the aortic and tricuspid valves with valvular regurgitation. He had additional symptoms and signs of a septic pulmonary embolus, presumably originating from the large tricuspid valve vegetation. The severity of his illness necessitated immediate treatment with broad-spectrum antibiotics after multiple blood cultures were taken. His treatment will include insertion of a Hickman line for frequent blood tests and antibiotic administration and he is likely to require valve replacement surgery, possibly urgently if he deteriorates haemodynamically, has further embolic events or fails to respond to 7–10 days of treatment. His prognosis will be very dependent upon his ability to overcome his drug addiction.

KEY POINTS

- Endocarditis should always be suspected in patients with fever and a heart murmur, particularly if the murmur is new or changing.
- Coexisting symptoms are usually wide ranging and non-specific, e.g. arthralgia, back pain (discitis) and weight loss. There is often a delay in diagnosis until a heart murmur is discovered or a complication such as acute heart failure or cerebral embolism occurs.
- The majority of endocarditis infections happen to native valves rather than prosthetic valves although many infected native valves have underlying disease such as a stenosed biscuspid aortic valve or mitral valve prolapse. The exception to this rule is the increasing number of intravenous drug users who typically get tricuspid valve endocarditis on a previously normal valve.
- Septic pulmonary embolism does not require treatment with anticoagulation; the appropriate treatment is antibiotics.

- Confirming the bacteraemia and identification of the infective organism is vital to the successful diagnosis and treatment of endocarditis. It is very important to take multiple sets of blood cultures before initiating antibiotic therapy, perhaps waiting as long as 24–48 hours, unless the patient is very unwell.
- Treatment is monitored by clinical progress and blood markers such as C-reactive protein.
- Recurrent embolic events from large vegetations, extension of infection beyond the valve and failure to respond to antibiotic therapy are all indications for valve replacement surgery, which happens in 30% of endocarditis cases.
- Guidelines for the use of antibiotic prophylaxis to prevent endocarditis have changed and there remains some debate of their use in the setting of dental work.

Case 15   A 22-year-old woman with faints

A 22-year-old woman comes to see her GP as she has begun to experience fainting episodes.

What are the most important questions to ask when taking a history for blackouts?

- How frequent are they?
  - Most blackouts, particularly in this young group, are very infrequent. Knowing how often they happen will be important when planning diagnostic tests.
- Is there any warning?
  - A lack of warning may carry a more sinister diagnosis. Severe cardiac arrhythmias may happen very suddenly, whereas more benign 'faints' often have a gradual onset or prodrome. Epileptic seizures may be preceded by an aura. Events with no warning are more likely to result in injury.
- Are there any particular triggers or situations that precede the blackouts?
  - Syncope during exercise is worrying as it may represent a mechanical outflow obstruction to the left ventricle or an exercise-induced arrhythmia. Syncope following pain or unpleasant stimuli may be neurally mediated faints. Orthostatic hypotension manifests after standing upright. Syncope after head rotation or neck pressure may be due to carotid sinus hypersensitivity.
- Was there a prompt or gradual recovery?
  - Short-lived arrhythmias usually result in prompt recovery whereas epileptic seizures or hypoglycaemic faints may be followed by periods with reduced conscious levels
- Were there any additional symptoms?

- Rapid palpitations may indicate an arrhythmia. Nausea and sweating may be associated with neurally mediated faints or hypoglycaemia.
- Is there an eye-witness account?
  - Were there seizure-like tonic–clonic movements consistent with epilepsy? Was the patient very pale and cold consistent with low cardiac output?
- Is the patient on any drugs?
  - Drugs such as diuretics and antihypertensives may lead to excessive blood-pressure reduction. Hypoglycaemic medications may lower blood sugar too much. Antiarrhythmic drugs may cause bradycardia. Recreation drug use may also cause arrhythmias or hypotension.

She tells you that she is a strict vegan. She has had four faints over the last 3 months. The first three happened while she was standing and were preceded by 30–60 seconds of nausea. They were not witnessed by anyone else. She was probably unconscious for no more than 2–3 minutes but felt groggy, unwell and drained for the rest of the day. The fourth, most recent, episode was more alarming. She was in a bar, standing talking to friends when she felt very light headed and unwell. As she slumped forward her friends caught her and lowered her into a chair. She was unresponsive and then had seizure-like activity with shaking limbs. They laid her on the floor in the recovery position where she became limp and flaccid before regaining consciousness after 4–5 minutes. Although she felt nauseated and unwell she refused an ambulance and instead arranged this visit.

There is no history of palpitations. In the past she has blacked out on a few occasions as a teenager, once during a vaccination. She has a sister who has also had a couple of blackouts and is currently under investigation. She is not on any medication.

Her physical examination shows she is pale. Her BP is 105/70 mmHg; pulse 60 bpm, slightly irregular; normal heart sounds and a soft systolic murmur at the upper left sternal edge. Respiratory examination is normal.

Cardiology: Clinical Cases Uncovered. By T. Betts, J. Dwight and S. Bull. Published 2010 by Blackwell Publishing.

<table>
<tr><td>

Box 15.1 Definition of syncope

The temporary loss of consciousness (awareness of oneself and surroundings) with spontaneous recovery. Commonly called faints or blackouts.

</td></tr>
</table>

Table 15.1 Life-threatening cardiovascular causes of syncope

Ischaemic heart disease
Cardiomyopathy
Severe valvular heart disease
Pre-excited atrial fibrillation
Long QT syndrome (LQTS)
Brugada syndrome
Catecholaminergic polymorphic ventricular tachycardia

What are the important findings? What are the differential diagnoses?

The relatively frequent blackouts are not obviously situational or caused by any particular stimulus but their severity and in particular the witnessed seizure-like activity are concerning. On the positive side they do not occur during exertion or when sitting or lying (factors that often indicate more worrying pathology). The family history may be of some concern (e.g. an inherited cardiac condition such as long QT syndrome). The 30–60 seconds warning are not typical of an aura but may be considered relatively short for neutrally mediated cardiogenic syncope.

Her physical examination reveals an irregular pulse and a systolic murmur. Underlying structural heart disease is more often associated with life-threatening causes of syncope.

The irregular pulse in a young woman like this could be due to:
• Sinus arrhythmia.
• Ectopic / premature beats.
• Atrial fibrillation.
    The murmur could be:
• An 'innocent' flow murmur.
• Aortic stenosis (AS).
• Left ventricular outflow tract obstruction (e.g. hypertrophic obstructive cardiomyopathy [HOCM], which can be associated with arrhythmias).
• Mitral regurgitation (MR) (most commonly the result of mitral valve prolapse).
• Increased pulmonary flow due to an atrial septal defect (ASD).
• A ventral septal defect (VSD).
    The differential diagnoses are:
• Epilepsy.
• An arrhythmia (tachycardia or bradycardia).
• Left ventricular outflow tract obstruction.
• Neurally mediated syncope (neurocardiogenic syncope, vasovagal syndrome).
• Psychogenic syncope.

Life-threatening cardiovascular causes of syncope are listed in Table 15.1.

What initial investigations should be performed?

• A 12-lead ECG: this will demonstrate the cardiac rhythm and may also show signs of underlying cardiac disease (e.g. left ventricular hypertrophy [LVH] in severe AS or HOCM).
• As she has an audible murmur and symptoms that may have a cardiac origin, an echocardiogram should be performed to look for structural heart disease.

A 12 lead ECG is performed. The results are shown in Figure 15.1.

What does the ECG show?

The 12-lead ECG shows sinus arrhythmia. Although the ventricular rate is not absolutely regular (it speeds up with inspiration and slows with expiration) each QRS complex is preceded by a P wave. There are large QRS complexes across the chest leads, but in a young, slim adult these cannot be used to indicate LVH (see p. 126, Figure 13.1). The corrected QT interval is 0.39 seconds.

Her transthoracic echocardiogram shows a structurally normal heart.

Does this narrow down the differential diagnoses?

The normal ECG makes inherited cardiac conditions such as long QT syndrome extremely unlikely. The normal echo rules out potentially serious conditions such as AS or HOCM. Sinus node and AV node disease are very rare in this age group, especially with a normal

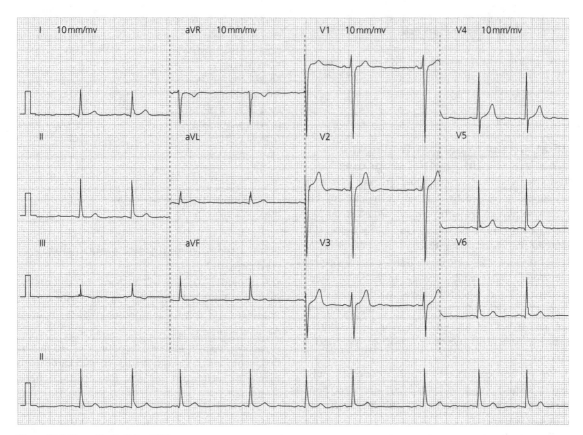

Figure 15.1 The patient's 12-lead ECG.

resting ECG and echo. Supraventricular and ventricular tachycardias remain a small possibility, although there are no symptoms of palpitations.

The most likely diagnoses, in descending order, are now:

- Neurally mediated syncope.
- Psychogenic syncope.
- An arrhythmia.
- Epilepsy.

Does the seizure-like activity make epilepsy the most likely diagnosis?

The seizure-like activity during the fourth blackout does not automatically indicate epilepsy. It may result from cerebral hypoxia due to lack of blood flow. It is important to note that during the fourth blackout she was held upright by her friends. If she was very hypotensive (resulting from an arrhythmia or profound vasodilatation), falling flat to the ground is a protective mechanism that allows gravity to distribute blood to the head.

Holding someone upright during a faint or arrhythmia exacerbates cerebral hypoperfusion.

What tests should be done next?
Cardiac monitoring

The frequency of events means a 24- or 48-hour Holter monitor is unlikely to be helpful. As her syncope occurs quite quickly, a 7- or 14-day loop recorder with a memory that can be activated after the event would be the most helpful.

An FBC

She has a soft systolic murmur and normal echocardiogram, suggesting a flow murmur. She is pale and is a vegan. She may be anaemic, resulting in a hyperdynamic circulation and the flow murmur.

Tilt table test (Figure 15.2)

This test is used to diagnose neutrally mediated syncope (vasovagal syndrome). The patient is secured to a table

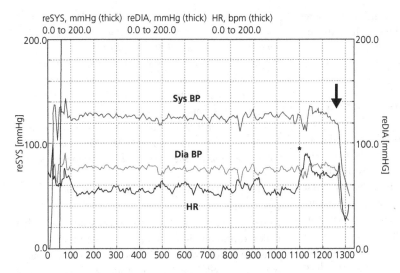

reSYS, mmHg (thick)   reDIA, mmHg (thick)   HR, bpm (thick)
0.0 to 200.0   0.0 to 200.0   0.0 to 200.0

Figure 15.2 Head-up tilt table test. Continuous non-invasive monitoring of the systolic (Sys BP) and diastolic (Dia BP) blood pressures and heart rate (HR) are depicted over a 22-minute period. After 18 minutes the vasovagal reflex begins with an increase in heart rate in an attempt to maintain the blood pressure, which begins to fall gradually (*). Two minutes later there is a dramatic fall in blood pressure to 50/30 mmHg in association with sudden reflex bradycardia of 30 bpm (arrow), resulting in syncope. The patient is quickly returned to the horizontal position.

with a footplate that is reclined back to an angle of 60–80 degrees (head up). There is constant ECG monitoring and either constant or very frequent non-invasive blood-pressure monitoring. The patient is left in that position for up to 45 minutes. In a positive result, there is a dramatic fall in blood pressure that may be accompanied by sinus tachycardia or profound bradycardia. This is accompanied by the usual symptoms of nausea, dizziness and possibly syncope. Laying the table flat allows for a quick recovery. The test is has a sensitivity of approximately 75% and a specificity of 90%.

Should she be referred to a neurologist?

Some rapid-access syncope clinics are staffed by a cardiologist and a neurologist to give a combined opinion. However, the low likelihood of epilepsy in this case should mean that a neurology referral need only occur if an arrhythmia is convincingly ruled out (normal sinus rhythm on a monitor during seizure-like activity) and a there is a negative tilt table test.

She has a loop recorder for 7 days. She has no blackouts but activates it on one occasion when she feels light headed and faint for a short time. The recording shows sinus tachycardia at 105 bpm then sinus bradycardia at 50 bpm.

The tilt table test is performed. After 18 minutes in the upright position she feels sweaty, clammy and nauseated and develops palpitations. Her heart rate increases from 60 to 90 bpm while her blood pressure hovers around 135/85 bpm. Shortly afterwards her pulse and blood

pressure drop dramatically to 60/30 mmHg and 30 bpm and she loses consciousness and starts to shake. The table is returned to the horizontal position and she quickly regains consciousness, although she continues to feel nauseated and clammy. Her blood pressure and pulse gradually increase back to baseline levels over the next 10 minutes, although she feels unwell for the next hour.

What do these results mean? What is the diagnosis?

The positive tilt table test with a recreation of symptoms with a profound fall in blood pressure diagnoses neutrally mediated syncope. Initially there was vasodilatation, causing a fall in blood pressure, reflex sinus tachycardia and the prodrome symptoms. The cardioinhibitory component then kicked in with profound bradycardia and hypotension, resulting in syncope. The Holter monitor recording probably represent a milder episode where syncope did not occur after the prodrome as the cardioinhibitory component did not occur.

The presence of syncope and seizure-like activity leads some authorities to classify this as 'malignant vasovagal syndrome'. The degree of cardioinhibition and bradycardia varies between patients. In many, the principle component is vasodilatation and there may not be any bradycardia but rather just a lack of reflex tachycardia. These patients are less likely to suffer syncope and just experience a long prodrome with nausea, seating, pallor, dizziness and malaise. A similar, overlapping condition is postural orthostatic tachycardia syndrome where there is profound compensatory sinus tachycardia in response to the vasodilatation which helps prevent a major drop in blood pressure but causes symptoms of rapid palpitations

What are the initial treatment options?
Lifestyle changes

The most important action is to keep well hydrated at all times. This means drinking a lot more fluids than most people are used to, i.e. 500 ml every 4 hours, starting on waking and carrying on through during the day (even more on hot days). Avoid potential diuretics such as caffeine and alcohol. Urine should be clear and the patient should never feel thirsty. Increase salt intake. Exercise to improve venous return through leg muscle action. Sometimes lower limb compression stockings to reduce venous pooling are advised. Avoid stimuli that provoke attacks and if a prodrome starts take immediate action by lying flat.

Medications

No medications have consistently been shown to be more effective than placebo in properly conducted randomised trials. Probably the most effective is the vasoconstrictor midodrine (an alpha agonist). Beta blockers are commonly prescribed (to suppress the sympathetic arm of the reflex) but are usually ineffective. Other drugs are fludrocortisone (a mineralocorticoid that retains salt and raises blood pressure) or SSRIs such as Seroxat®. In extremely severe cases, blood volume expanders such as erythropoietin have been tried.

She asks if this condition is life threatening and should she avoid any activities such as driving. What should you tell her?

This condition is common and is not life threatening. Rarely the 'malignant' form, with syncope after little warning, can result in injury due to falling, so it is important to recognise the prodrome and take evasive or preventative action. In the UK, driving is allowed without restriction if the 'three Ps' are present, i.e. a prodrome, posture (it is unlikely to occur during sitting or lying) and there is provocation (pain, fright, dehydration). She does not have all three Ps as there is no obvious provocative element. Also, it is recurrent, occurring more than once every 6 months. However, it is a benign condition and she otherwise has a healthy heart, so she has to wait 4 weeks after a blackout before being able to drive.

She starts increasing her fluid and salt intake but continues to suffer pre-syncope once a month and syncope every 2–3 months. She subsequently tries a beta blocker, but feels extremely fatigued and lethargic on a low dose. She then tries fludrocortisone but it caused a headache and dizziness. Seroxat® was ineffective. Midodrine possibly reduced the frequency of the attacks but also caused a headache. She returns for further advice and treatment. Her main worry is the syncope, which frightens her and her friends, particularly if she has a seizure. She also wants to be able to drive again.

Is there anything else that can be offered?

In severe cases of malignant vasovagal syndrome with a major cardioinhibitory component (manifest as sinus arrest and pauses of >5 seconds) a permanent pacemaker may be offered. The most appropriate pacemaker is a dual chamber device with atrial and ventricular leads to overcome simultaneous sinus arrest and AV nodal block. A pacemaker will overcome the bradycardia component but have little impact on the vasodilatory component. Some pacemakers have specific algorithms that initiate rapid atrial and ventricular pacing when they detect rapid or sudden drops in heart rate in an attempt to try and keep the blood pressure up and prevent the worse symptoms. A pacemaker in this woman may prevent syncope from occurring although she is likely to continue to experience her prodrome and feel unwell, nauseated and light-headed during attacks as well as potentially experiencing palpitations during rapid pacing. The down-side of a pacemaker is the life-long need for generator changes and the risk of infection or lead failure. A summary of treatment options is given in Table 15.2.

Table 15.2 Summary of treatment options for neurocardiogenic syncope

High-volume fluid intake
Exercise training
Tilt training
Increase salt intake
Support stockings
Beta blockers, e.g. metoprolol
Mineralocorticoids, e.g. fludrocortisone
Alpha agonists, e.g. midodrine
Selective serotonin reuptake inhibitors, e.g. Seroxat®
Plasma volume expanders, e.g. erythropoetin
Dual-chamber pacemaker

CASE REVIEW

This 22-year-old woman presented with fainting episodes, one of which was associated with seizure-like activity. The seizure was the result of prolonged cerebral hypoperfusion when she was kept in an upright position during her hypotensive faint. The key features in her history that indicate a neurocardiogenic cause included the presence of a prodrome and their situational and postural nature. Her audible flow murmur, the result of anaemia secondary to a vegan diet, rightly prompted a full cardiovascular assess-ment as many cardiac causes of syncope carry a poor prognosis unless identified and treated. Provocative testing with a tilt table test recreated the symptoms and demonstrated mixed bradycardia and vasodilatory components. Treatment is often challenging and she failed to respond well to hydration, beta blockers and mineralocorticoids. A pacemaker could potentially attenuate symptoms, preventing syncope, by addressing the cardioinhibitory component.

KEY POINTS

- Syncope accounts for 1 in 30 visits to A&E. In patients with underlying heart disease, syncope may be associated with a high rate of recurrence and a poor prognosis. The purpose of investigations is therefore to assess whether the person is at increased risk of sudden death by looking for the presence of cardiac disease.
- The most common cause in the general population is the 'simple faint', i.e. neurocardiogenic syncope (vasovagal syndrome). The recurrent nature, prodrome and associated 'autonomic' symptoms and appearance (nausea, pallor, etc.) are typical of neurocardiogenic syncope.
- The normal ECG and echocardiogram also point to a benign cause.

- Seizure-like activity is uncommon but can happen with cardiovascular causes due to transient cerebral anoxia. This may lead to a misdiagnosis of epilepsy.
- A positive tilt table test not only confirms the diagnosis but also guides treatment as it indicates the role of the vasomotor and cardioinhibitory components. Neurocardiogenic syncope is treated in most instances by prevention through life-style changes. Good hydration is the cornerstone of treatment. Drug therapy has limited success. Rarely, pacemakers are used to treat severe cardioinhibitory responses that cause frequent syncope and seizures.
- In patients who present with syncope it is important to give recommendations regarding driving. In the UK the Driver and Vehicle Licensing Agency (DVLA) produce a guide on medical standards of fitness to drive.

Case 16   A 76-year-old woman with blackouts

A 76-year-old woman is referred urgently to the Cardiology clinic. She had a myocardial infarction 4 years earlier, percutaneous coronary intervention with a stent for angina 12 months earlier and has had two blackouts in the last month, 3 weeks apart.

What are the key questions in the initial history?

• In what setting did the blackouts occur? Were they exertional or at rest? Were they postural?

• Was there a prodrome or was there no warning?

• What was she like on recovery? Groggy or alert?

• Were there any associated symptoms, e.g. palpitations?

• Does she have any other symptoms, e.g. angina, breathlessness, dizzy spells, etc.?

• Are there any witnesses who can describe the attack?

• Was there any tongue-biting or incontinence to suggest a seizure?

She tells you that on one occasion she was gardening and trying to lift a heavy plant pot and on the other occasion she was carrying shopping from her car into the house. She had no warning and suddenly found herself on the ground. She was alert on recovery. There was no seizure-like activity. There were no other associated symptoms. She does have exertional breathlessness although she can manage 400 m on the flat and a single flight of stairs. She has not had angina since her coronary stent 12 months earlier. Occasionally, she feels light-headed if she stands up too quickly. She is currently taking aspirin, a beta blocker, an angiotensin-converting ezyme (ACE) inhibitor, a loop diuretic and a statin.

Her physical examination reveals blood pressure 130/55 mmHg; resting pulse 55 bpm, regular, normal

volume. The JVP is raised by 2 cm, her apex beat is displaced to the lateral clavicular line, sixth intercostal space and there is a systolic murmur heard all over the precordium and in the carotids. The lung fields are clear and there is mild pitting oedema at the level of her shins.*

What are the differential diagnoses?

• **A bradycardia.** 'Stokes-Adams' attacks are the result of ventricular standstill during intermittent complete heart block. They typically occur with no warning, are short-lived and have a prompt recovery with the return of AV-node conduction. Sinus pauses or sinus arrest can result in similar symptoms. Patients typically appear very pale at the onset and then flushed on recovery. Long episodes of asystole may result in seizure-like activity due to cerebral hypoxia. The elderly are more prone to conduction disease, particularly if there is a history of ischaemic or other heart disease. Bradycardia may be made worse by medications such as beta blockers, verapamil, diltiazem and antiarrhythmic drugs.

• **A tachycardia.** Ventricular tachycardia may cause syncope, particularly if it is very rapid, occurs in the upright position or during exertion. Syncope tends to occur at the onset before compensatory vasoconstriction can occur, therefore there may not be any associated awareness of palpitations. Ventricular tachycardia is usually (although not always) associated with structural heart disease, particularly myocardial infarction. It may be sustained (in which case if the patient does not suffer a cardiac arrest they recover consciousness and develop immediate symptoms such as palpitations, breathlessness, chest pain and shock) or non-sustained (in which case they regain consciousness within a few seconds with the return to sinus rhythm).

• **Aortic stenosis (AS).** She has a systolic murmur that radiates to the carotids and has exertional syncope, features consistent with severe AS. However, the reasonable exercise capacity, normal pulse character and the lack of a narrow pulse pressure argue against this.

Cardiology: Clinical Cases Uncovered. By T. Betts, J. Dwight and S. Bull. Published 2010 by Blackwell Publishing.

• **Orthostatic hypotension.** Postural drops in blood pressure are particular common in the elderly and those taking antihypertensive or heart failure medications. The clue is usually the sudden move to an upright, standing position preceding the collapse and often there is a short prodrome. Lying and standing blood pressures should be performed.

Her description is typical of a cardiovascular cause rather than a neurological cause. In patients with known heart disease a cardiac cause should always be sought first, as syncope in this group carries a worse prognosis and a high likelihood of recurrence, necessitating prompt diagnosis and treatment.

Witness accounts to syncopal episodes are extremely useful as patients often have poor recollection of the event. Features such as pallor, flushing, twitching or seizure-like activity, impaired consciousness before or after the event are all helpful in making a diagnosis and some witnesses may even feel and record a pulse.

KEY POINT

Syncope accounts for 11% of A&E visits and up to 6% of acute hospital admissions. Around 10% of all syncope cases have a cardiac cause – such cases have an increased mortality risk. Syncope in patients with NYHA class III or IV heart failure is associated with a 1-year mortality of 45%.

What are the appropriate immediate investigations?

The following tests should all be performed during the consultation

• **12-lead ECG.** Perform to look for signs of old or recent myocardial infarction, left ventricular hypertrophy and strain and evidence of conduction disease (bundle branch block, heart block, sinus pauses or bradycardia).

• **Chest X-ray (CXR).** Look for cardiomegaly and pulmonary congestion (signs of heart failure and left ventricular failure) and heavy calcification of the aortic valve (suggesting significant aortic stenosis)

• **Echocardiogram.** This is an important test as the risk of this being due to a life-threatening arrhythmia are directly related to left ventricular function. It will also reliably report on aortic valve function.

• **Lying and standing blood pressure** to assess for orthostatic hypotension.

• **Carotid sinus massage.** This is a test for carotid sinus hypersensitivity, which is an abnormally strong bradycardia reflex that results in sinus pauses, sometimes complete heart block and a fall in blood pressure with stimulation in the neck region. Carotid sinus massage is performed by massaging the carotid pulse for 5 seconds with the patient in a supine position, recording the ECG and blood pressure. A positive result is a 3-second pause or 50 mmHg drop in blood pressure. Care should be taken if there is a carotid bruit and massage should probably not be performed.

What does her ECG show?

The 12-lead ECG (Figure 15.1) shows sinus bradycardia at 54 bpm. There are anterior Q waves with poor R-wave progression across the chest leads consistent with her old anterior myocardial infarction. There is left-axis deviation. The PR interval is prolonged (0.24 seconds) indicating first degree heart block. The QRS of 120 ms is at the upper limit of normal, although the morphology suggests incomplete left bundle branch block (LBBB).

A CXR shows mild cardiomegaly (cardiothoracic ratio [CTR] 0.54), some upper lobe blood diversion and minor calcification in the aortic valve region.

The transthoracic echocardiogram shows a dilated left ventricle. The anterior wall and septum are thin and akinetic (i.e. do not contract), consistent with an extensive old anteroseptal myocardial infarction. The left ventricular ejection fraction is estimated as 27% (severely impaired). The aortic valve is calcified but opens well. The peak gradient is 20 mmHg with an estimated valve area of 1.6 cm². There is moderate central mitral regurgitation (MR).

Lying and standing blood pressures showed only a mild drop in systolic pressure (135 mmHg to 125 mmHg) immediately after and 3 minutes after standing.

Carotid sinus massage did not result in any significant pauses.

How do these tests impact on the differential diagnoses? Do further tests need to be performed or can appropriate therapy be given?

• The ECG confirms the prior myocardial infarction. The first-degree heart block and left-axis deviation are relatively common findings in this situation and do not necessarily suggest a bradycardia cause although they do increase the likelihood.

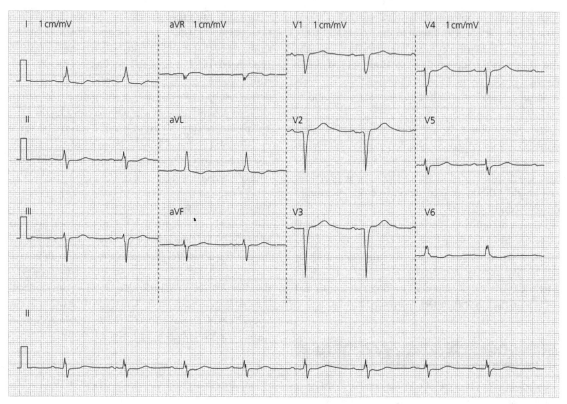

Figure 16.1 The patient's 12-lead ECG.

- The echocardiogram rules out severe AS and identifies significant left ventricular scarring and dysfunction. This increases the likelihood of a ventricular arrhythmia being the cause.
- The likely differential diagnoses now rest between intermittent complete heart block or ventricular tachycardia.

If the country and health service in which this is taking place follows American and European Cardiovascular Society guidelines, the patient satisfies the criteria for a primary prevention implantable cardioverter defibrillator (ICD). The Multicenter Automatic Defibrillator Implantation Trial 2 (MADIT 2) trial showed a survival benefit in patients with ischaemic heart disease and left ventricular ejection fraction (LVEF) <30% who were given a prophylactic ICD by preventing sudden cardiac death from ventricular arrhythmias. ICDs also provide bradycardia pacing therapy, so both the potential diagnoses would be addressed.

However, in the UK primary prevention ICDs are only approved for patients with ischaemic heart disease, LVEF <30% and a QRS duration >120 ms, which this woman does not have. Further evidence of ventricular arrhyth-

mias is required before an ICD is indicated. It is therefore important to try and correlate rhythm with symptoms (which requires a further episode of syncope) or perform provocative or diagnostic tests that strengthen a particular diagnosis. Empirical implantation of a pacemaker would not protect her from ventricular arrhythmias and increasing antiarrhythmic drug therapy could worsen bradycardia.

What tests should be performed next?

Correlation of rhythm with symptoms:

- **24- or 48-hour Holter monitor.** This is unlikely to record another syncopal episode as her attacks are infrequent. However, it may demonstrate asymptomatic intermittent heart block or non-sustained ventricular tachycardia.
- **7-day event monitor.** Patient-activated recorders in this situation would be unhelpful unless the recorder has a memory loop so that activation after the event documents the rhythm at the time of collapse.
- **Implantable loop recorder.** This is the most useful method, but also the most invasive and expensive.

The concern with prolonged recording is that the next attack may be fatal and an opportunity to prevent this has been missed. An alternative strategy is provocative testing.

• **Exercise testing.** Both her events occurred with physical exertion, albeit mild. A carefully supervised treadmill test (now that AS has been excluded) may provoke a further event and may also reveal critical ischaemia (despite the lack of angina symptoms). The risk is that the treadmill provokes an attack with syncope that causes collapse with subsequent injury.

• **Electrophysiological study (ventricular stimulation study).** This is an invasive study performed in a cardiac catheterisation laboratory. Under sedation a pacing wire is inserted into the right ventricle via a femoral vein. The ventricle is paced at a constant rate and additional paced premature beats are added at progressively shorter intervals to try and provoke ventricular tachycardia. It is a moderately sensitive and specific test, particularly if sustained monomorphic ventricular tachycardia is induced. It is less specific if ventricular fibrillation is induced. It is also more sensitive and specific in ischaemic heart disease compared with non-ischaemic cardiomyopathies. During the same procedure, AV node and His bundle conduction can also be assessed; however, this is not very sensitive or specific for heart block as a cause of syncope.

How urgently should further testing be performed?

There remains concern about the urgency to obtain a diagnosis. There have been two events in the past month already and the likely diagnosis is an arrhythmia. The patient should be offered immediate hospital admission for telemetry and subsequent provocative testing with an electrophysiological study. At the very least, these should be organised as urgent outpatient and day-case investigations. As the patient has no exertional symptoms consistent with angina (whereas her previous coronary stent was inserted for exertional angina) it is unlikely that there is significant myocardial ischaemia precipitating her syncopal attacks. Repeat coronary angiography is not mandatory; however, as she is being scheduled to have an invasive catheter laboratory procedure it may be prudent to image the coronary arteries at the same time, just in case there is a critical coronary AS that should be treated

to try and reduce the frequency or consequences of subsequent events.

The patient refuses immediate hospital admission but agrees to have a 24-hour Holter monitor attached and is scheduled for an elective day-case electrophysiological study the following week.

What additional advice should be given?

She should be told to call an ambulance and be brought straight to hospital if she has a further syncopal episode. She should be told not to drive her car until a diagnosis has been reached and appropriate treatment given.

She returns the Holter monitor 2 days later. There is not significant bradycardia (no pauses >3 seconds). There is infrequent ventricular ectopy and one asymptomatic four-beat salvo of non-sustained ventricular tachycardia.

She attends for her invasive electrophysiology study 5 days later. Coronary angiography demonstrates a chronically occluded LAD artery (present at the time of her stent insertion and the cause of her myocardial infarction) and a patent stent in her RCA. AV node and His bundle conduction is within normal limits. Programmed ventricular stimulation is then performed (Figure 16.2), inducing monomorphic ventricular tachycardia at 200bpm with loss of consciousness and is promptly cardioverted with a single external 150J biphasic shock.

What is the most appropriate treatment and is there any additional adjunctive treatment that could be offered?

The presence of inducible haemodynamically compromising sustained monomorphic ventricular tachycardia in a patient with syncope of unknown origin, ischaemic heart disease and poor left ventricular function is a class I indication for ICD implantation. Even if she had not suffered syncope as a presenting complaint, she would now satisfy primary prevention criteria as she has ischaemic heart disease, LVEF <35%, non-sustained ventricular tachycardia on a Holter and inducible VT with programmed stimulation (entry criteria for the original MADIT trial and an indication recognised by American, European and UK guidelines). ICDs (Box 16.1) are superior to standard drug treatment and amiodarone treatment at preventing sudden cardiac death in these patients.

ICDs treat ventricular arrhythmias after they occur, but do not stop them from happening in the first place.

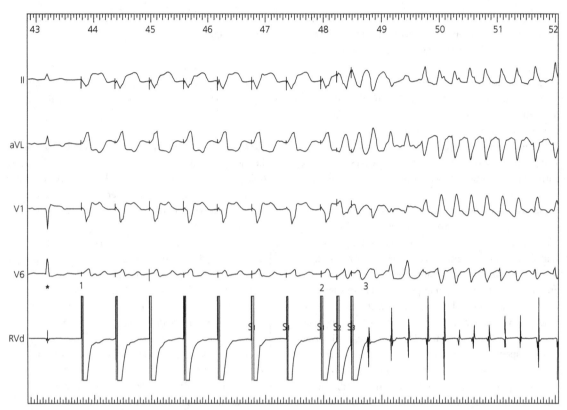

Figure 16.2 VT stimulation study showing induction of ventricular tachycardia. Four ECG leads are shown (II, aVL, V1 and V6) and the electrogram from the bipolar catheter placed in the right ventricular apex (RVd). The tracing shows a single beat of sinus rhythm (*) followed by eight paced beats (1) and two extra stimuli (paced premature beats, 2), which initiate ventricular tachycardia (3).

Box 16.1 Implantable cardioverter defibrillators (ICDs)

ICDs can be inserted under local anaesthesia. They consist of a generator (or 'can') that is implanted subcutaneously above the pectoralis muscle. One or two leads then enter the subclavian vein and are attached to the inside of the right ventricle (and right atrium if a dual-chamber device), which allows the device to monitor the heart rate. They are typically programmed to act if the ventricle exceeds a programmed heart rate, e.g. 180 bpm. When this happens there may be a choice of therapies delivered, depending upon the rate. Antitachycardia (overdrive) pacing is painless and terminates ventricular tachycardia in 75–80% of events. It is ineffective for polymorphic ventricular tachycardia or ventricular fibrillation. Shock therapy (typically 35 J) is painful but

terminates ventricular tachycardia and ventricular fibrillation in over 97% of events. If the first treatment is unsuccessful, the device recognises this and has further attempts often using more aggressive treatments. Occasionally, the ventricular rate may exceed the programmed detection rate due to sinus tachycardia or atrial arrhythmias (e.g. atrial fibrillation). The ICD will try to discriminate between a ventricular tachycardia and supraventricular tachycardia but if in doubt will administer a shock inappropriately rather than withhold treatment for a potentially life-threatening ventricular arrhythmia. ICD battery life lasts for 4–6 years, after which the generator needs to be changed. There are also small risks of lead fracture or device infection.

There remains a role for beta blockers and amiodarone therapy to try and reduce the frequency of device therapies. All patients should take beta blockers; however, the benefits of amiodarone need to be weighed up against the potential risks (thyroid dysfunction, photosensitivity, pulmonary and hepatic toxicity and peripheral neuropathy).

What lifestyle issues need to be addressed in ICD recipients?

Most patients can continue to lead active and fulfilling lives. The UK DVLA imposes driving restrictions (e.g. no driving for 1 month after primary prevention ICD or 6 months after secondary prevention ICD implant, or for 6 months after appropriate shock therapy from an ICD). Patients need to avoid strong electromagnetic fields, but cellular phones and microwave ovens do not present any problems if used sensibly. Patients can travel and pass through airports but should declare their device to avoid going through large metal detectors. If a patient receives a shock therapy while in contact with another individual there is no danger to that other person. Following a shock, patients usually make a prompt recovery. As treatments occur within 10–12 seconds of the arrhythmia onset, many may not have been aware of the tachycardia preceding the therapy. Patients require regular follow-up, usually at device clinics on a 6-month basis.

CASE REVIEW

This 76-year-old woman with a known history of ischaemic heart disease and prior myocardial infarction was referred after suffering two episodes of syncope. Both blackouts had worrying features, such as a lack of prodrome and occurrence during exertion, that make arrhythmias a likely cause. The physical examination and echocardiogram demonstrated poor left ventricular function resulting from her old myocardial infarction and excluded significant valvular heart disease. The potential severity of her symptoms necessitated prompt investigation using coronary angiography and provocative testing with a ventricular stimulation study. The finding of easily-inducible haemodynamically-compromising ventricular tachycardia led to insertion of an implantable cardioverter defibrillator.

KEY POINTS

- Syncope in a patient known to have heart disease should always be viewed with concern. Cardiac causes carry a worse prognosis.
- Usually the key to getting a diagnosis is to correlate rhythm with symptoms using Holter recordings or loop recorders; however, high-risk cardiac patient require urgent specialist referral.
- Secondary prevention with a defibrillator is advised in all heart failure patients who present with successful resuscitation from a cardiac arrest or haemodynamically-compromising ventricular tachycardia

as there is a high chance of a recurrent event and no antiarrhythmic drugs have been shown to improve prognosis.
- No test has been shown to be an ideal predictor of sudden death. Perhaps the best risk-stratifier is left ventricular function and a history of myocardial infarction. The MADIT II trial showed that an ICD reduces total mortality by a third (20% to 14%) during an average follow up of 20 months.
- ICDs treat ventricular arrhythmias after they occur, but do not stop them from happening in the first place.

Reference

Moss AJ *et al*. Multicenter Automatic Defibrillator Implantation Trial 2 (MADIT 2). *New Eng J Med* 2002; **346**: 877–83.

Case 17   A 35-year-old woman with palpitations

A 35-year-old woman attends her local medical centre with a 3-month history of an intermittent unpleasant sensation in her chest.

What key questions should be asked?
• What is the nature of the chest sensation? Is it a pain or discomfort (if so, what are its characteristics), or an awareness of her heart beat?
• Where in the chest is it and does it spread/radiate?
• Are the palpitations fast or slow, sustained or intermittent, regular or chaotic?
• Do they have a gradual or sudden onset and offset?

The patient describes intermittent pounding, which often feels like her heart beat is missing or skipping a beat. This can be accompanied by sudden, very short-lived 'lurches' in her chest. Sometimes she wakes at night and thinks her heart beat is quite chaotic and irregular, although not particularly fast.

What are the key characteristics of the main differential diagnoses?
It is now apparent that by 'chest discomfort' she means an unpleasant rhythm sensation rather than chest pain or tightness. Therefore an arrhythmia is the most likely diagnosis.

Sinus rhythm and increased heart beat awareness
Although most people have no perception of their resting heart beat, some patients have increased heart-beat awareness and can feel normal sinus rhythm. Underlying anxiety or depressive symptoms are frequently associated. The palpitations are usually regular, less than 100 bpm at rest and patients can accurately tap out their heart rate. Sinus tachycardia (>100 bpm) associated with stress and anxiety often has a gradual onset and offset with subtle variations in rate.

Intermittent heart block/bradycardia
Rarely, conduction defects such as Mobitz type I Wenckebach (in which there are intermittent non-conducted P waves and ventricular pauses) may be felt as slow palpitations.

Atrial or ventricular ectopic beats
Ectopic beats are premature atrial or ventricular contractions (extrasystoles) that occur earlier than the next sinus beat should occur. As they occur prematurely the ectopic beat is often weak and hard to detect as the ventricles have not had time to fill properly. There is then a compensatory pause before the next sinus beat, during which the ventricles over-fill, thus causing the sensation of a missed then heavy heart beat. They usually happen as single events, although occasionally alternate with normal sinus beats (bigeminy) (Box 17.1). They are more frequently felt at rest and at night, probably because the heart rate is slower (creating a longer window of opportunity) and there are fewer distractions. They typically disappear during physical exertion.

> **Box 17.1 Frequently used terms**
>
> • Bigeminy – paired complexes, ventricular premature contraction (VPC) alternating with a normal beat.
> • Trigeminy – VPC occurring every third beat (two sinus beats followed by VPC).
> • Quadrigeminy – VPC occurring every fourth beat (following three normal beats).
> • Couplet – two consecutive VPCs.
> • Non-sustained VT – three or more consecutive VPCs (<30 seconds).

Cardiology: Clinical Cases Uncovered. By T. Betts, J. Dwight and S. Bull. Published 2010 by Blackwell Publishing.

Atrial fibrillation

The hallmark of atrial fibrillation is a chaotic 'irregularly irregular' heart rate. Many patients with atrial fibrillation do not experience palpitations. Those who do typically have faster ventricular rates (i.e. rapid and irregular). If paroxysmal, the palpitations will have a sudden onset and offset. There are usually no obvious precipitating factors although sometimes paroxysms are exercise-induced (sympathetic/catecholaminergic) or occur after food or at night (vagal)

Supraventricular tachycardia (SVT)

SVTs cause very rapid, regular palpitations, often too fast for a patient to count, which have a sudden onset and offset. They can be accompanied by chest pain, breathlessness, dizziness and sometimes syncope.

Ventricular tachycardia

Ventricular tachycardia is rapid and regular with a sudden onset and offset. It can be accompanied by chest pain, breathlessness, dizziness and sometimes syncope or cardiac arrest. It is most commonly associated with structural heart disease, particularly ischaemic cardiomyopathy. There are rarer forms of 'benign' ventricular tachycardia occurring in structurally normal hearts that are brought on during exercise or stress.

KEY POINT

It is always important to understand what a patient means by palpitations. The true definition is 'an unpleasant awareness of the heart beat' and does not necessarily mean that the heart beat is rapid (tachycardia).

What is the best way to ask a patient to describe the nature of their palpitations?

A useful technique is to ask the patient to tap out their palpitations to give an indication of speed and regularity. Alternatively, tap out a variety of rhythms (ectopics, atrial fibrillation with a rapid ventricular rate, a regular SVT) and see which the patient feels is most similar to their sensations.

The patient taps out a rhythm that is part regular and part irregular at a rate of around 60–70 bpm. The description of 'missed' and 'skipped' beats and their irregular nature fit more with ectopics or atrial fibrillation and make SVT or ventricular tachycardia very unlikely.

What other questions should be asked?

- Are there any provoking factors?
- Does anything help them go away?
- Do the palpitations occur at any particular time of day?
- Does she have any other cardiac symptoms?
- Is there a family history of heart disease?

Provoking factors may be useful to help identify the cause and also indicate risk. Exercise-induced palpitations and arrhythmias may cause more concern. Caffeine and alcohol may provoke ectopics or atrial fibrillation. 'Vagal' manoeuvres may terminate SVTs. Benign ectopics are more frequently noticed at rest or at night and may disappear with exertion. Chest pain, breathlessness and syncope may indicate underlying structural heart disease, which in turn makes a serious arrhythmia more likely. Inherited arrhythmia syndromes (such as LQTS or Brugada syndrome) usually result in syncope or sudden death, rather than palpitations.

She gets symptoms most days. She notices them more frequently in the evening and particularly when trying to go to sleep or lying on her left-hand side. She is in the process of changing jobs and feels quite stressed at present. She drinks a bottle of wine every night and often more at weekends. She has cut out coffee as she found that the palpitations were worse after this. Her exercise capacity is not impaired. She has not had syncope. There is no family history of note. Her physical examination is unremarkable. She has a regular pulse of 72 bpm, blood pressure of 110/65 mmHg and no murmurs.

Are any immediate investigations required?

12-lead ECG

A 12-lead ECG should be performed to look for evidence of underlying heart disease (Q waves from previous myocardial infarctions, left ventricular hypertrophy, conduction abnormalities, etc.). As a 12-lead ECG only records 12 seconds of heart rhythm it is extremely unlikely to offer a diagnosis unless the patient is experiencing symptoms at the time or is in a permanent abnormal rhythm.

Echocardiogram

The ready availability of echocardiography and its non-invasive nature means that there is often a very low threshold for requesting this investigation. The principle role is to look for structural heart disease although not only is it unusual to find this in patients presenting with palpitations, it is rare to find an abnormal echo in the setting of a normal physical examination and 12-lead ECG. For patients with atrial fibrillation, the decision to anticoagulate is made on clinical risk factors and is not normally influenced by echo findings. In many instances, the main benefit of an echocardiogram is the ability to tell the patient they have a structurally normal heart and offer reassurance.

Exercise test

A treadmill test is only indicated if the symptoms are brought on by physical exertion, or there are separate exertional symptoms, such as dyspnoea or chest pain. In this particular example a treadmill is not indicated.

Blood tests

The most important blood test to perform is thyroid function as thyrotoxicosis may manifest as sinus tachycardia, feelings of stress and anxiety and sometimes atrial fibrillation. Electrolyte abnormalities (potassium, calcium and magnesium) should also be looked for.

Her 12-lead ECG shows sinus arrhythmia with no other abnormalities. Sinus arrhythmia is a common finding in younger individuals at rest, particularly those who exercise regularly. It is due to changes in autonomic vagal tone during inspiration and expiration causing slowing and quickening of the sinus rate. Her echocardiogram reveals a structurally normal heart. In this particular example a treadmill is not indicated. Thyroid function is normal.

What additional investigation is the most appropriate?

The key to a diagnosis is to correlate her symptoms with her rhythm. This is best done with an appropriate form of prolonged cardiac monitoring (Table 17.1). Options include the folllowing.

12-lead ECG during symptoms

Patients who have sustained symptoms lasting more than an hour or so should be encouraged to attend their GP or local A&E for a 12-lead ECG during the next episode. A 12-lead ECG during symptoms is the gold standard diagnostic test.

24-hour Holter monitor

This is simple to perform. It is attached using three or four electrodes and worn continuously over a 24-hour period. It records every heart beat, thus detects symptomatic and asymptomatic rhythm disturbances. Patients

Table 17.1 Appropriate use of different types of cardiac monitor

Frequency	Symptoms	Recorder
Daily – at least once a week	Palpitations or syncope	24-hour Holter
Weekly – monthly	Palpitations lasting hours at a time	12-lead ECG at A&E or GP surgery
Weekly – monthly	Short-lived palpitations	Patient-operated event monitor Transtelephonic monitor Loop recorder
Weekly – monthly	Syncope	Loop recorder
Monthly – 2–3 x per year	Syncope (or rapid palpitations too short lived for 12-lead ECG)	Implantable loop recorder (Reveal)

record a diary, thus rhythm can be correlated with symptoms. It is ideal for symptoms that occur on a daily basis but is usually unhelpful for symptoms that occur less than once week. Only 5% of all Holter recordings reveal a diagnosis.

Event recorder

These are used over a 7–30 day period. They are attached using two or three electrodes but can be removed during baths or showers or other activities. When symptoms are experienced, a button is pressed and a recording is made. More sophisticated devices (loop recorders) have a constantly updated internal memory that record and remember the rhythm 1–3 minutes before the time the button was pressed and 3–5 minutes after it was pressed. Some even have automated recording if the heart rate goes above or below preset limits. Multiple recordings can be made. Transtelephonic event monitors allow the rhythm to be transmitted over a phone line. These event recorders are suitable for symptoms that occur once every few weeks.

Implantable loop recorder (Reveal)

These are small devices that are implanted subcutaneously and perform continuous ECG monitoring, recording a continuous loop. When activated they store rhythm 1–3 minutes before and 3–5 minutes after the episode. They may be activated manually by using a handset, which the patient carries with them, or automatically if the heart rate drops below or exceeds preset limits. Battery life is usually 15–18 months. They are idea for infrequent symptoms that are concerning (i.e. syncope).

The most appropriate test for this woman is a 24-hour Holter monitor as she is experiencing symptoms on a daily basis. This is duly performed and according to her diary card she experienced symptoms at 23:00 hours.

What does the Holter monitor recording show? (Figure 17.1)

The Holter monitor shows sinus rhythm with atrial and ventricular ectopic beats. The ectopic beats are premature, causing the heart beat to come sooner than expected. There is then a corresponding pause before sinus rhythm resumes at the expected point in time. Atrial ectopic beats cause premature P waves, which are subsequently conducted through the AV node and bundle branches. The QRS complexes are therefore usually narrow, unless they are so premature that there is transient bundle branch block. Ventricular ectopics originate in ventricular myocardium outside of the normal conducting system and produce wide QRS complexes.

What should you tell the patient regarding the diagnosis, prognosis and treatment?

The correlation of ectopic beats with her typical symptoms confirms the diagnosis. The fact that she is otherwise healthy and active without limitation, has a normal physical examination, ECG and echocardiogram means that these are benign ectopics and the prognosis is good. They are extremely common (>50% of healthy medical students have atrial ectopy and 12–20% have ventricular ectopy on Holter monitoring). Ectopics typically come and go in patches and may be more noticeable at times of stress or anxiety. Many people are asymptomatic; however, those with increased heart beat awareness may suffer considerable symptoms. Reassurance that the heart is normal and the condition is benign and often self limiting can offer great comfort. Reducing stress, caffeine and alcohol may facilitate improvement.

It is unusual to need to prescribe medications. Often the side-effects outweigh the benefits and medications may not successfully suppress the ectopy. Although there is little evidence to support their use, beta blockers are sometimes prescribed.

PART 2: CASES

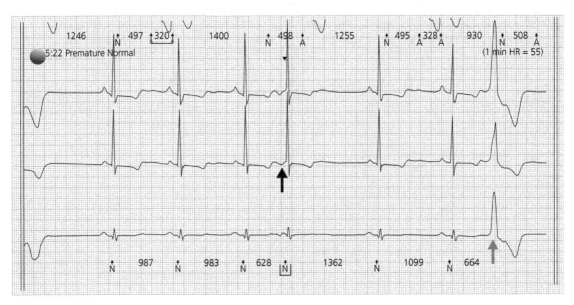

Figure 17.1 A Holter recording demonstrating both an atrial premature beat with an inverted P wave (black arrow) and narrow QRS complex and also a wide complex ventricular premature beat (grey arrow).

CASE REVIEW

This 35-year-old, healthy woman presents with a history of palpitations, which on close questioning are not rapid, but rather an awareness of 'missed' and 'extra' beats. Her symptoms had appeared in the setting of stressful life events with an increased alcohol and caffeine intake. A resting 12-lead ECG showed sinus arrhythmia (a normal variant) and a transthoracic echocardiogram revealed a structurally-normal heart, putting her in a good prognostic group. The diagnosis of benign ectopy was confirmed by performing a 24-hour Holter monitor and correlating her rhythm with her symptoms. No specific treatment, other than reassurance and life-style modification, was required.

KEY POINTS

- The most common form of abnormal heart rhythm is ectopic beats (also called premature beats or extrasystoles).
- Care needs to be taken when asking questions to make sure the patient's understanding of 'palpitations' is the same as the physician's, i.e. it is an unpleasant awareness of the heart beat and not necessarily rapid.
- Ectopic beats typically occur mainly at or at night, are associated with stress and caffeine and are described as 'missed' or 'skipped' beats.
- Atrial and ventricular ectopics in younger patients with structurally normal hearts have a normal prognosis and should be considered benign. Ectopics in older patients with structural heart disease may indicate an unfavourable prognosis, e.g. >10 ventricular ectopics per hour after myocardial infarction is associated with an increased risk of sudden cardiac death.
- The key to getting a definitive diagnosis is correlation of rhythm with symptoms. It is vital that the correct for of ambulatory monitoring is used, which is often determined by the frequency of symptoms.
- In patients with structurally normal hearts, it is symptoms that need addressing rather than the absolute number of benign ectopics, and in patients with abnormal hearts there is no evidence that suppression of ectopics with drugs improves prognosis.
- In a structurally normal heart, reassurance is often all that is required and symptoms settle spontaneously. Rarely, beta blockers can be tried. In extreme examples (a very high burden and severe symptoms), radiofrequency ablation of the ectopic focus can be performed.

A 42-year-old man with palpitations

A 42-year-old man who is a keen triathlete is brought to his local A&E. He had just returned home from a 10-km training run when he suddenly became aware of breathlessness, rapid palpitations and felt light headed. His wife brought him to the A&E but during the car journey he began to feel better.

His initial assessment shows a resting pulse of 48 bpm, which is irregular. His blood pressure is 110/65 mmH; O₂ saturations are 98% on air and he is comfortable and well perfused.

What are the key questions in the initial history?

- In which order did his symptoms appear?
- Was it a sudden or gradual onset?
- Was it a sudden or gradual offset?
- Has he ever had this before?

It is important to establish cause and effect, i.e. did rapid palpitations lead to dizziness and breathlessness, or did it start with breathlessness and gradually palpitations appeared?

He was resting and doing some stretches 5–10 minutes after finishing his run. He suddenly became aware of rapid, irregular palpitations and immediately felt light headed. As the dizziness improved over the next minute he began to feel breathless and unwell. This persisted for 10 minutes and he and his wife became concerned enough to bring him to A&E. Ten minutes into the car journey he noticed that his palpitations had disappeared, which coincided with him feeling better and he was no longer breathless. This has never happened before.

He is otherwise healthy with no significant past medical history. As part of a 'well-man' check 12 months earlier he had a fasting total cholesterol measured at 6.5 mmol/L. His father had coronary artery bypass grafting at the age of 48 years, following a myocardial infarction. His father had been a heavy smoker and it was in reaction to his father's surgery that he had taken up regular sports including triathlons, a low-fat diet and he has never smoked.

A 12-lead ECG shows sinus arrhythmia. A routine CXR is normal. Basic blood tests (FBC, biochemistry, troponin) are also normal

What are the differential diagnoses?

- Sinus tachycardia.
- A paroxysmal arrhythmia:
  - SVT.
  - Atrial fibrillation.
  - Ventricular tachycardia.
- ACS.
- Acute respiratory compromise:
  - Pulmonary embolism.
  - Pneumothorax.

From the history, the sudden onset and cessation of rapid palpitations followed by dizziness and breathlessness make a paroxysmal arrhythmia the most likely diagnosis. The fact that they were described as irregular makes atrial fibrillation the most likely arrhythmia. Sinus tachycardia is usually a response to other pathology and typically is regular and has a gradual onset and offset.

The lack of chest pain makes an acute coronary syndrome (ACS) unlikely and the family history and hypercholesterolaemia risk factors are counterbalanced by his healthy life style and young age. The normal ECG is reassuring. The rapid improvement in symptoms and normal physical findings and investigations effectively rule out pulmonary embolism or pneumothorax.

Cardiology: Clinical Cases Uncovered. By T. Betts, J. Dwight and S. Bull. Published 2010 by Blackwell Publishing.

He is discharged from A&E without a clear diagnosis. As it was a single, self-limiting episode and there were no other worrying findings, the A&E doctors decided not to instigate any treatments or outpatient investigations.

Two weeks later he has a similar episode, which wakes him from sleep and lasts 5 minutes. As it stops spontaneously he does not seek medical attention. One month later he has a further episode immediately after a large evening meal. He waits 20 minutes but as it did not stop spontaneously he is brought to A&E again. On arrival, he describes rapid, irregular palpitations, feels light-headed, breathless and has chest discomfort that feels like a tight band. He is alert and orientated. His blood pressure is 95/70 mmHg; pulse 130–140 irregular; lung fields clear; O_2 saturations 99% on room air.

What does the 12-lead ECG show?

The 12-lead ECG (Figure 18.1) shows atrial fibrillation with a rapid ventricular response of approximately 150 bpm.

What treatment options are there and which would you choose and why?

The treatment options are:

- Do nothing.
- Urgent external DC cardioversion.
- Pharmacological cardioversion.
- Pharmacological rate control.

His previous episodes have both stopped spontaneously after a short time and 40–50% of presentations to A&E with new-onset atrial fibrillation stop within 24 hours of onset. If he had minimal symptoms it would be reasonable to wait a short while; however, he is very symptomatic so something needs to be done. NICE guidelines for the rhythm-control management of paroxysmal atrial fibrillation are shown in Figure 18.2.

External DC cardioversion is an option. If he was severely compromised then it would be the treatment of choice; however, he appears stable with reasonable blood pressure and perfusion and no pulmonary oedema. He does however have mild chest tightness. DC cardioversion would require general anaesthesia and as he has just

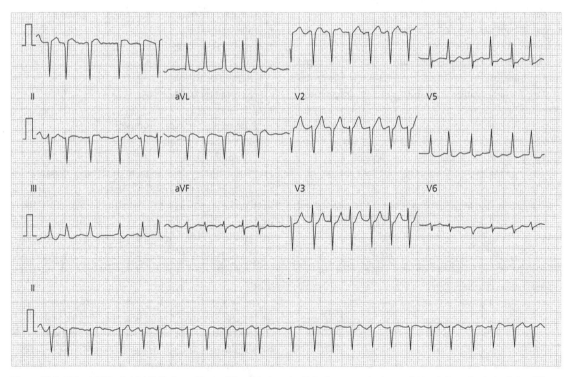

Figure 18.1 12-lead ECG of atrial fibrillation with a rapid ventricular rate. Note the unusual extreme right axis (negative in leads I and II). The most common cause for this is incorrect attachment of the limb leads.

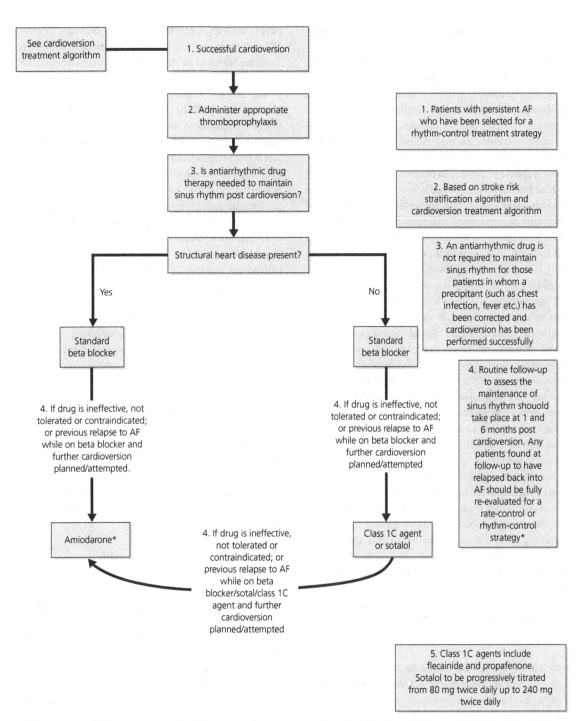

*If rhythm-control fails, consider the patient for rate-control strategy, or specialist referral for those with lone atrial fibrillation (AF) or ECG evidence of underlying electrophysiological disorder (e.g. Wolff–Parkinson–White [WPW] syndrome).

Figure 18.2 NICE guidelines for the rhythm-control management of paroxysmal atrial fibrillation.

finished a large meal this should be postponed and other strategies tried in the short term.

Pharmacological cardioversion with a class IC drug such as flecainide has been shown to increase the chance of returning to sinus rhythm within 8 hours of taking the medication. Flecainide may be administered as a slow i.v. injection (2 mg/kg over 15 minutes, maximum 150 mg) or single oral dose (300 mg). Patients need to be on bed rest while waiting for it to act. As it has a negative inotropic effect it should be avoided in patients known or suspected to have heart failure, impaired left ventricular function or who are haemodynamically compromised. The beneficial effects of pharmacological cardioversion with intravenous amiodarone do not appear until after 8–12 hours of the infusion, so there is little point in administering this drug in the acute setting, particularly as it should ideally be given through central venous access.

Pharmacological rate control is also an option as it may reduce symptoms while waiting for the paroxysm to stop spontaneously. Rapid control (and titration against blood pressure) can be obtained with intravenous infusions of esmolol (a beta blocker) or diltiazem (a calcium-channel antagonist); however, these are rarely necessary and are very expensive. Oral beta blockers or calcium-channel blockers are the most appropriate. Digoxin is less effective and slower to act. Amiodarone, even when given intravenously (requiring central venous access) can take longer to work.

For this patient the best option is probably a combination of flecainide 300 mg orally for pharmacological cardioversion, which if unsuccessful after 60 minutes could be followed by metoprolol 25 mg tds for rate control (can be increased on a dose-by-dose basis). It is also sensible to start anticoagulation with low-molecular-weight heparin. If sinus rhythm does not return using drug treatment within 48 hours it means external DC cardioversion can be performed without the need for transoesophageal echocardiography to exclude left atrial thrombus. If sinus rhythm is restored within 24 hours, it can be stopped.

He is given flecainide and metoprolol orally; 55 minutes later he goes back into sinus rhythm and his symptoms ease off. His thyroid function tests are normal. His troponin I comes back as 1.3 μg/L (normal values < 0.01).

How should this be interpreted and what should be done?

Elevated troponins are usually associated with ACSs; however, they may be elevated for other reasons. Tachycardias may sometime cause small troponin rises in people with angiographically normal coronary arteries. DC cardioversion itself does not cause elevated troponins. The significance of an elevated troponin is based upon the likelihood of underlying coronary artery disease, i.e. risk profile and pre-existing symptoms. This patient has a medium risk profile but no pre-existing symptoms and is therefore unlikely to have coronary artery disease. The troponin rise is probably a consequence of the arrhythmia and is not prognostically important. It is usually sensible to ignore it; however, if ongoing treatment with a class IC antiarrhythmic drug is going to be considered, these are contraindicated in the presence of coronary artery disease and further testing is required. A non-invasive test such as an exercise stress test, dobutamine stress echo or exercise Myoview may be indicated; however, many such patients are automatically entered into the ACS pathway and end up with coronary angiography.

He is admitted and undergoes coronary angiography the following day. This demonstrated normal coronary arteries. Transthoracic echocardiography shows normal atrial and ventricular size and function and no valve abnormalities. He is ready for hospital discharge

What are the drug treatment options? What are the advantages and disadvantages of each?

As he has had three episodes in a relatively short time period (including two A&E attendances), has no reversible underlying cause and is very symptomatic, a trial of drug therapy is indicated. The following antiarrhythmic drug options are available:

'Pill in the pocket' approach with flecainide 300 mg

In people who respond well to oral flecainide, this is an alternative to regular daily prophylactic medication. Flecainide 300 mg orally is taken at the onset of a paroxysm and the person rests until sinus rhythm is restored. This avoids daily drug treatment (with its potential side effects) and is useful for infrequent paroxysms that are stopped early in response to flecainide. It should not be used in people with heart failure, coronary artery disease or significant structural heart disease or people known to have atrial flutter.

Daily prophylactic drug therapy with beta blockers

Standard beta blockers (metoprolol, bisoprolol, etc.) are the first-line choice but have little antiarrhythmic effect.

They may be most useful in patients with 'adrenergic' atrial fibrillation, i.e. paroxysms that come on during physical exertion or emotional stress. This particular patient appears to have 'vagal' atrial fibrillation that comes on at rest or after food. Beta blockers may cause fatigue and lethargy and should be avoided in patients with bronchospasm. They reduce exercise capacity, which would not be tolerated by this keen sportsman.

Daily prophylactic therapy with flecainide

This is an alternative for patients who do not have contraindications (see above). Side-effects may include rashes, nausea, visual disturbances, hypoaesthesia and tinnitus. In a small proportion of patients, flecainide converts fibrillation into flutter and may slow the atrial rate enough to allow one-to-one conduction through the AV node, leading to a very rapid ventricular rate (often with aberrancy, manifest as a broad complex tachycardia that often causes significant haemodynamic compromise). It should not be prescribed to patients known to have atrial flutter, unless additional AV-nodal blocking drugs are prescribed.

Daily prophylactic therapy with sotalol

Sotalol is a beta blocker with additional class 3 antiarrhythmic properties. These class 3 properties are only manifest at high doses (>160 mg per day); however, these doses are seldom reached due to beta-blocker side-effects.

Daily prophylactic therapy with amiodarone

This class 3 drug is the most potent but also has a wide range of potentially serious side-effects (photosensitivity, thyroid dysfunction, ocular deposits, pulmonary fibrosis, liver dysfunction and peripheral neuropathy). Although probably the most efficacious, it is often restricted to use only when other options have failed and when non-pharmacological treatment are also being considered.

Anticoagulation

Anticoagulation with aspirin is indicated as his CHAD2 score (see Box 19.1) is 0.

He initially tries the 'pill-in-the-pocket' approach with flecainide. He continues to get paroxysms every 2–3 weeks which last 10 minutes to 2 hours in duration. It becomes apparent that the flecainide is having little effect on acute termination of the arrhythmia. He tries daily sotalol but feels tired and fatigued even on the low dose of 80 mg bd. He then tries daily flecainide 100 mg bd. Two weeks after

starting this therapy he is brought to the A&E by ambulance after collapsing during a training run. On arrival he is conscious; blood pressure is 95/60 mmHg; pulse 115 bpm, regular.

What does his 12-lead ECG show?

His 12-lead ECG (Figure 18.3) shows typical atrial flutter. Typical flutter usually has an atrial rate closer to 300 bpm – the slower atrial (and therefore ventricular) rates in this instance are due to treatment with flecainide.

What is the likely cause of his collapse?

His collapse happened during physical exertion in the setting of atrial flutter. In a small proportion of patients, flecainide converts atrial fibrillation into atrial flutter. Atrial flutter usually has an atrial rate of 300 bpm, which is just too fast for the AV node to conduct, so it is usually associated with 2:1 conduction and a ventricular rate of 150 bpm. Flecainide may also slow the atrial rate enough (e.g. to 260 bpm) to allow one-to-one conduction through the AV node, particularly in the setting of physical exertion and high sympathetic tone, as it is a drug with very little AV-node blocking properties. This can lead to a very rapid ventricular rate (often with aberrancy, manifest as a broad complex tachycardia), which causes significant haemodynamic compromise. It should not be prescribed to patients known to have atrial flutter unless additional AV-nodal-blocking drugs are prescribed.

Paroxysmal atrial fibrillation can be accompanied by sinus node dysfunction. Sometimes at the end of a paroxysm there is a long pause before the first sinus beat. These pauses, if long enough, can cause pre-syncope or syncope.

He is admitted and started on a beta blocker. A DC cardioversion is carried out 8 hours later. He is discharged on bisoprolol 1 mg od. Over the next month he has two further episodes of paroxysmal atrial fibrillation and becomes depressed and frustrated as he cannot continue his triathlon training. His GP refers him to a cardiac electrophysiologist.

What remaining treatment options are there? What are the advantages and disadvantages of each?
Amiodarone

If other drug options have failed, amiodarone may be attempted but it has a long list of side-effects (see above) and is frequently ineffective.

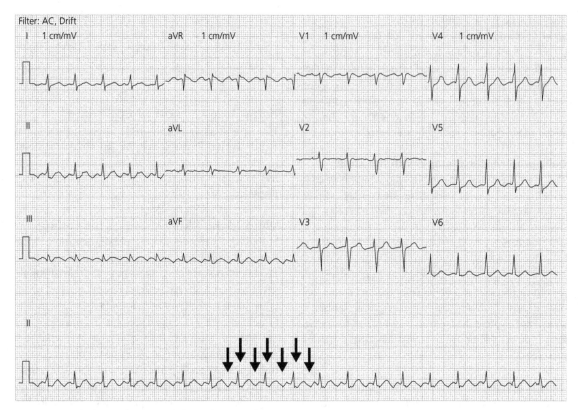

Figure 18.3 12-lead ECG of typical atrial flutter. The ventricular rate is 115 bpm and regular. There is a 'sawtooth' baseline with negative flutter waves in leads II, III and aVF. The atrial rate is 230 bpm and there is 2:1 AV block with alternate F waves obscured by the QRS complexes (arrows).

AV-node ablation and pacemaker insertion

The 'ablate and pace' option has been available for over 15 years. A radiofrequency ablation catheter is inserted into the femoral vein and passed up into the right atrium under X-ray guidance. The AV node is identified and cauterised, producing complete heart block. A permanent ventricular pacemaker is required to control the ventricular rate. The procedure is simple, low risk and can be done under local anaesthesia. It does not prevent atrial fibrillation from happening and the atriums continue to fibrillate intermittently but there is no longer a rapid ventricular rate. Symptoms such as palpitations are usually abolished; however, if the loss of atrial contractile function also causes symptoms (lethargy, fatigue, reduced exercise capacity), these will remain. Although the pacemaker can increase its pacing rate in response to movement, it will not be as efficient as the normal sinus node and conduction system. Pacemaker generator batteries last 5–8 years before being replaced and pacemaker-lead

revisions are not unusual after 10–15 years. This treatment is most suited to elderly, less active patients with atrial fibrillation and rapid ventricular rates and would not suit this particular patient.

Left atrial ablation (pulmonary vein isolation):

This patient would be an ideal candidate for left atrial ablation (pulmonary vein isolation). Over the past 7 years, left atrial ablation has emerged as a therapy for paroxysmal or persistent atrial fibrillation. It has been recognised that atrial fibrillation is often initiated and maintained by ectopics or bursts of rapid tachycardia that originate from muscle inside the pulmonary veins where they connect to the left atrium. Burning around the veins creates barriers to electrical conduction and prevents these 'triggers' from entering the atrium, thus preventing atrial fibrillation. Other 'trigger' sites in the right and left atrium may also be targeted. Overall, the procedure has a 70–80% chance of achieving good rhythm control, often off drug therapy, although a significant proportion of patients, perhaps as many as 60%, require more than one procedure to achieve a good result. Each procedure carries a 1% risk of stroke and a

2–3% risk of serious bleeding such as cardiac tamponade. Ablation is usually reserved for highly symptomatic patients, preferably <75 years of age, who have failed at least two drug therapies.

CASE REVIEW

This fit 42-year-old man presents with rapid irregular palpitations that cause significant symptoms. His rhythm has returned to normal by the time his first ECG is performed; however, his description is typical of atrial fibrillation. He has further paroxysms, followed by a persistent episode that leads to an A&E visit and ECG documentation. Treatment with flecainide and metoprolol is followed by reversion to sinus rhythm. There is a small rise in cardiac troponin which leads to admission for coronary

angiography; however, his coronary arteries are normal. A transthoracic echocardiogram shows a structurally normal heart. He is prescribed daily flecainide and aspirin, but subsequently collapses due to atrial flutter and a rapid ventricular rate, an uncommon side-effect of flecainide therapy. He remains symptomatic despite drug therapy and is presented with the options of non-pharmacological treatments, the most appropriate being pulmonary vein isolation ablation.

KEY POINTS

- Rapid irregular palpitations help distinguish atrial fibrillation form other supraventricular and ventricular arrhythmias.
- In the presence of a structurally normal heart, most palpitations and tachycardia mechanisms are benign.
- Approximately 30% of patients with paroxysmal atrial fibrillation have no coexisting disease and are described as 'lone' or idiopathic atrial fibrillation.
- Although there is a vast spectrum of clinical presentations and symptoms, younger, more active patients tend to have faster ventricular rates and worse symptoms.
- After a single episode, prophylactic drug therapy is not normally recommended as it may be many years before the next paroxysm, particularly if there is a provoking cause (infection, high alcohol consumption, trauma, etc.).
- Once multiple episodes occur, the decision to treat depends upon the frequency and duration and the symptoms associated with them.
- Unfortunately, antiarrhythmic drugs rarely completely suppress paroxysms of atrial fibrillation, although they

may reduce the frequency and duration and make the attacks more tolerable.
- Although they are well tolerated in most individuals, class 1C drugs may organise atrial fibrillation into atrial flutter. Unfortunately, this may cause worse symptoms due to a persistent rapid rate at 150bpm due to 2:1 conduction, or transient 1:1 conduction, which can cause very severe symptoms.
- Class 1C drugs should be avoided in heart failure and ischaemic heart disease as in these situations they may cause dangerous ventricular arrhythmias.
- A variety of non-pharmacological treatments for atrial fibrillation have emerged over the last few years. AV-node ablation and pacemaker insertion is ideally suited to older patients (or those with a bradycardia pacing indication) whose principle symptoms are due to a rapid ventricular rate that cannot be controlled with drugs. Left atrial ablation is now emerging as a major treatment for symptomatic, drug-refractory patients.

Case 19 A 64-year-old man with fatigue and palpitations

A 68-year-old man visits his GP for a check-up. He has been feeling non-specifically unwell for the last 2–3 weeks with fatigue, breathlessness and difficulty walking up hills. He is previously active and usually plays 18 holes of golf twice a week.

What initial questions should be asked?

• What causes him to stop walking? Is it breathlessness, fatigue, chest tightness, leg pains or another symptom?
• Are there any other associated symptoms?

Sometimes patient give a clear description of what is limiting them (e.g. 'I get chest tightness whenever I walk up a flight of stairs', or 'I run out of breath whenever I walk my dog up a particular hill'), but often initial descriptions are more vague (e.g. 'I don't feel quite right when I walk', or 'I can't keep up with my wife'). It is important to ask clearly what the limiting factor is. Although someone might appear to have cardiac or respiratory symptoms, remember that arthritis, peripheral vascular disease and poor balance or muscle weakness may limit exertion as much as breathlessness, fatigue or chest pain.

On closer questioning he says that for 3 weeks he has felt constantly fatigued. When he has tried to play golf or performed similar physical exertion he gets short of breath very quickly. He has no chest pain but with heavy exertion does feel tight around the chest, light headed and 'jittery', as if his heart is beating very fast. It would appear that there is a probable cardiorespiratory cause to his symptoms.

What further questions should be asked?

• Can he lie flat?
• Does he wake up at night breathless?

Cardiology: Clinical Cases Uncovered. By T. Betts, J. Dwight and S. Bull. Published 2010 by Blackwell Publishing.

• Have his ankles started swelling?
• Is he wheezy?
• Does he have a cough?
• Does he have any past history of cardiac or respiratory disease?

It is important to elicit symptoms typical for heart failure (orthopnoea, paroxysmal nocturnal dyspnoea, peripheral oedema) or lung disease (bronchospasm, infection, allergic).

He has always slept with two pillows. He has woken up at night twice in the last week feeling breathless. There is no ankle swelling. He does not smoke and has no known past medical history. On physical examination his blood pressure is 150/95 mmHg. His pulse is 140 bpm and irregular. His JVP is raised by 3 cm. His apex beat is displaced laterally. There is a soft pansystolic murmur heard best at the apex. His lung fields have a few sparse crackles at the bases. There is very mild pitting oedema at the lower shins.

What is the most likely diagnosis?

The appearances are consistent with congestive cardiac failure together with atrial fibrillation and MR.

What are the possible causes of his symptoms?

• Ischaemic heart disease – the lack of significant chest pain would mean silent ischaemia or infarction – with the subsequent development of atrial fibrillation and mitral regurgitation (MR).
• Severe MR causing heart failure and atrial fibrillation.
• Dilated cardiomyopathy with the subsequent development of atrial fibrillation and MR.
• Tachycardia cardiomyopathy: Atrial fibrillation with a rapid ventricular rate that eventually results in a dilated cardiomyopathy, MR and heart failure.

The aetiology of the heart failure needs to be found in case there is a reversible cause that can be treated.

The GP sends the patient to A&E where he is seen and admitted by the medical team.

What investigations need to be performed next?

• **12-lead ECG.** Confirm the rhythm, document the rate at rest, look for evidence of previous damage (LVH from hypertension, Q waves from previous myocardial infarction, etc.).

• **Chest X-ray (CXR).** Confirm pulmonary venous congestion and cardiomegaly and look for respiratory disease.

• **Transthoracic echocardiography.** To assess cardiac function (in particular left ventricular systolic function and mitral valve structure and function).

• **Blood tests.** Biochemistry and renal function to assess electrolytes, etc.; thyroid function to look for thyrotoxicosis; cardiomyopathy screen, such as ferritin; etc.), cholesterol, glucose.

What does his 12-lead ECG show?

The ECG (Figure 19.1) shows an irregular, rapid narrow complex ventricular rhythm with no discrete P waves. This is the hallmark of atrial fibriliation. The deep S waves in V1 and V2, and tall R waves in VS and V6, suggest left ventricular hypertrophy (LVH). There is lateral ST depression too (leads V4-V6).

CXR revealed cardiomegaly (CTR 0.55) and upper lobe blood diversion. O_2 saturations are 96% on room air.

An echocardiogram shows a dilated left ventricle with poor systolic function although the rapid rate makes it hard to assess. The left ventricular wall thickness is at the upper limit of normal. The left atrium is also dilated (4.5 cm). The mitral leaflets fail to coapt with a central regurgitant jet but there is no leaflet prolapse. There is mild–moderate 'central' MR, suggesting it is a consequence of left ventricular dilatation rather than the cause of his heart failure. Blood tests are all within the normal range.

What is the most important abnormality to address?

The rapid ventricular rate is probably the single most important abnormality to correct. Not only will it be compromising cardiac output and contributing to his current symptoms and signs of left ventricular failure, it is quite likely that it is the cause of his underlying cardiomyopathy as there is no evidence of previous myocardial infarction or severe valve dysfunction.

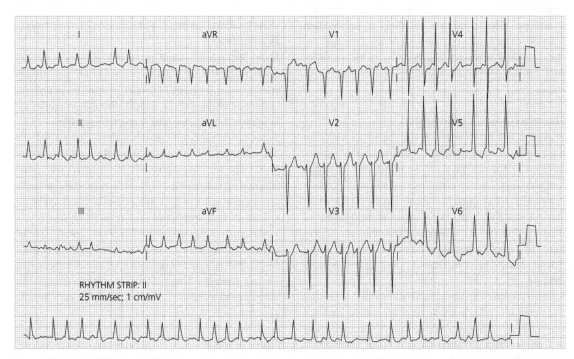

Figure 19.1 12-lead ECG of atrial fibrillation with a rapid ventricular rate of 140 bpm. The QRS complexes are irregular and the baseline is fibrillatory with no discrete P-wave activity.

PART 2: CASES

What treatment is required?

• There is evidence of mild pulmonary oedema so an intravenous dose of **diuretic** may help by clearing the lung fields (improving oxygenation) and reducing left ventricular end diastolic pressure (pre-load). **Oxygen** may also be administered.

• The atrial fibrillation may be addressed by a number of approaches. A rapid ventricular rate may sometime be the result of severe hypoxia (crashing pulmonary oedema, severe pain or significant ischaemia) and therefore correcting these will slow the ventricular rate; however, in this example the heart failure symptoms are chronic and the signs relatively mild and his rate will probably continue to be rapid, despite the diuretic and oxygen. If the atrial fibrillation was thought to be of acute onset and the cause of all his symptoms, **urgent DC cardioversion** could be undertaken; however, its duration is not known and he is not on anticoagulants and, importantly, he is not severely compromised.

What are the different treatments available?

External direct current cardioversion

External DC cardioversion is a very effective method for restoring sinus rhythm in atrial fibrillation, particularly if of recent onset (<3 months' duration). It requires deep sedation or general anaesthesia. It is the treatment of choice if there is severe acute haemodynamic compromise (cardiogenic shock) resulting from the rapid ventricular rate.

Pharmacological cardioversion

Pharmacological cardioversion may be performed with intravenous or oral flecainide. Flecainide is a negative inotrope and in the setting of impaired left ventricular function may be pro-arrhythmic (causing dangerous ventricular arrhythmias) or cause significant hypotension. Amiodarone may also promote restoration of sinus rhythm but its beneficial effect may not appear until 24 hours of administration; intravenous amiodarone should be administered via a central venous cannula.

Both forms of cardioversion should only be attempted if it is known that atrial fibrillation has been present for <48 hours. After 48 hours' duration there is a chance that left atrial thrombus may have developed, which could be dislodged by the restoration of sinus rhythm. In addition, cardioversion should only be attempted for atrial fibrillation if the patient is known to have been therapeutically anticoagulated for the previous 3 weeks, or a transoesophageal echocardiogram is performed to exclude left atrial thrombus. Anticoagulation is then required for at least 6 weeks post-cardioversion.

Pharmacological rate control

Pharmacological rate control is therefore the best approach. The most effective drugs are usually beta blockers or calcium-channel blockers. Some caution may be required as there is poor left ventricular function and signs of left ventricular failure; however, his blood pressure is good. The alternative is digoxin but this takes longer to work and is less effective, particularly in the setting of increased sympathetic drive (exercise, stress, etc.). Amiodarone can be used but may result in pharmacological cardioversion, which needs to be avoided in this patient until appropriately anticoagulated, and also takes some time to work.

Therefore, in this setting of clinical heart failure the most appropriate treatment is oral digoxin, with the introduction of a shorter-acting beta blocker such as metoprolol 25 mg tds when his lung fields are clear and oxygenation is good.

What other investigation and treatment is required?

Many institutions would perform diagnostic coronary angiography to look for the presence of severe coronary artery disease as a cause of his cardiomyopathy. If present, there may be prognostic benefit through revascularisation, even if he does not have angina symptoms.

Anticoagulation with warfarin should be started. He has a CHADS2 (Box 19.1) score of at least 1 (congestive heart failure) but probably 2 (congestive heart failure + hypertension). If DC cardioversion is eventually going to be performed, then therapeutic anticoagulation is required for a minimum of 3 weeks in advance.

Standard heart failure medications should also be introduced, such as an angiotensin-converting enzyme (ACE) inhibitor and beta blocker (if not already started for rate control). This will also treat hypertension (his blood pressure is raised despite the cardiac compromise and there is ECG evidence of LVH).

Over the next 48 hours his ventricular rate slows to 70 bpm at rest and 110 bpm on walking up a flight of stairs. He is no longer breathless on exertion and has no more

---

Box 19.1 CHADS2 scoring system

1 point for each of **C**ongestive cardiac failure, **H**ypertension, **A**ge >75 years and **D**iabetes

2 points for a prior ischaemic cerebrovascular event (**S**troke or transient ischaemic attack)

Score	% annual stroke risk without anticoagulation	Long-term warfarin?
0	1.9 (1.2–3.0)	No
1	2.8 (2–3.8)	Debatable
2	4.0 (3.1–5.1)	Yes
3	5.9 (4.6–7.3)	Yes
4	8.5 (6.3–11.1)	Yes
5	12.5 (8.2–17.5)	Yes
6	18.2 (10.5–27.4)	Yes

The stroke risk is balanced against annual risk of serious bleeding (e.g. haemorrhagic stroke) of 1% providing the INR is maintained within the therapeutic range. Warfarin will reduce the ischaemic stroke risk to one third.

---

palpitations. Coronary angiography shows normal coronary arteries. A repeat echocardiogram with the controlled ventricular rate shows that left ventricular function is actually only moderately impaired. He still feels fatigued. He is ready for hospital discharge.

Should outpatient DC cardioversion be performed in 4–6 weeks time? What additional preparation should be considered? What are the arguments for and against cardioversion?

DC cardioversion may be performed to regain sinus rhythm. The advantages of this are that his symptoms (e.g. fatigue) may improve further with the restoration of atrial contractile function and if sinus rhythm is maintained his thromboembolic risk is reduced. If he has a tachycardia cardiomyopathy then restoration of sinus rhythm (or very good ventricular rate control during atrial fibrillation) should allow the return of normal left ventricular function. If he has a dilated cardiomyopathy and the atrial fibrillation is secondary to this, then it is quite likely that atrial fibrillation will return at some point in the near future. Over 60% of patients undergoing DC cardioversion have a recurrence by 12 months. Recurrence rates may be reduced by ongoing treatment with antiarrhyth-

mic agents such as amiodarone, but still remain around 40% and of course drugs such as amiodarone have a long list of potential side-effects. If patients have no symptoms and adequate rate control, then remaining in permanent atrial fibrillation (with appropriate thromboembolic prophylaxis) is an appropriate treatment.

As this is the first detected episode of atrial fibrillation the probable diagnosis is tachycardia cardiomyopathy and he still has some symptoms of fatigue (either due to fibrillation or beta blockers) then elective DC cardioversion is warranted. As he is only beginning anticoagulation it is decided not to prescribe amiodarone.

Six weeks after discharge he has an elective day-case external DC cardioversion, which successfully restores sinus rhythm with a single 150J biphasic shock. He is then reviewed 3 months later in the outpatient clinic with a 12-lead ECG that shows sinus rhythm and a repeat echocardiogram that shows normal left ventricular size and function. The left atrium remains dilated (4.2 cm) and there is mild central MR. He is comfortably playing golf and has no symptoms.

What should he do regarding his medications (digoxin, beta blocker, ACE inhibitor and warfarin)? What are the relevant concerns?

- **Digoxin.** The digoxin was prescribed purely for ventricular rate control. Now he has been in sinus rhythm for 3 months it is no longer required. It is not an antiarrhythmic and will not reduce the risk of atrial fibrillation recurrence.
- **Beta blocker.** The main argument to continue the beta blocker is that he requires it as part of his hypertension treatment. Whether he still requires it for heart failure treatment is debatable as he has successfully 'remodelled'.
- **ACE inhibitor.** Likewise, the argument to continue the ACE inhibitor is that he requires it as part of his hypertension treatment as well as for his recent heart failure.
- **Warfarin.** He is now beyond the conventional 3 month post-cardioversion window for anticoagulation

The main concern is that his atrial fibrillation will return. It is likely that his atrial fibrillation had been present for weeks, if not months, before he developed the tachycardia cardiomyopathy and subsequent heart failure symptoms that led to his eventual presentation. How will he know if his atrial fibrillation returns if he is not symptomatic? Should he continue to take the beta blocker and warfarin in case it does return? The beta blocker would hopefully control the ventricular rate so tachycardia cardiomyopathy would not occur. The warfarin would reduce the thromboembolic risk; however, now that his heart failure is gone he only has a CHADS2 score of 1 at worse and the role of warfarin is debatable.

These decisions are often influenced by the patient's attitude to warfarin, the risk of a stroke and perceived side-effects from ongoing drug therapy. In this case the added concern of an asymptomatic atrial fibrillation recurrence going undetected would suggest that indefinite drug treatment is the preferred option, especially as the recurrence rate is estimated at 60%.

CASE REVIEW

This 64-year-old man presented with fatigue and lethargy. Physical examination revealed atrial fibrillation, confirmed by 12-lead ECG. History and examination also revealed symptoms and signs of heart failure. Echocardiography demonstrated severely impaired left ventricular function. At this stage it was not known whether the atrial fibrillation is a consequence or the cause of the cardiomyopathy. His ventricular rate is controlled with digoxin and heart failure medication is commenced. Subsequent coronary angiography reveals normal coronary arteries. He is discharged and after 6 weeks of anticoagulation with warfarin undergoes elective DC cardioversion back to sinus rhythm. Three months after this his left ventricular function has returned to normal, confirming an original diagnosis of tachycardia-mediated cardiomyopathy.

KEY POINTS

- Not all patients with atrial fibrillation and a rapid ventricular rate present with palpitations. Some have less specific symptoms, such as fatigue and breathlessness, whereas a few may be asymptomatic.
- A constant rapid ventricular rate (mean 24 heart rate >110 bpm) over a period of days or weeks can result in tachycardia-mediated cardiomyopathy in susceptible individuals. For this to happen they are generally asymptomatic from the arrhythmia and present eventually with heart failure.
- Atrial fibrillation with a rapid ventricular rate that causes acute, decompensated heart failure should be treated with urgent cardioversion. In this situation the arrhythmia duration is usually <48 hours. Persistent episodes lasting >48 hours need appropriate anticoagulation before DC cardioversion (or a transoesophageal echocardiogram to exclude left atrial thrombus) and therefore rate control is often preferred.
- Rate control is best achieved with beta blockers or calcium-channel blockers; however, in the setting of overt heart failure and low blood pressure, digoxin may be preferred initially.

- If cardioversion is planned, anticoagulation should be started with warfarin. A minimum of 3–4 weeks within the therapeutic range is required before cardioversion, with 6 weeks minimum afterwards.
- The role of additional drug therapy (e.g. amiodarone) to facilitate cardioversion and maintenance of sinus rhythm is debatable. The chance of recurrence is reduced with amiodarone; however, there are potential side-effects to consider and also pharmacological cardioversion needs to be avoided until therapeutic anticoagulation has been present for 3–4 weeks.
- If DC cardioversion is unsuccessful yet there is good pharmacological ventricular rate control, asymptomatic patients can be left in atrial fibrillation. If patients have good rate control but remain symptomatic due to the loss of atrial contractile function, pulmonary vein isolation ablation may restore and maintain sinus rhythm. If the rate is not well controlled (due to ineffective or poorly tolerated drugs), the choice is between extensive pulmonary vein isolation ablation to restore sinus rhythm or AV-node ablation (to create complete heart block) and insertion of a permanent pacemaker.

A 24-year-old man with palpitations

A 24-year-old man is brought to A&E with sudden-onset rapid palpitations associated with chest tightness, breathlessness and feeling dizzy and unwell. It started 30 minutes earlier, while playing football.

What is your initial approach?

The initial approach is to record the patient's vital signs and assess the degree of haemodynamic compromise. This will tell you how quickly you need to act. Warning signs include:

- Decreased conscious level.
- Peripherally shut down (pale, cold, clammy).
- Hypotension (systolic blood pressure < 90 mmHg).
- Crackles in lung fields and low oxygen saturations, indicating pulmonary oedema.

He is uncomfortable but alert and orientated. He is warm to touch and looks well perfused. His blood pressure is 92/55 mmHg, pulse 200 bpm, O_2 saturations on 5 L/min via a face mask are 99% and his lung fields are clear.

In the setting of tachycardia and chest pain or breathlessness it is important to establish the primary problem and the consequences. Very rapid pathological tachycardias may result in symptoms such as chest pain and breathlessness and may even cause pulmonary oedema, myocardial ischaemia or syncope due to poor perfusion in patients with underlying structural heart disease. Conversely, acute ischaemia, pulmonary oedema, sepsis or pain may cause a reflex sinus tachycardia or atrial fibrillation with a rapid ventricular rate, which is a normal stress response and a consequence rather than the primary problem. It is always important to address the underlying cause.

In this young, otherwise fit (he plays regular football) patient the tachycardia is so rapid (200 bpm) that it is likely to be the cause of his symptoms. Sinus tachycardia rarely exceeds 150–160 bpm in A&E patients.

What investigation should be performed next?

As tachycardia is the problem, a 12-lead ECG should be performed immediately. Although telemetry or a cardiac monitor may give an indication of rate and regularity it cannot be relied on to clearly show whether the tachycardia is broad complex or narrow or distinguish the presence or absence of P waves.

What does the 12-lead ECG show?

The 12-lead ECG (Figure 20.1) shows narrow complex tachycardia. It is regular with a rate of 200 bpm. It is narrow complex, as the QRS duration is <120 ms (three small squares) There is also lateral ST segment depression (leads V4–V6).

What is the likely ECG diagnosis?

If a tachycardia is narrow complex, it must travel through the ventricles using the normal conduction system (His bundle and bundle braches), therefore the tachycardia must involve travel through the AV node from atrium to ventricle. This rules out ventricular tachycardia, which is always broad (QRS complexes >three small squares or 120 ms).

The differential diagnoses are therefore as follows:
- **Sinus tachycardia.** Usually 100–150 bpm. A P wave before each QRS (upright in lead II) with a normal PR interval. Slight variations in the heart rate but basically regular.
- **Atrial fibrillation.** 100–170 bpm. Irregularly irregular ventricular rate with no discrete P-wave activity. There may be coarse atrial fibrillatory activity, which is particularly obvious in lead V1.

Cardiology: Clinical Cases Uncovered. By T. Betts, J. Dwight and S. Bull. Published 2010 by Blackwell Publishing.

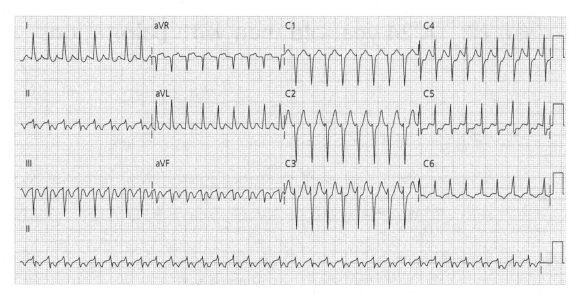

Figure 20.1 12-lead ECG of narrow complex tachycardia.

- **Atrial flutter.** Classically, 300 bpm in the atriums and 150 bpm in the ventricles due to 2 : 1 AV block, producing a regular ventricular rate. Flutter waves (one every large square) produce a 'saw-tooth' baseline in leads II, III and aVF and positive waves in V1. Alternate flutter waves may be obscured by QRS complexes making them hard to see.
- **Atrial tachycardia.** Usually regular, 100–180 bpm. A P wave before each QRS complex. The shape of the P wave depends upon the site of the tachycardia focus, therefore may be upright, flat or negative in lead II. There may be a QRS after each P wave or there may be intermittent conduction through to the ventricles (e.g. 2 : 1 AV block).
- **Atrioventricular nodal reciprocating tachycardia (AVNRT).** Regular at 150–220 bpm. There is simultaneous atrial and ventricular activation so the P waves are usually hidden in the QRS complexes. Occasionally, this may manifest as a 'pseudo-R wave' in the QRS complex in lead V1.
- **Atrioventricular reciprocating tachycardia (AVRT).** Orthodromic direction: regular at 170–240 bpm. The arrhythmia circuit travels through the AV node, then the bundle braches, then the ventricular muscle, then the accessory pathway back to the atrium. If visible, the P wave is therefore in the ST segment, just after the end of the QRS complex.

All of the above are classified as supraventricular arrhythmias. Convention is that supraventricular tachycardias (SVTs) are the subgroup of supraventricular arrhythmias

that use the AV node as a critical part of a re-entrant circuit, i.e. AVNRT and AVRT.

What is the most appropriate treatment?

Prompt restoration of sinus rhythm is required. This may be done in a variety of ways depending upon the arrhythmia mechanism:
- 'Vagal manoeuvres', i.e. carotid sinus massage, ocular massage, the Valsalva manoeuvre.
- Adenosine administered as an intravenous bolus injection.
- Verapamil administered as an intravenous bolus injection.
- Other antiarrhythmic drug infusions (e.g. flecainide).
- External DC cardioversion.

A narrow complex regular tachycardia, which is likely to be a SVT, may be terminated with vagal manoeuvres in a minority of people. If not, first-line therapy should be intravenous adenosine. In patients who do not respond to this, and/or are extremely compromised, urgent external DC cardioversion should be performed.

How should adenosine be administered? Are there any contraindications and what should the patient be told to expect?

Adenosine should be administered as a rapid bolus. Start with 6 mg but if that has no effect, give 9 mg, then 12 mg.

It is metabolised by blood-vessel endothelium and red blood cells, which is why its effect is extremely transient and short lived and needs to be given rapidly through a large bore cannula, preferably in an antecubital fossa vein and followed immediately by a saline flush. As well as causing transient AV-node block there is short-lived flushing, sweating and chest tightness.

Its effect is antagonised by theophylline and caffeine and exacerbated by dipyridamole and carbamazepine. Avoid in people on exacerbating drugs and those with moderate or severe asthma.

The effects of adenosine on different arrhythmias mechanisms are shown in Table 20.1. The effect of adenosine on supraventricular arrhythmias depends upon the arrhythmia mechanism. No visible effect on a narrow-complex tachycardia usually means the dose is not high enough. In 5% of patients adenosine may trigger atrial fibrillation. In <1% it may trigger polymorphic ventricular tachycardia, so defibrillator back-up is required.

Table 20.1 Effects of adenosine of different arrhythmias mechanism

Arrhythmia	Effect of adenosine
Sinus tachycardia	Slowing of tachycardia rate, rarely with intermittent heart block, before return of sinus tachycardia
Atrial tachycardia	Usually transient AV block with ongoing atrial tachycardia unmasking rapid P-wave activity. Tachycardia may terminate in 30–50% of cases, restoring sinus rhythm
Atrial flutter	Transient AV block, unmasking rapid flutter waves
AVNRT	Tachycardia terminates and sinus rhythm restored
AVRT	Tachycardia terminates and sinus rhythm restored
Ventricular tachycardia	Usually no effect. May rarely terminate idiopathic ventricular tachycardias

AV, atrioventricular; AVRT, atrioventricular reciprocating tachycardia; AVNRT, atrioventricular nodal reciprocating tachycardia.

If adenosine fails, or there is immediate tachycardia reinitiation, SVTs may be terminated by intravenous verapamil 5–10 mg slow bolus.

I *A 12-mg dose of adenosine terminates the tachycardia.*

The ECG is then recorded. What does it show?

The ECG (Figure 20.2) shows sinus rhythm with a short PR interval and slurred upstroke (delta wave) at the onset of the QRS complexes, i.e. ventricular pre-excitation through an accessory pathway. The large R wave in lead V1 indicates that the accessory pathway is on the left side of the heart, crossing the mitral valve annulus and connecting the left atrium with the left ventricle. The combination of ventricular pre-excitation and SVT is called Wolff-Parkinson-White syndrome.

On further questioning the patient says he has previously had short-lived rapid palpitations occurring two or three times a year for as long as he can remember but they have always stopped on their own after 1 or 2 minutes or with breath-holding. He has no other medical history of note and there is no family history of arrhythmias, heart disease or sudden death. He has never lost consciousness. His physical examination is unremarkable with no cardiac murmurs. His pulse is 72 bpm and blood pressure 135/78 mmHg.

What should be done next? Does he require hospital admission?

A satisfactory diagnosis has been reached, i.e. Wolff-Parkinson-White syndrome. The arrhythmia has been successfully treated and the history suggests it is an infrequent occurrence that usually terminates on its own. There are no worrying features in his history (such as syncope or family members with sudden cardiac death). Hospital admission is therefore not required.

A daily prescription of prophylactic medication should be considered. The arguments for medication are that it may prevent further attacks, particularly those requiring A&E treatment. The arguments against medication are that it would be required every day, yet his attacks are infrequent and until today stopped on their own. Antiarrhythmic drugs frequently have limiting side-effects and may only have limited efficacy.

He should be referred as an outpatient to a cardiologist with a special interest in arrhythmias.

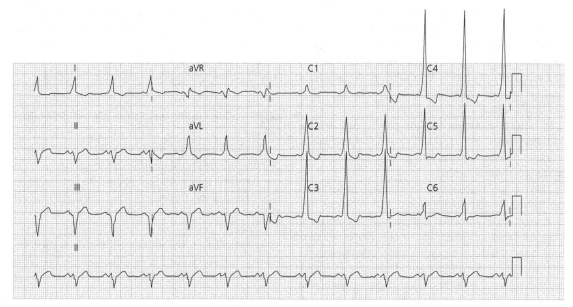

Figure 20.2 The 12-lead ECG after a 12 mg dose of adenosine.

He is referred to the local tertiary referral centre to see a cardiac electrophysiologist. He attends the outpatient clinic 4 weeks later.

What additional cardiac investigations are required?

• It is standard practice to perform **transthoracic echocardiography** to look for structural heart disease that may be associated with Wolff-Parkinson-White syndrome. These include Ebstein's anomaly of the tricuspid valve or hypertrophic cardiomyopathy.

• **Exercise testing** may be used for risk stratification purposes (see below).

• A Holter monitor is not required as the resting 12-lead ECG shows ventricular pre-excitation and helps to localise the position of the accessory pathway and the A&E ECG documents the tachycardia.

Is his condition dangerous or life threatening? What discussions should take place?

SVT is not life threatening and does not cause harm, unless it is allowed to go on for many hours (in which case heart failure may gradually develop) or there is syncope due to hypotension at the tachycardia onset that results in injury. For most patients with SVT therefore, treatment is for symptoms rather than prognosis. This is not necessarily the case for people with ventricular pre-excitation however. Regardless of whether they get SVT or not, there is a risk that they may develop pre-excited atrial fibrillation. In most people with atrial fibrillation the ventricles are activated entirely through the normal conduction system. Although the atriums fibrillate at 500–600 bpm the AV node is a protective filter and it is very rare for the ventricular rate to exceed 170 bpm. If there is an accessory pathway present that can conduct from atrium to ventricle (i.e. ventricular pre-excitation) this provides another route for atrial fibrillation to excite the ventricle. An accessory pathway does not have the same filtering properties as the AV node and may in some individuals have very short refractory (recovery) periods producing extremely rapid ventricular activation through the pathway at irregular rates >300 bpm. This in turn may precipitate ventricular fibrillation, thus patients with pre-excitation (regardless of whether they have SVT or not) are at risk of sudden cardiac death (SCD). The annual risk averages out at 0.1%. The risk is probably higher in patients with symptomatic SVT. Low-risk pathways are ones that do not conduct well from atrium to ventricle and have long recovery times. These low-risk pathways may be identified non-invasively by spontaneous disappearance of the delta wave and pre-excitation on Holter monitoring or ECGs, or by abrupt disappearance of pre-excitation on a treadmill once the sinus rate increases.

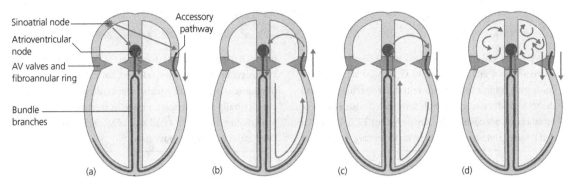

Sinoatrial node

Atrioventricular node

AV valves and fibroannular ring

Bundle branches

Accessory pathway

(a)   (b)   (c)   (d)

Figure 20.3 Diagrams of arrhythmia circuits resulting from an accessory pathway. (a) Sinus rhythm with ventricular pre-excitation, resulting in a short PR interval and delta wave. (b) Orthodromic atrioventricular reciprocating tachycardia (AVRT). As conduction from atrium to ventricle is only through the atrioventricular (AV) node during this tachycardia, the QRS complexes are usually narrow unless there is coexisting bundle branch block. (c) Antidromic AVRT. As conduction from atrium to ventricle is only through the accessory pathway during this tachycardia the QRS complexes are very pre-excited, i.e. broad with a slurred onset. (d) Pre-excited atrial fibrillation. The very rapid atrial rates are conducted to the ventricles through the AV node and accessory pathway, producing very rapid ventricular rates with varying amounts of pre-excitation and a combination of narrow and wide QRS complexes.

The accessory pathway refractory period may be more formally assessed with an invasive electrophysiological study, during which it is also possible to test whether the accessory pathway can support AV-reciprocating tachycardia. The different arrhythmias that result from an accessory pathway are illustrated in Figure 20.3.

What treatments options are available?

As described above treatment options are:

• **Do nothing.** Accept a 0.1% annual risk of sudden cardiac death, avoid drugs as the SVT is infrequent and do nothing unless symptoms become worse.

• **Drug therapy: trial of beta blockers.** These may prevent SVT attacks but will have no effect on the annual SCD risk. Side-effects may occur.

• **Drug therapy: flecainide or propafenone.** These class IC antiarrhythmic drugs affect accessory pathway conduction and may reduce the risk of SCD from pre-excited atrial fibrillation as well as preventing SVT.

• **Diagnostic invasive electrophysiology study for risk stratification purposes.** Assessing the accessory pathway refractory period and its precise location may help identify low-risk accessory pathways where prognosis is not an issue and also indicate whether there are risks associated with radiofrequency ablation treatment.

• **Invasive electrophysiological study and radiofrequency ablation.** This represents the definitive treatment and can provide a cure, removing the need for drugs and abolishing the risk of SCD. Procedures are normally performed as day cases under sedation. Success rates are approximately 95% although 5–10% of patients may need two procedures to achieve a cure. Significant complications include pneumothorax (<1%), cardiac tamponade (1%), heart block and pacemaker (1% depending upon the accessory pathway location), stroke (0.2–0.5% left-sided pathways only) and death (0.1%). Patients need to avoid strenuous activity for 1 week after and in the UK the DVLA prohibit driving for 1 week.

He asks if it is OK to continue playing sports. What should you tell him?

There is a small risk that pre-excited atrial fibrillation may develop during high-intensity sports. If his accessory pathway is high risk (has a short refractory period) he should either avoid such sports or have the accessory pathway ablated. The only way to formally assess the pathway's properties is with an invasive electrophysiological study. If a diagnostic study is being performed, many would argue that it would be sensible to go ahead and ablate the pathway regardless as catheters are already *in situ*, as long as it is not a mid-septal pathway with a significant risk of complete heart block. Therefore, low-intensity recreation sports are probably fine to continue; high-intensity, very competitive sports should be avoided unless cleared after an electrophysiology study or ablation.

CASE REVIEW

This 24-year-old man was rushed to A&E with a regular tachycardia of 200 bpm. The ECG showed narrow QRS complexes, indicating a supraventricular mechanism, and the tachycardia was successfully terminated with a bolus of intravenous adenosine. The sinus rhythm ECG showed a delta wave and short PR interval indicating ventricular pre-excitation, giving a diagnosis of Wolff-Parkinson-White syndrome. He was referred to a cardiac electro-physiologist where subsequent echocardiography showed a structurally normal heart. Different treatment strategies were discussed and the small risk of SCD due to pre-excitated atrial fibrillation was raised.

KEY POINTS

- Many patients with infrequent short-lived, self-terminating episodes of SVT learn to live with their symptoms or may even have them dismissed as panic attacks until ECG documentation is achieved.
- A regular, narrow complex tachycardia is either a SVT (usually rates 160–220 bpm), atrial flutter (150 bpm), atrial tachycardia (120–180 bpm) or sinus tachycardia (100–140 bpm with slight variation).
- SVTs use the AV node as part of the re-entrant circuit, which is why they can be terminated with i.v. adenosine. Automatic, focal atrial tachycardias are also terminated in 30–50% of cases.
- Adenosine i.v. needs to be given very rapidly, into a large cannula in a brachial or central vein, immediately followed by a saline flush. Always record a continuous ECG rhythm strip when administering adenosine.
- SVTs that do not respond to adenosine or immediately reinitiate may successfully be treated with i.v. verapamil, as long as the blood pressure is not too low.
- Ventricular pre-excitation is important to recognise as this is the one situation in which atrial fibrillation may be life threatening due to extremely rapid, irregular ventricular rates degenerating into ventricular fibrillation. The risk approximates to 0.15% per annum.
- Radiofrequency catheter ablation is now the treatment of choice for people with symptomatic SVTs. However, there remains much debate about what to do with asymptomatic ventricular pre-excitation discovered on ECGs.

A 77-year-old woman with fatigue and bradycardia

A 77-year-old woman, well known to her GP, with a history of hypertension, attends the surgery with a 3-week history of fatigue, lethargy and diminished exercise capacity. She has had one episode when she felt light-headed and pre-syncopal. She denies chest pain or palpitations.

Her blood pressure is 140/90 mmHg. Her pulse is 40 bpm, regular. The rest of her cardiovascular, respiratory and abdominal examination is unremarkable.

What are the most likely differential diagnoses?

The striking feature is her bradycardia (Box 21.1). Other common causes of fatigue are tachycardias such as atrial fibrillation, anaemia, endocrine disorders such as hypothyroidism, depression, and sleep disorders such as obstructive sleep apnoea.

A very simple test would be to ask the patient to walk briskly around the room or ideally up a flight of stairs, then re-examine the pulse. If the rate increases (even if only by 10 or 20 bpm) it is likely to be sinus node disease. If the rate stays the same or increases by <10 bpm it is more likely to be AV-node disease and heart block. The most important test is a 12-lead ECG.

A 12-lead ECG is performed in the surgery. What does it show?

The 12-lead ECG (Figure 21.1) shows there is sinus rhythm, indicated by P-wave activity at a rate of 80 bpm. There is complete dissociation between the atriums and ventricles with the broad QRS complexes marching through independently at a slow rate of 45 bpm.

Cardiology: Clinical Cases Uncovered. By T. Betts, J. Dwight and S. Bull. Published 2010 by Blackwell Publishing.

What are the potential causes? What questions should be asked and what additional tests need to be done?

• Degenerative changes in the His–Purkinje system (age-related).
• Acute myocardial infarction – typically occurs with inferior myocardial infarctions and is transient.
• Drugs, particularly toxic levels and combinations of beta blockers, non-dihydropyridine calcium-channel blockers and digoxin.
• Infections such as Lyme disease.
• Systemic diseases such as sarcoid and amyloid.
• Congenital complete heart block.

Questions should be asked about recent chest pain (for evidence of myocardial infarction), weight gain and cold intolerance (hypothyroidism, although this typically causes sinus bradycardia rather than AV block) and drug history.

She takes a diuretic and angiotensin-converting enzyme (ACE) inhibitor for her hypertension and has no features of recent myocardial infarction, systemic disease or hypothyroidism.

What action needs to be taken? How soon should it be done?

Her heart block is irreversible and from her history has probably been present for a few weeks. She has not had syncope but has had one pre-syncopal episode. The wide QRS complexes and rate of 40 bpm suggests that the escape rhythm originate from ventricular muscle rather than the His bundle or proximal bundle branches and is therefore not reliable. Treatment with a permanent pacemaker is required, not only to improve symptoms but also to improve prognosis as there is a risk of the escape rhythm failing and ventricular standstill and an asystolic cardiac arrest. Slow, wide escape rhythms and syncope are worrying features that would warrant urgent pacemaker implant.

> **Box 21.1 Definition of bradycardia: a heart rate of <60 bpm**
>
> What are the different mechanisms of bradycardia and what simple tests can be performed in the surgery to obtain a diagnosis?
>
> - **Physiological bradycardia.** Young patients and athletic patients often have a resting bradycardia due to high vagal tone. It is not uncommon for elite athletes to have resting heart rates in the 40s and evidence of first- and second-degree block during sleep. This is not prognostically important and the key feature is the lack of symptoms and a normal increase in heart rate and conduction with physical exertion.
> - **Drug-induced sinus bradycardia.** Some cardiovascular drugs, particularly beta blockers but also diltiazem, verapamil and other antiarrhythmic drugs result in slowing of the sinus node rate at rest and during physical exertion. This may or may not result in symptoms.
> - **Sinus node dysfunction.** This may manifest as sinus pauses (causing pre-syncope or syncope), sinus bradycardia (causing lethargy and fatigue) and chronotropic incompetence on exercise (impaired exercise capacity) or tachy–brady syndrome (sinus pauses and paroxysmal atrial fibrillation). It may occur spontaneously in elderly patients and be exacerbated by drugs such as beta blockers.
> - **AV-node disease (heart block).** Second-degree (Mobitz type II) or third-degree (complete) heart block is the result of AV node or His–Purkinje disease. The ventricular rate is slower than the atrial rate and in the case of complete heart block is completely dissociated.
> - **Bigeminy or frequent ectopy.** Although not a true bradycardia, premature beats may be so weak (as the ventricles have not had time to fill) that they are not felt when palpating the radial pulse. In the case of atrial or ventricular bigeminy this will lead the examiner to think the heart rate is only half the actual ventricular rate.

The decision is therefore between urgent hospital admission for monitoring and inpatient pacemaker implant or arranging urgent day-case pacemaker implant for sometime in the next week.

She is sent to the local A&E for hospital admission. On arrival, her ECG is repeated and still shows complete heart block with a ventricular rate of 40 bpm. The A&E junior doctor wishes to insert a temporary pacing wire.

Should temporary pacing be performed?

No. Temporary pacing should only be performed if the bradycardia is causing significant haemodynamic compromise at rest (heart failure, chest pain, renal failure) or there are frequent or long episodes of ventricular standstill, resulting in syncope. Temporary pacing wires have a tendency to become infected or displaced and are often inserted by inexperienced individuals. These complications may result in significant morbidity and subsequently delay of permanent pacemaker implant. As long as she is on a cardiac monitor, significant bradycardia or an asystolic arrest can be witnessed and treated promptly. A permanent pacemaker needs to be organised.

What immediate action could be taken if an asystolic arrest occurred while awaiting permanent pacemaker implant?

An asystolic arrest should be treated with prompt cardiopulmonary resuscitation and basic life-support measure. Resuscitation guidelines recommend 1 mg adrenaline and 3 mg atropine i.v. It may be possible to perform transcutaneous pacing through an appropriately equipped defibrillator – this requires a very high output and also causes skeletal muscle contraction. If the patient regains consciousness it can be painful and distressing but it may provide respite while an urgent temporary pacing wire is inserted.

After an uneventful 48 hours, a permanent pacemaker is implanted. The operator implants a single right ventricular lead and programs the device to a heart rate of 60 bpm.

How does a pacemaker work? What complications need to be consented for?

A pacemaker system consists of a relatively small pulse generator (containing a battery, capacitor and the computer processor) and one or more pacing leads. Under local anaesthesia, the generator is implanted subcutaneously above the pectoralis muscle through a 3–5 cm incision. The leads are inserted into the cephalic or subclavian vein and passed under X-ray guidance into the right atrium and/or right ventricle where they become passively or actively attached to the endocardial surface. The pulse generator is attached to the lead(s) and the wound sutured shut.

A single-lead pacemaker is often called a 'demand' pacemaker. It is able to sense events within the paced chamber and deliver pacing stimuli to that chamber. They are programmable through wireless communication. The

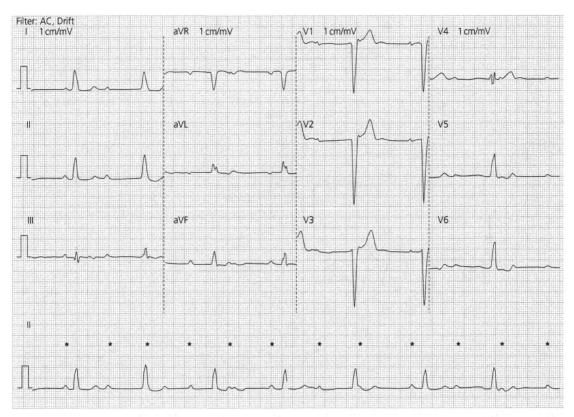

Figure 21.1 12-lead ECG of complete heart block. There is sinus rhythm, indicated by P-wave activity at a rate of 80 bpm (*).

pacemaker will not allow the heart rate to drop below the programmed minimum rate. Dual chamber pacemakers have two leads, one in the atrium and one in the ventricle. This allows atrial events to be sensed and the ventricle paced if the impulse does not conduct through the AV node, thereby keeping the two chambers in synchrony. Pacemakers may also have a rate-response function. Vibrations such as those caused by movement and exercise cause the pacemaker to increase the minimum heart rate, simulating the normal physiological response.

Complications include those at the time of the implant (haematoma 1–2%, infection 1%, pneumothorax 1%, cardiac tamponade <1% and lead dislodgement 2–5%) and late after implant lead fracture or infection.

As this woman received a single chamber ventricular pacemaker, rate response must be turned on otherwise the pacemaker will be a constant 60 bpm whether she is resting or active and walking. An alternative would have been to implant a dual-chamber pacemaker, which would increase the ventricular pacing rate as her sinus rate increased naturally.

She was successfully discharged from hospital. At her first pacemaker clinic follow-up appointment 4 weeks later she says that her exercise capacity had improved a little but she was aware of uncomfortable pulsation on fullness in the neck, dizziness and still some fatigue. Interrogation of the pacemaker shows normal sensing and pacing function.

As part of the check a 12-lead ECG is performed. What does it show?

The 12-lead ECG (Figure 21.2) shows single chamber ventricular pacing in VVI mode. Each QRS complex is preceded by a pacing spike (arrow). The ventricular rate is 60 bpm. There are also P waves visible which are dissociated from the ventricular paced rhythm. Note the right bundle branch block (RBBB) shape to the QRS complex, indicating a left ventricular pacing site.

What are the two diagnoses? What procedure will correct both of them?

• **Pacemaker syndrome.** This is due to the dissociation between atrial and ventricular contraction during

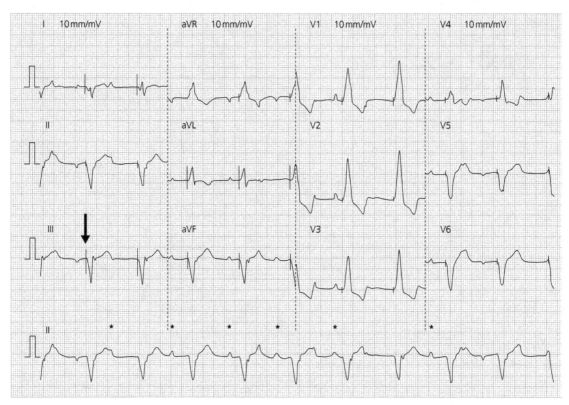

Figure 21.2 12-lead ECG showing single chamber ventricular pacing in VVI mode. Each QRS complex is preceded by a pacing spike (arrow). The ventricular rate is 60 bpm. P waves (*) are visible.

ventricular pacing. As the atriums are not synchronised to the ventricles they do not always contract during ventricular filling (diastole). There is reduced filling and therefore reduced cardiac output, resulting in fatigue and sometime dizzy spells. Intermittently, the atriums will actually contract at the same time as ventricular systole, when the tricuspid and mitral valves are shut. This sends pressure waves up into the internal jugular vein causing unpleasant neck pulsation. Between 7 and 20 % of patients with sinus rhythm and complete heart block who receive single lead ventricular pacemakers will suffer pacemaker syndrome. It can be overcome by implanting a dual-chamber pacemaker with atrial and ventricular leads, which allows the pacemaker to make sure atrial contraction is always followed by ventricular contraction after a programmable PR interval. Dual-chamber pacemakers are more expensive and are more likely to suffer complications; however, it is usually best to save single-chamber ventricular pacemakers for patients with atrial fibrillation, where atrial

pacing, sensing and synchronisation is no longer relevant.

• **The pacing lead is in the left ventricle.** This rare complication is usually due to the presence of an atrial septal defect or patent foramen ovale. The pacing lead accidentally crosses from the right to left atrium, then through the mitral valve into the left ventricle. At the time of implant this may give a normal fluoroscopic appearance. Although sensing and pacing may be normal, the presence of a pacing lead in the systemic circulation is a risk for thrombus formation and therefore a stroke. It may also cause ventricular tachycardia.

The appropriate treatment is removal of the ventricular pacing lead (which should be possible at this early stage using gentle traction), repositioning it in the right ventricle, insertion of an atrial lead and upgrading the generator to a dual-chamber device.

Examples of an ECG and CXR following dual-chamber pacemaker insertion are shown in Figures 21.3 and 21.4.

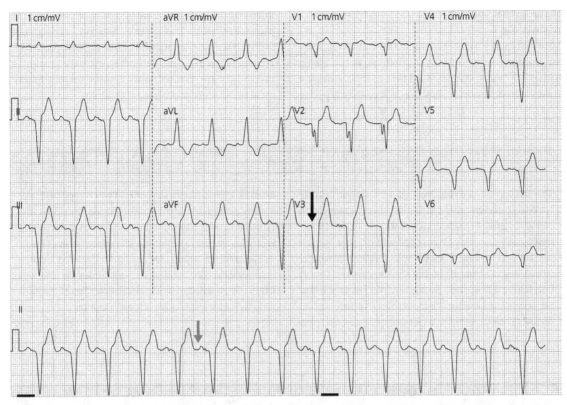

Figure 21.3 12-lead ECG showing correct atrial and ventricular pacing with a dual-chamber pacemaker in DDD mode. There is a P wave before every QRS complex. There is a small pacing spike in front of each P wave (seen best in lead II, grey arrow) and in front of each QRS complex (seen best in lead V3, black arrow). Note the left branch bundle block (LBBB) shape to the QRS complex, indicating a right ventricular pacing site.

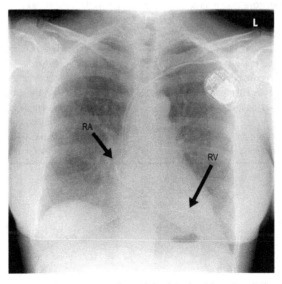

Figure 21.4 Chest radiograph showing a dual-chamber pacemaker with leads in the right atrium (RA) and right ventricle (RV) and a left pre-pectoral generator.

How often will she require outpatient follow-up?

Most pacemaker patients require an annual visit for interrogation of the device. As well as documenting battery life (and a recommended time to replacement) it is important to check lead function as occasionally pacing thresholds increase over time or sensing diminishes. The pacemaker may also detect hitherto undiagnosed arrhythmias, such as atrial fibrillation. Most pacemaker generators last 5–8 years depending upon the amount of pacing they are required to do and the use of sophisticated monitoring and pacing algorithms.

CASE REVIEW

This 77-year-old woman presents with fatigue and an episode of pre-syncope. Her basic physical examination reveals a resting bradycardia and complete heart block is subsequently confirmed with a 12-lead ECG. Her age and the lack of coexisting illness point to the cause being age-related degeneration of the His–Purkinje system. Urgent insertion of a temporary pacing wire was not required as her symptoms were not life threatening. As there was no reversible cause to treat, a permanent pacemaker was inserted. Unfortunately, she suffered two complications of a permanent pacemaker: the use of a single ventricular lead caused a failure of synchronisation between the atria and ventricles and led to symptoms known as pacemaker syndrome; and her ventricular pacing lead crossed a previously undiagnosed intra-atrial communication and was left in the left-sided, systemic circulation. These complications were corrected with a second operation

KEY POINTS

- Complete heart block may present with an insidious history of fatigue and lethargy or a dramatic, acute presentation of syncope and collapse.
- Complete heart block is usually irreversible, although occasionally conduction may improve after inferior myocardial infarction or if the heart block is the consequence of drugs or abnormal electrolytes.
- During heart block, the systolic and diastolic blood pressure readings are not a good measure of perfusion. The conscious level, peripheral perfusion, presence of symptoms and urine output are a better indicator of whether the escape rhythm is adequate to perfuse the vital organs.
- Temporary pacing wire insertion requires skills in both central venous access and manipulation of temporary pacing wires and should only be performed if absolutely necessary.
- Permanent pacing is the treatment of choice in complete heart block, usually with a dual-chamber pacemaker unless the patient has permanent atrial fibrillation or is infirm and immobile.
- Single-chamber pacemakers in patient with sinus rhythm cause adverse effects (pacemaker syndrome) in a significant minority.
- Post-operative checks after pacemaker implant include interrogation with the programmer to check lead parameters (including lead stability, pacing and sensing), a 12-lead ECG to document appropriate function and QRS morphology, and a CXR to record lead position and exclude pneumothorax.

Case 22   A 57-year-old man with collapse

The wife of a 57-year-old man calls an emergency ambulance when her husband collapses at home. He was unconscious for 30 seconds but when the paramedics arrived he had regained consciousness but felt extremely unwell with breathlessness, chest pain and dizziness. They rush him to A&E, which is only 5 minutes away.

What should be done on arrival?

Initially, vital signs should be assessed to decide how promptly any treatment is required.
• General appearance and conscious level. Is he pale, sweaty, peripherally shut down and cool to touch? Is he alert and orientated and able to communicate?
• Pulse, blood pressure, respiratory rate and oxygen saturations.
If someone appears to be shocked and severely compromised, urgent action is required.

His pulse is 210 bpm; blood pressure 80/50 mmHg; O₂ saturations on 4 L/min via a face mask are 90%. He is pale, clammy, cool and very breathless, only able to speak single words rather than whole sentences. His chest is uncomfortable. There are a few sparse inspiratory crackles at his lung bases.

What is the likely cause of his condition? What is the next step?

He has a tachycardia that is too fast to be sinus tachycardia and is therefore likely to be an abnormal rhythm resulting in severe haemodynamic compromise. A 12-lead ECG should be performed to diagnose the rhythm and guide treatment. A cardiac monitor can be used to confirm the heart rate and help identify the rhythm;

however, 12-lead ECGs are more detailed and better at distinguishing broad-complex from narrow-complex tachycardia and determining the underlying tachycardia mechanism.

What does his 12-lead ECG show?

The 12-lead ECG (Figure 22.1) shows a wide-complex tachycardia. The QRS duration is 150 ms, rate 210 bpm, with independent P-wave activity (VA dissociation, the P wave indicated by the arrows). There is positive concordance across the chest leads (all QRS complexes are positive). The regular rhythm rules out atrial fibrillation.

What are the differential diagnoses of broad-complex tachycardia?

The differential diagnoses of broad-complex tachycardias are:
• **Ventricular tachycardia**.
• **Supraventricular arrhythmias** (SVTs, atrial tachycardia, atrial flutter) with aberrant conduction (bundle branch block).
• **Antidromic tachycardia in Wolff-Parkinson-White syndrome**.

The heart rate and degree of compromise do not help to distinguish ventricular tachycardia from SVT. There are certain ECG characteristics (Box 22.1) that help to make the diagnosis of ventricular tachycardia from SVT with bundle branch block; however, these are often hard to remember. It is easier to assume that a broad-complex tachycardia is ventricular in origin and 90% of the time you will be correct. The likelihood of it being ventricular tachycardia increases if there is a history of heart disease, particularly prior myocardial infarction. It is better to mistreat SVT as ventricular tachycardia, than the other way round.

The independent P waves give a diagnosis of ventricular tachycardia

Cardiology: Clinical Cases Uncovered. By T. Betts, J. Dwight and S. Bull. Published 2010 by Blackwell Publishing.

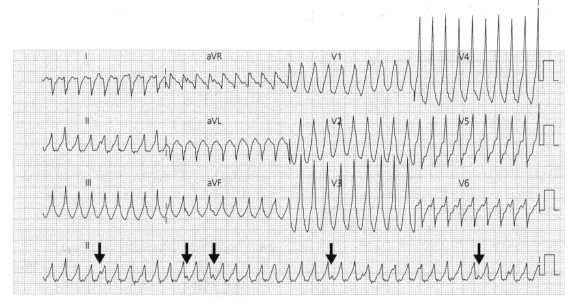

Figure 22.1 12-lead ECG of a wide-complex tachycardia. The QRS duration is 150 ms, rate 210 bpm, with independent P-wave activity (ventricular–atrial dissociation, the P wave indicated by the arrows).

> **Box 22.1 Broad-complex tachycardia features that indicate a ventricular origin**
>
> - Independent P wave activity (dissociated P waves).
> - Fusion or capture beats.
> - Negative concordance across chest leads.
> - Onset of QRS to nadir of S wave >0.1 second in any chest lead.

What are the immediate treatment options?

- **Adenosine i.v.** This may be administered if it is felt that SVT is the most likely diagnosis as it may terminate the tachycardia; however, it will have no impact on ventricular tachycardia.
- **Verapamil i.v.** This may terminate SVT but will cause severe haemodynamic compromise if the diagnosis is ventricular tachycardia. Verapamil should **not** be given.
- **Lidocaine i.v. bolus.** This is no longer in up-to-date resuscitation guidelines and is generally ineffective. Lidocaine is a negative inotrope and may cause a further fall in blood pressure.
- **Amiodarone i.v. 300 mg bolus over 20–60 minutes.** Although this does appear in guidelines it is

not evidence based and only 15–20% of patients will go back into sinus rhythm within 1 hour of administration. Amiodarone is also a negative inotrope.

- **External DC cardioversion.** This is the treatment of choice for severely compromised patients as it will promptly restore sinus rhythm whether the tachycardia is ventricular, junctional or atrial in origin.

A 12-mg bolus of i.v. adenosine has no effect. The patient's blood pressure is now 70/40 mmHg and he is so breathless he can no longer speak. It is elected to perform urgent DC cardioversion.

How should urgent cardioversion be performed?

External cardioversion is a painful therapy and requires deep sedation or general anaesthesia if the patient is conscious. In a compromised patient, expert airway management is required, which usually requires an anaesthetist. The anaesthetic team should be summoned urgently. Defibrillation takes place using external paddles that may be stuck on to the chest and operated remotely or held there by the operator. They should be positioned with one on the right of the sternum below the clavicle and the other in the left mid-axillary line. A single 150 J biphasic or 200 J monophasic synchronised shock should be delivered, making sure no one is in contact with the patient and that any oxygen delivered through a face mask is turned off.

A single synchronised 150 J biphasic shock restores sinus rhythm at 90 bpm. His blood pressure increases to 95/55 mmHg.

What should be done next? What are the potential causes of his arrhythmia?

Further supportive measures may be required. If there is still cardiogenic shock despite restoration of sinus rhythm, then inotrope infusions may be required (although positive inotropes may provoke further arrhythmias). A basic history and examination should be undertaken to identify the cause of the tachycardia. A 12-lead ECG should be performed. Bloods should be taken for electrolytes and cardiac enzymes.

Potential causes of the tachycardia are:
• **Acute myocardial infarction.** If there is evidence of acute infarction or ischaemia, prompt treatment may be required. This would be suggested by a history of chest pain *prior to* the onset of collapse and tachycardia, and the presence of ST-segment elevation or depression on the sinus rhythm ECG. If ST-segment elevation is present, particularly if there is a history of preceding chest pain, then reperfusion with thrombolysis or primary angioplasty is indicated. Although monomorphic ventricular tachycardia can happen in the setting of acute ischaemia, ventricular fibrillation is the more common ventricular arrhythmia.
• **Old myocardial infarction.** Left ventricular scarring from prior myocardial infarction (ischaemic cardiomyopathy) is probably the most common cause of monomorphic ventricular tachycardia. A minority of patients will not have a known history of myocardial infarction as they did not present to hospital at the time (mistaking the pain for indigestion) or had silent infarctions (e.g. diabetics).
• **Non-ischaemic cardiomyopathy.** Dilated, right ventricular and hypertrophic cardiomyopathies may have their initial presentation as a ventricular arrhythmia or with sudden cardiac death.
• **Idiopathic ventricular tachycardia.** There are two forms of idiopathic ventricular tachycardia that occur in structurally normal hearts – right ventricular outflow tract tachycardia (a LBBB morphology with inferior axis on ECG) and fascicular tachycardia (also known as verapamil-sensitive idiopathic left ventricular tachycardia or

Belhassen's ventricular tachycardia with a RBBB morphology and left-axis deviation on ECG). Typically, they would present in young adults who are otherwise fit and well.
• **Severe electrolyte abnormalities.** Profound hypo- or hyperkalaemia may present as a ventricular arrhythmia although usually this is polymorphic ventricular tachycardia or ventricular fibrillation.
• **Drug toxicity.** Certain classes of drugs (class I antiarrhythmics, digoxin, antidepressants, etc.) may cause ventricular arrhythmias at toxic doses.

A brief history reveals that the patient is a diabetic on regular insulin injections and has hypertension treated with a thiazide diuretic. Although there is no known history of ischaemic heart disease, 2 months earlier he had 2 days of intermittent chest pain with nausea that he attributed to indigestion and he did not seek medical advice. Since then he has had less energy and mild exertional breathlessness, despite having a sedentary life style. His collapse today occurred without warning and with no preceding chest pain. On examination, there are no murmurs or bruits; however, there is a third heart sound and there are a few crackles in his lung bases. O₂ saturations are 90% on the face mask. The 12- lead ECG shows sinus rhythm with anterior Q waves and poor R-wave progression across the chest leads. His blood tests show sodium 132 mmol/L (normal range 3.5–5.0); potassium 3.6 mmol/L (normal range 3.5–5.0); urea 7.8 mmol/L (normal range 2.5–6.7); creatinine 132 μmol/L (normal range 70–150).

Would you administer any other immediate treatment? What is the next step? Which investigations will you request?

• He still has signs of pulmonary oedema (low oxygen saturations and crackles in his lung bases) and it is important to maximise myocardial oxygen delivery so a bolus of **loop diuretic** such as furosemide should be given. His serum potassium is relatively low, possibly as a consequence of his thiazide diuretic although a hyperadrenergic state can also lower it.
• The role for **immediate drug therapy** is debatable. At some point he will require beta-blocker therapy but as he has signs of pulmonary oedema it would be sensible to wait until he is more stable before starting. There is often a reflex action to administer a bolus of amiodarone after successful cardioversion, 'just in case' the arrhythmia returns. There are no guidelines or recommendations to

support its use in this instance and the majority of patients will only suffer a single episode of ventricular tachycardia in one admission. Intravenous Amiodarone may lower his blood pressure further.

• He should be transferred to a high-dependency monitored bed, such as a coronary care unit, where he can be placed on **telemetry** whilst awaiting further investigations.

• Subsequent inpatient investigations should be:

   ○ An **echocardiogram** to assess cardiac structure and function, particularly the left ventricle.

   ○ **Coronary angiography** to look for evidence of ischaemic heart disease, not only to obtain a diagnosis but to see whether revascularisation using stents or surgery is appropriate

On arrival at the CCU an echocardiogram is performed and shows a dilated left ventricle with anterolateral thinning and hypokinesia (consistent with an old infarction) and no significant valve disease. During the echocardiogram he suddenly feels faint, breathless and has chest tightness. His cardiac monitor shows a broad-complex tachycardia identical to that in A&E at 210 bpm. His blood pressure falls to 75/40 mmHg.

How should this be treated? Is there anything different you would do from the previous episode? Which drugs would you consider?

Another DC cardioversion is required, necessitating another urgent call for the anaesthetic team. As the ventricular tachycardia is now recurrent, it is advisable to start antiarrhythmic therapy to prevent more attacks. The drug of choice is amiodarone as it is probably slightly more effective than lidocaine and less of a negative inotrope in someone you now know has impaired left ventricular function. Amiodarone can be administered while waiting for the anaesthetic team to arrive to perform the cardioversion. It is also important to check that the potassium has been corrected and is in the upper portion of the normal range (i.e. 4.5–5.0 mmol/L). Magnesium may also be administered as an antiarrhythmic, particularly if patients take potassium-losing diuretics. It is given as i.v. magnesium sulphate 8 mmol (4 mL of a 50% solution)

How should the amiodarone be administered?

Intravenous amiodarone can cause severe skin necrosis if it leaks from a peripheral cannula into the subcutaneous

tissues, thus it is usually recommended that it is administered through a central venous line. However, in an emergency there may not be time or the expertise available to insert a central line so the initial bolus can be administered through a newly sited large-bore cannula. It may be given as 300 mg over 1 hour or 150 mg over 20 minutes, repeated if necessary. After 300 mg is given, a maintenance infusion of 900 mg over the next 23 hours can be set up, ideally through a central line.

A 150-mg bolus of amiodarone and 8 mmol magnesium is administered with no effect. A second DC cardioversion is performed, which restores sinus rhythm. A right internal jugular central venous line is inserted and the second 150-mg bolus and maintenance infusion of amiodarone is given.

The patient is stable for the next 12 hours; however, ventricular tachycardia occurs once again with a similar degree of haemodynamic compromise. The anaesthetic team are called again and a third DC cardioversion performed.

What further action needs to be considered? What additional preventative and therapeutic treatments can be offered?

The patient now has what is classified as a 'ventricular tachycardia storm', i.e. more than two episodes in the space of 24 hours. This is despite amiodarone therapy. He has required three external cardioversions, each with anaesthetic support. He needs to be treated in a specialist cardiac unit.

The following treatment strategies should be considered.

Additional drug therapy

• A further bolus of amiodarone 300 mg while continuing the maintenance infusion.

• Oral beta blockers, providing his blood pressure will tolerate them and there is no overt pulmonary oedema.

Insertion of a transvenous right ventricular temporary pacing wire

This may be performed through the internal jugular, subclavian or femoral vein under X-ray guidance. Being able to pace the right ventricle means that overdrive (anti-tachycardia) pacing can be used to terminate ventricular tachycardia at the bedside, avoiding the need for general anaesthesia or external shocks. During tachycardia the pacemaker box is programmed to a rate 20–30 bpm faster than the ventricular tachycardia at a high output. Pacing is initiated until the QRS morphology changes and the monitored heart rate increases to the pacing rate, indicating capture. Once there have been 8–12 captured paced beats the pacing is abruptly terminated. Overdrive pacing can terminate 80–85% of monomorphic ventricular tachycardias; however, it is ineffective against polymorphic ventricular tachycardia or ventricular fibrillation. There is a small risk that overdrive pacing may accelerate the tachycardia into one that causes loss of consciousness or ventricular fibrillation, therefore a defibrillator must be immediately available. After ventricular tachycardia has been terminated, constant ventricular pacing at 90–100 bpm may prevent ectopy and ventricular tachycardia initiation; however, this will also result in the loss of synchrony between the atriums and ventricles, which may reduce cardiac output.

Urgent coronary angiography

Recurrent ventricular tachycardia may be a manifestation of critical ischaemia due to a severe stenosis in the proximal portion of a coronary artery. If so, revascularisation with a stent or surgery is appropriate. It is advisable only to undertake angiography in this situation if immediate revascularisation is available if required.

Insertion of an intra-aortic balloon pump

Not only will this improve coronary artery flow, it will also reduce the afterload. Both of these effects will improve the ration of myocardial oxygen delivery to myocardial oxygen demand, which in turn may help prevent arrhythmias.

Intubation and ventilation

This may serve a number of purposes. If the patient is in persistent pulmonary oedema with poor oxygenation, ventilation may improve oxygen delivery. Patients receiving frequent shocks are usually in a hyperadrenergic state, which may be pro-arrhythmic, and deep sedation may reduce circulating catecholamine levels. Also, if there is a need for frequent external cardioversion it may be appropriate to have the patient under constant general anaesthesia. The downside of general anaesthesia is that there may be a further decrease in blood pressure. Intubation and ventilation is usually reserved for patients

with ventricular fibrillation storms or ventricular tachycardia that does not respond to overdrive pacing.

Ventricular tachycardia ablation

Ventricular tachycardia ablation can be performed in specialist centres. This is best performed when there is a single, monomorphic tachycardia.

He is given 25 mg of oral metoprolol, a further 300 mg of amiodarone over 1 hour and a temporary pacing wire is inserted from the right femoral vein. Coronary angiography demonstrates a chronically occluded LAD artery that is filled retrogradely by collaterals from the RCA. The left Cx artery and RCA have only minor plaque disease. There is no scope for revascularisation.

Over the next 24 hours he has two episodes of ventricular tachycardia that are successfully terminated with overdrive pacing. He then goes 72 hours without any further arrhythmias. The temporary pacing wire is removed and his amiodarone infusion is stopped and oral amiodarone (200 mg tds) is commenced. His metoprolol is increased to 5 mg tds and his thiazide diuretic is stopped and an ACE inhibitor successfully started.

What should be done before hospital discharge?

This patient satisfies the secondary prevention criteria for an ICD as he has had haemodynamically-compromising ventricular tachycardia, has ischaemic heart disease and poor left ventricular function and has no reversible cause that can be treated. This should be inserted before hospital discharge. One of the contraindications for ICD implant is incessant or very frequent ventricular arrhythmias as it will result in the patient receiving frequent shocks, perhaps on a daily basis. If his ventricular tachycardia had not settled, adjunctive treatment would have been required to target the problematic ventricular tachycardia. When drugs have failed to do this, the alternative is catheter ablation. In experienced hands, this offers a 70–80% chance of eradicating or dramatically reducing the incidence of that particular tachycardia; however, as the ventricle is scarred ablation does not guarantee that another ventricular tachycardia circuit will not arise and cause subsequent life-threatening arrhythmias. Ablation and drugs are not a substitute for the ICD in this setting.

CASE REVIEW

This 57-year-old man presented in severe shock as a result of a sudden-onset broad-complex tachycardia. The ECG had typical features of ventricular tachycardia. Intravenous adenosine had no effect and sinus rhythm was initially restored with a 150 J biphasic shock. His history suggested a background of ischaemic heart disease with remote myocardial infarction but no acute ischaemia. An echocardiogram later that day confirmed poor left ventricular function. He had two further episodes of ventricular tachy-cardia within the next 24 hours, all requiring cardioversion. Administration of beta blockers and amiodarone and correction of any electrolyte imbalance was not immediately effective, so he underwent urgent coronary angiography to look for critical coronary artery disease and insertion of a temporary pacing wire to use for overdrive pacing of further ventricular tachycardia episodes. Once the ventricular tachycardia storm had settled he underwent insertion of an ICD.

KEY POINTS

- More than 90% of broad-complex tachycardias (QRS interval >120 ms) are ventricular in origin. If the patient is known to have ischaemic heart disease or heart failure, that percentage is even higher.
- If in doubt, assume a broad-complex tachycardia is ventricular.
- Tachycardia treatment should be guided by the patient's clinical status. With ventricular tachycardia however, stable patients may deteriorate rapidly.
- For any haemodynamically-compromising broad-complex tachycardia the most appropriate treatment is restoration of sinus rhythm with external DC cardioversion. Pharmacological cardioversion with intravenous antiarrhythmic medication should not be attempted in this situation. In very stable patients, i.v. adenosine may be administered for diagnostic purposes, although it will be ineffective for ventricular tachycardia.

- The definition of a 'ventricular tachycardia storm' varies, but can be taken to be three or more episodes of sustained ventricular tachycardia in a 24-hour period. Nowadays, it is most commonly encountered in patients with ICDs who receive multiple shocks.
- During ventricular tachycardia storms, any reversible underlying cause should be identified and treated. Cardiac function and myocardial oxygen delivery should be optimised.
- Ventricular tachycardia storms may settle with drug therapy (amiodarone and beta blockers) and shocks for ventricular tachycardia may be avoided by the use of overdrive pacing.
- Ventricular tachycardia storms should be managed in specialist cardiac centres where invasive procedures such as intra-aortic balloon pump insertion, coronary intervention or, if necessary, radiofrequency ablation are readily available.

Case 23 — A 36-year-old woman with a family history of sudden death

A 36-year-old woman is referred to the cardiology clinic by her GP. Her brother, who was 2 years older, was recently found dead in his home gym. He had been fit and well and exercised regularly. She and her GP are concerned that there may be a familial problem.

What are the important questions to ask in the initial history?

First ask questions about her history:
• Does she have any cardiovascular symptoms, i.e. palpitations, chest pain or breathlessness? In particular, has she ever had syncope? Does she have any past medical history?

Then ask about her brother:
• Did he have any history of cardiac symptoms, including blackouts? Was he a smoker or have any known risk factors for cardiovascular disease?
• Was an autopsy done? What was the official cause of death?

Then ask about her other family members:
• Has anyone else died unexpectedly? Are there any medical conditions that other family members have?

Sudden unexplained death in adults is often called (and assumed to be) sudden cardiac death (SCD). In people over 60 years, the most common cause is ischaemic heart disease and acute myocardial infarction causing a ventricular arrhythmia; however, this is less common in younger people, when other forms of cardiac disease are more likely. It is extremely important to get autopsy data. An autopsy should have been performed as the death was unexpected and the cause unknown and therefore required for issue of a death certificate. If no structural heart disease is seen (coronary artery disease, myocardial disease or valvular heart disease) and the

heart appears to be structurally normal, a primary arrhythmia is assumed to be the cause of death. Autopsies will also uncover other causes such as aortic dissection, pulmonary embolism and subarachnoid haemorrhage.

She tells you that she is fit and healthy with no symptoms. She is a keen runner and has completed two marathons. She does not smoke or drink alcohol. Her brother had also been very fit and well. She vaguely remembers him fainting once or twice at school when he was younger. Her brother did have an autopsy and she thinks that nothing out of the ordinary was found. Her father died unexpectedly at the age of 32 years (when she was only 3 years old) and thinks that they were told he had suffered a heart attack. Tragically, her first child, who was born 3 years ago, died at the age of 4 months from a 'cot death'. She has one other older sister who is well and has two healthy children and a younger step-brother (her mother subsequently remarried).

Her physical examination is unremarkable.

What are the important points in her history and how should they be interpreted?

Often a patient's knowledge of family member's medical history is vague and they use lay terminology that could be misrepresentative. The fact that she is fit and asymptomatic is initially reassuring, but then again, so was her brother. His previous faints could be important as they may represent a more sinister cardiac cause such as an arrhythmia (which subsequently resulted in his death). He was in his home gym when he died so the mechanism could be exercise related. If her understanding of the autopsy is correct then it effectively rules out conditions with structural heart disease, such as coronary artery disease, cardiomyopathies or valve disease, providing the autopsy was conducted by an experienced pathologist with a knowledge of cardiac conditions causing sudden death.

Cardiology: Clinical Cases Uncovered. By T. Betts, J. Dwight and S. Bull. Published 2010 by Blackwell Publishing.

Her father's death at an early age is also very unusual. Thirty years ago a post-mortem may not have been done and it was more common to assume sudden deaths were due to myocardial infarction. Even if an autopsy was done and an alternative cardiac diagnosis made, the explanation to the family and subsequent description to the children could have been mislabelled as a 'heart attack' due to its general application as a lay term.

The death of her child is also very worrying. As an isolated event, the term 'cot death' or 'sudden infant death syndrome' is appropriate, but when put into the context of her full family history, an inherited condition is more likely.

On the assumption that this may be an inherited cardiac condition, what are the differential diagnoses?
Cardiomyopathies
• Hypertrophic cardiomyopathy is the commonest cause of SCDs in people <35 years of age. Its prevalence is 1:500, and many are asymptomatic and SCD can be the first presentation. Symptoms include exertional breathlessness, chest tightness and palpitations. There may be a systolic murmur, either from an associated left ventricular outflow tract gradient or mitral regurgitation (MR). There may be left ventricular hypertrophy (LVH) or T-wave changes on the ECG. The diagnostic test is echocardiography. It may be inherited in an autosomal dominant fashion.

• Arrhythmogenic right ventricular cardiomyopathy/dysplasia is the second most common cause of sudden cardiac death in the young. This disease is characterised by fibrous and fatty infiltration of the right ventricle. It may cause heart failure and ventricular arrhythmias. It is often inherited in an autosomal dominant fashion. Diagnosis can be difficult and requires a combination of clinical, ECG and imaging (MRI or echocardiogram) findings and histology from tissue biopsy or autopsy.

• Dilated cardiomyopathy may be familial in as may as 20–30% of cases through a wide variety of gene abnormalities. It typically presents with heart failure symptoms but may also result in ventricular arrhythmias (and rarely heart block). It is diagnosed on imaging (usually echocardiography) and the exclusion of coronary artery disease by angiography.

Coronary artery disease
• Familial hyperlipidaemia or hypercholesterolaemia is associated with extremely high cholesterol and LDL levels, resulting in premature atherosclerosis. It is autosomal dominant. Heterozygous familial hypercholesterolemia is found in 1:500 people. Common signs are peripheral stigmata, such as corneal arcus, xanthelasmatas and xanthomas.

Arrhythmias (ion channelopathies) (Table 23.1)
• LQTS has a number of variants (types 1–5), the most common being long QT types 1 (which include Romano-Ward syndrome) and 2. It is due to abnormalities in cardiac myocyte potassium channels (or in long QT type 3 in the sodium channel), resulting in prolonged ventricular repolarisation. It is often autosomal dominant, although a rare form associated with deafness (Jervell Lange-Nielsen syndrome) is autosomal recessive. The classic arrhythmia is Torsades de Pointes (a form of polymorphic ventricular tachycardia) that can cause syncope or death. The heart is otherwise structurally normal on examination. Arrhythmias in types 1 and 2 are associated with exertion or stress, whereas type 3 is associated with sleep.

• Brugada syndrome is a rare abnormality of the cardiac myocyte sodium channel than can cause ventricular tachycardia or fibrillation. It typically affects males in their fourth or fifth decade and manifests as blackouts or cardiac arrest during sleep. There is a characteristic ECG pattern of incomplete RBBB and ST-segment elevation in leads V1–V3; however, this appearance may be intermittent or latent. The heart is otherwise structurally normal. It is a highly lethal condition that does not respond to drug therapy and if symptomatic, patients require an ICD.

• Other, much less common familial conditions are catecholaminergic polymorphic ventricular tachycardia (blackouts or death during exertion), Lev-Lenegre's syndrome (gradual development of heart block) and Wolf-Parkinson-White syndrome with pre-excited atrial fibrillation (although this is rarely familial).

If one of these familial conditions is present in the family, what is the likelihood that she has the abnormal gene?
If her father and brother died of one of the above conditions it is likely to be inherited in an autosomal dominant fashion, therefore she has a 50% chance of having the gene. If her own baby died of the same condition, it must have received the gene from her, meaning she must also be affected.

Table 23.1 Arrhythmias (ion channelopathies)

Condition	Prevalence	ECG abnormality	Classic features	Genetic abnormality	Drug challenge or provocative tests to diagnose and guide treatment	Treatment options
LQTS	1:10000	QTc >0.44 (men) or 0.45 (women) +/- abnormal T-wave morphology	Syncope or cardiac arrest due to Torsades de Pointes, occurring with exertion (LQT1), loud noises or startles (LQT2) or rest (LQT3)	LQT1: KCNQ1 LQT2: HERG, KCNH2 LQT3: SCN5A Usually autosomal dominant	Adrenaline challenge or exercise test may show abnormal prolongation of QT interval rather than shortening in LQT1. Genetic testing has a 70% yield	Beta blockers for LQT1 and 2. Pacemaker for bradycardia-dependent arrhythmias and LQT3. ICD for high-risk patients (see Table 23.2). Left cervicothoracic stellectomy for LQT1 with recurrent events despite treatment
Brugada syndrome	Unknown. Possibly causes 4–10 sudden deaths per 100000 per year	Incomplete RBBB and ST-segment elevation in leads V1–V3. May be manifest, dynamic or latent	Male female. Usually middle aged. Syncope or cardiac arrest, often at rest or sleep	20–30% have SCN5A mutation. 50% familial with autosomal dominant	Class 1C antiarrhythmics (ajmaline, flecainide) may unmask latent ECG changes. EP study to induce ventricular arrhythmias may help risk stratify	ICD in high-risk patients
Catecholaminergic VT	Unknown, but rare	Usually normal at rest	Exercise or stress-induced polymorphic VT, syncope or death, usually in children	30% familial. Autosomal dominant (cardiac ryanodine receptor gene) or recessive (calsequestrin gene)	Exercise test. Adrenaline challenge	Beta blockers +/- ICD

ECG, electrocardiogram; EP, electrophysiology; ICD, implantable cardioverter defibrillator; LQTS, long-QT syndrome; QTc, corrected QT calculated by Bazett's formula; RBBB, right branch bundle block; VT, ventricular tachycardia.

What investigations and enquires need to be made?

• It is very important to see the official **autopsy** report on the brother. The father's cause of death on his death certificate needs to be confirmed and an enquiry made to see if he had an autopsy.

• A **12-lead ECG** to look for a prolonged QT interval (LQTS]), left ventricular hypertrophy (hypertrophic cardiomyopathy), ST elevation and incomplete RBBB in leads V1–V3 (Brugada syndrome), ventricular pre-excitation (Wolf-Parkinson-White syndrome), an Epsilon wave (arrhythmogenic right ventricular cardiomyopathy) or conduction disease.

• A **transthoracic echocardiogram** to look for cardiomyopathies, in particular hypertrophic cardiomyopathy.

What does her 12-lead ECG show?

The 12-lead ECG (Figure 23.1) shows sinus rhythm, a normal QRS morphology and duration but abnormally shaped and prolonged T waves. The QT interval should be measured from the beginning of the QRS complex to the end of the T wave in the lead that gives the longest value. As the QT interval naturally shortens at faster heart rates it should be corrected using Bazett's formula (the QT interval measured in seconds is divided by the square root of the preceding R–R interval measured in seconds).

The QT interval in this 12-lead ECG, measured from the beginning of the QRS to the end of the T wave, is 0.52 seconds. When corrected for the rate (divided by the square root of the R–R interval of 1.22 seconds) the corrected QT interval is 0.47 seconds. The upper limit of normal is 0.44 for men and 0.45 for women.

The echocardiogram is normal.

What is the diagnosis and how sure can you be?

The diagnosis is LQTS (Box 23.1). There is not an absolute cut-off between normal and abnormal, but the greater the corrected QT is above 0.45 seconds, the more likely it is due to a gene abnormality. If it is >0.5 seconds, it is definitely very abnormal. Conversely, a small proportion of people with an abnormal gene will have a corrected QT interval of 0.4–0.45 seconds. If this was an isolated finding with no symptoms or family history, there may be some doubt as to its relevance; however, the terrible family history of sudden death makes the diagnosis extremely likely. Table 23.2 gives some markers of high risk of LQTS.

Where there is uncertainty due to a corrected QT interval of 0.43–0.47, additional testing may be helpful. Holter monitoring, particularly at night when the heart rate is slow, may show more dramatic QT prolongation when corrected for rate. An adrenaline infusion challenge or exercise test may cause abnormal prolongation of

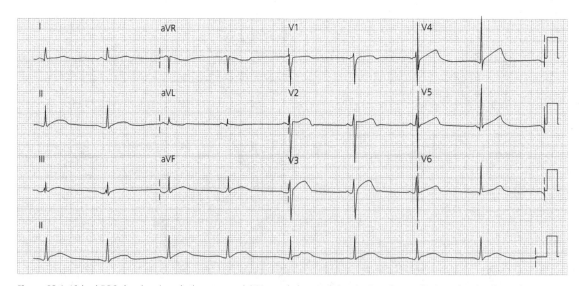

Figure 23.1 12-lead ECG showing sinus rhythm, a normal QRS morphology and duration but abnormally shaped and prolonged T waves.

Box 25.1 Long-QT syndrome (LQTS)

LQTS is present in approximately 1 : 10 000 of the population. Some patients may be asymptomatic through life; others may have their first arrhythmia episode as an infant. Indeed, long QT syndrome may be one of the causes of cot death. The diagnosis is not always straight-forward as there are many causes of syncope; some people have longer than normal QT intervals but no gene abnormality, whereas some long-QT-gene carriers have near normal QT intervals on their ECGs. Patients with the most common form, long QT type 1 (a potassium channel abnormality), tend to have the most frequent arrhythmia events, which tend to occur with exertion, stress or swimming, but only a minority result in sudden death, so they often present with multiple syncopal episodes. Patients with long QT type 3 (a sodium channel abnormality) have very infrequent episodes, which tend to occur at rest or sleep but a significant proportion are fatal.

Criterion		Points
*ECG findings**		
QTc (ms) †	>480	3
	460–470	2
	450 in male patient	1
Torsades de Pointes ‡		2
T-wave alternans		1
Notched T waves in three leads		1
Low heart rate for age §		0.5
Clinical history		
Syncope	With stress‡	2
	Without stress	1
Congenital deafness		0.5
Family history¶		
A. Family members with definite LQTS #		1
B. Unexplained sudden cardiac death <30 years in an immediate family member		0.5

*In the absence of medications or disorders known to affect these electrocardiographic features.
† QTc is corrected QT calculated by Bazett's formula.
‡ Torsades de Pointes and syncope with stress are mutually exclusive.
§ Resting heart rate below the second percentile for the age.
¶ The same family member cannot be counted in A and B.
# Definite LQTS is defined by an LQTS score of more than 3 (>4).

Table 23.2 Markers of high risk in long-QT syndrome (LQTS) patients

QT-interval duration for patients with type 1 or 2 – longer intervals are higher risk, especially if >500 ms

Homozygous syndromes such as Jervell Lange-Nielson syndrome

Syncope

Prior cardiac arrest (relative risk of 12.9 of experiencing another cardiac arrest)

Male sex in long QT type 3

the QT interval in patients with long QT types 1 and 2.

What should be done next? What treatment can be offered?

Drug treatment

Beta blockers, principally nadolol, have been shown to be very effective in the most common forms of LQTS, types 1 and 2, where symptoms are often associated with exercise, emotional outbursts or being startled. It is important to prescribe a dose that achieves an effect, as measured by a blunting of the heart rate response to exercise. Unfortunately, many patients do not like the side-effects of fatigue and reduced exercise capacity that may accompany beta blockers.

ICD

Although beta blockers may dramatically reduce events, they cannot guarantee freedom from cardiac arrest. An ICD can offer life-saving shock therapy in the event of a lethal arrhythmia. Unfortunately, they come at a cost, particularly in young people where there will be a life-long need for generator changes and potentially lead revisions. They also have a significant chance of inappropriate shocks for sinus tachycardia, despite programming and beta blocker use. The decision to implant an ICD in a long-QT patient is influenced by a number of factors (Table 23.3).

Advice regarding physical activity

Certain sports are associated with ventricular arrhythmias in LQTS, particularly water sports. Patients should never swim unobserved. High-intensity exercise (sprinting, squash, tennis, football) should be avoided. Light jogging or cycling and use of treadmills and exercise bikes

Table 23.3 defibrillator (ICD) implantation in patients with long-QT syndrome (LQTS)

Previous cardiac arrest.

Syncope or ventricular tachycardia while taking beta blockers.

Possibly as primary prevention for patients with higher-risk genotypes, e.g. type 2 or especially type 3.

---

is probably alright and walking and golf are considered safe.

Advice regarding drug interactions

Patients with LQTS should avoid QT-prolonging drugs (various antibiotics, antipsychotics and antiarrhythmics). A comprehensive list is available through patient organisations and on websites, e.g. www.sads.org.uk/drugs_to_avoid.htm.

Family screening

Having identified a familial condition, other family members need to be screened. Her older sister requires an ECG. If obviously normal, she is not a carrier and her children do not need screening. If her late brother has children, they also need screening with ECGs. It is extremely likely that the gene came from her father; however, it would be prudent to screen her mother with an ECG to rule her out. Her step-brother is probably not affected as he has a different father and only needs screening if the mother's ECG is abnormal. If her late father has any siblings, they too should be screened.

Genetic testing

This is not always readily available but fortunately is emerging as a useful tool. It is most useful when there are a number of affected family members (as demonstrated by symptoms or phenotypic appearances) and a condition in which a few simple gene abnormalities are known. In this particular setting it may help identify which type of LQTS she has, which would guide the use of beta blockers or an ICD. If a gene abnormality was identified, then it could be used to screen all current and future family members, giving a definite yes or no answer as to whether they were carriers. This would be important for any future children she may have.

She starts regular nadolol 80 mg od. She is unhappy about the mild side-effects but agrees to continue taking the medication. She declines to have an ICD as she is

asymptomatic and now on beta-blocker treatment and she is concerned about the risk of inappropriate shocks. She no longer runs competitively but attends a gym for light aerobic exercise instead. Six months later she returns to clinic and says she is 12 weeks' pregnant. She is feeling very tired and lethargic and asks about stopping her medication.

What would you advise about beta blockers in pregnancy?

The protective benefits of beta blockers in preventing life-threatening arrhythmias need to be balanced against the potential harm to the foetus. Beta blockers have been reported to cause intrauterine growth retardation; however, it is extremely rare. There are published registries of long-QT patients taking beta blockers through pregnancy, none of which reports harm to the foetus. As the potential consequences of an arrhythmia could be fatal, for LQTS women continuation of treatment is advised. Increased monitoring of foetal growth with ultrasound would hopefully identify any problems early on so action could be taken. After delivery it should be mentioned that beta blockers will be secreted in breast milk; however, it is usually in such small concentrations that the baby is unaffected.

She is unsure and due to side-effects and concern for her child she subsequently chooses to stop her beta blocker. The baby is delivered at term without complication. She does not restart the beta blocker as she feels more energetic off them. Two weeks later she has a nocturnal cardiac arrest when her baby (who sleeps in her bedroom) cries. Her husband is woken by her convulsions and calls an ambulance and performs cardiopulmonary resuscitation. The ambulance crew arrive and successfully defibrillate her back to sinus rhythm. She is admitted to the ITU and ventilated for 48 hours. She is recommenced on her beta blockers. She suffers a degree of mild anoxic brain damage but makes a good recovery.

What is the next step in her management?

• She has suffered a cardiac arrest (albeit when off drug treatment). Although her compliance may now be better, an ICD is recommended and should be implanted before hospital discharge.

• Her baby needs to be screened. An ECG should be performed to measure the corrected QT interval. If a gene abnormality is found, then genetic screening can be performed. If the baby has LQTS then beta-blocker therapy (e.g. with propranolol syrup) is required.

CASE REVIEW

This completely asymptomatic 36-year-old woman comes for a consultation because of the sudden, unexpected death of her brother. Sudden death often has a cardiovascular cause. On close questioning it is discovered that her father also died unexpectedly at a young age and she had an infant that died a cot death. A familial condition is sus-pected and a 12-lead ECG shows a prolonged QT interval. As she is asymptomatic she is started on beta blockers but declines to have an ICD. The then becomes pregnant and decides to stop her beta blocker. In the post-partum period she suffers a cardiac arrest but fortunately is resuscitated and subsequently receives an ICD implant.

KEY POINTS

- Sudden unexpected death in a young person should always be investigated thoroughly including a post-mortem. If there is any suggestion of a potential familial condition, all first-degree relatives should be screened.
- If the deceased persons heart is found to be abnormal (dilated or hypertrophic cardiomyopathy, fatty infiltration of the right ventricle, premature coronary atheroma) then family members should be screen with ECGs and echocardiograms. If the deceased person's cardiovascular system appears to be structurally normal, a primary arrhythmia due to an ion channelopathy is a possible diagnosis that may only be revealed by detecting it in family members through 12-lead ECGs and drug challenges.
- The corrected QT interval (QTc) is calculated by dividing the QT interval by the R–R interval.
- Pregnancy is associated with increased risk of events in women with LQTS.
- Owing to the potentially severe consequences, it is usually advised that long-QT patients who normally take beta blockers should continue them throughout pregnancy and the post-partum period.
- Patients who have a strong family history of sudden death, have symptoms despite beta blockers or have LQT3, should undergo ICD implant.
- Genetic testing will identify 70–80% of long-QT patients and is useful for screening family members once an affected proband has been identified. It is not a good test for screening purposes in individuals with syncope of unknown origin.
- Many drugs cause prolongation of repolarisation and need to be avoided in patients with congenital LQTS. Overdose of some drugs (class III antiarrhythmics such as amiodarone or sotalol, antibiotics such as erythromycin and antipsychotics such as haloperidol), may result in pathological QT prolongation and cause Torsades de Pointes. Any patient on such drugs who presents with syncope or a cardiac arrest should have their corrected QT interval calculated on a 12-lead ECG.

Case 24 — A 60-year-old man with high blood pressure

A 60-year-old Caucasian man decides it is time to have a health check and attends his local GP surgery 'well man clinic'. As part of the assessment the practice nurse takes his blood pressure, which is recorded as 172/88 mmHg. He is 1.73 m tall, weighs 86 kg and has no past medical history. His basic physical examination is unremarkable with no audible murmurs on cardiac auscultation.

How do you interpret this blood pressure reading?

A simple definition of hypertension is a blood pressure consistently above 160/100 mmHg in an adult. Conversely, a normal blood pressure is one below 140/90 mmHg. The area in between is abnormal (Table 24.1); however, the decision to treat is based on overall cardiovascular risk.

It is often inappropriate to base management on a single blood pressure reading. It is conventional to assess the blood pressure on three separate occasions before making a confirmed diagnosis. It is also advisable to measure the blood pressure twice at each visit, once at the beginning and once at the end of the consultation.

What additional questions need to be asked as part of the basic assessment?

It is important to ask about all cardiovascular risk factors as well as life-style issues that may contribute to hypertension:
• Ask if there is a history of coronary artery disease or known hyperlipidaemia.
• Ask if there is a history of diabetes.
• Ask if there is a family history of hypertension or coronary artery disease, especially in relatives under the age of 60 years.

• Take a smoking history.
• Ask about alcohol consumption.
• Ask about diet (including salt intake) and exercise habits.

He has no history of cardiac symptoms or diabetes. His 86-year-old mother is currently on blood pressure tablets and his father died at the age of 74 years from a heart attack. He stopped smoking 20 cigarettes a day 20 years ago. He drinks 2–3 units of alcohol most days, sometimes more at weekends. His only exercise is walking the dog. He says he eats well and usually adds salt to his meals after they are cooked.

What is your advice and management plan?

He needs to have his blood pressure taken again in 4 weeks and 8 weeks time. Meanwhile there are some sensible life-style measures that should be undertaken. His body mass index (BMI) is 28.7, which means he is overweight. He needs to exercise more, reduce his calorie intake and stop adding salt to his food. His alcohol intake is also too high.

He returns to the surgery to have his blood pressure measure 4 weeks and 8 weeks later. The measurements are 168/94 mmHg, then156/95 mmHg. Over that time period he has started exercising more and taken the dietary advice and has lost 2 kg in weight.

What would you recommend?

He has had three successive readings with systolic blood pressures greater than 140 mmHg (two above 160 mmHg) and three diastolic readings above 90 mmHg.

Certainly, if he has had three readings greater than 160 mmHg despite his life-style changes, he should start drug therapy. It is important to assess his cardiovascular risk. This takes into account diabetes, renal disease, cholesterol and evidence of end-organ damage. Perform the following tests:

Cardiology: Clinical Cases Uncovered. By T. Betts, J. Dwight and S. Bull. Published 2010 by Blackwell Publishing.

- Urine dipstick testing for protein.
- Plasma glucose, electrolytes, creatinine, serum total cholesterol (TC) and HDL cholesterol.
- 12-lead ECG to look for evidence of LVH and previous myocardial infarction. In people <40 years of age the ECG voltage criteria for LVH may be unreliable and an echocardiogram may be a more specific measure of LVH.

Table 24.1 blood pressure definitions

Blood pressure classification	Systolic blood pressure (mmHg)	Diastolic blood pressure (mmHg)
Normal	<120	<80
Pre-hypertension	120–139	80–89
Stage 1 hypertension	140–159	90–99
Stage 2 hypertension	≥160	≥100

If his 10-year cardiovascular disease risk is calculated as ≥20%, or there is existing cardiovascular disease or target organ damage, it is important to treat a blood pressure consistently above 140/90 mmHg (Figure 24.1). As his mean systolic blood pressure is around 165 mmHg and he is over 60 years, his 10-year risk will be >20%, regardless of his TC:HDL ratio, therefore he requires treatment for blood pressure >140/90 mmHg. His 10-year cardiovascular risk can be assessed using a number of published calculators, such as the Framingham equation (http://hp2010.nhlbihin.net/atpiii/calculator.asp?usertype=prof), the ASSIGN score (www.assign-score.com/) or the Joint British Societies calculator (http://cvrisk.mvm.ed.ac.uk/calculator/calc.asp). The different calculators assess the risk of developing ischaemic heart disease, stroke and/or death from cardiovascular disease.

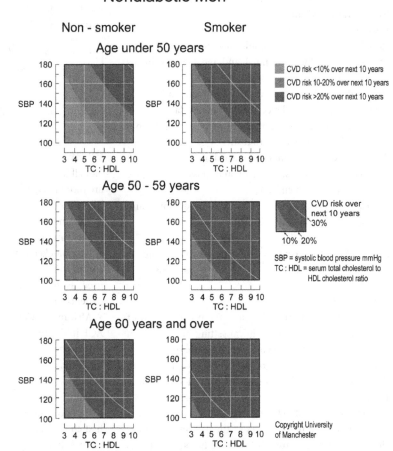

Nondiabetic Men

Figure 24.1 Example of a 10-year cardiovascular risk chart for a non-diabetic male. By plotting the total cholesterol (TC): high-density lipoprotein (HDL) ratio against the systolic blood pressure, the risk of developing cardiovascular disease over the next 10 years can be estimated.

He asks you why he has high blood pressure. What do you tell him and would you perform any additional tests or examinations?

Hypertension is extremely common and usually asymptomatic to begin with, therefore is often detected using screening or when blood pressure is taken for other reasons. The majority of patients have essential (primary) hypertension. A small minority have secondary hypertension that results from other diseases or conditions, the most common being renal disease and pregnancy. Secondary causes are more likely in younger patients and/or those with more severe hypertension and may have accompanying symptoms rather than being a coincidental finding.

Causes of hypertension include:
• Intrinsic renal disease (glomerulonephritis, polycystic kidneys, polyarteritis nodosa, etc.).
• Renovascular disease (renal artery stenosis).
• Endocrine causes (Cushing's syndrome, Conn's syndrome, phaeochromocytoma, acromegaly, hyperparathyroidism).
• Coarctation of the aorta.

Additional investigations should include:
• Auscultation for abdominal and renal artery bruits (renovascular disease).
• Radiofemoral delay and weak pulses (coarctation).
• Fundoscopy for evidence of target organ damage.
• Plasma sodium and potassium (Conn's syndrome) and calcium (hyperparathyroidism).

And if there is a high index of suspicion:
• Renal ultrasound scan (size) and possibly Doppler scans (renal artery stenosis).
• Urinary catecholamines (phaeochromocytoma) and free cortisol (Cushing's syndrome).

He is reluctant to accept that he has high blood pressure. He asks you why this cannot be 'white coat hypertension'.

What is your answer?

White coat hypertension describes the phenomenon of raised blood pressure in a clinical setting but not when the patient takes their own blood pressure at home. It may be found in 20–50% of the general population. To diagnose this, he needs to take his own blood pressure using a home monitor. These are accepted as being reliable and accurate. Blood pressure should be recorded 3–4 times a week at different times of the day on each occasion, to get a true picture. If his home blood pressure is consistently <140/90 mmHg then white coat hypertension can be diagnosed. An alternative way of differentiating white coat hypertension from true hypertension is ambulatory blood pressure monitoring.

White coat hypertension is probably not entirely benign and may result in a prognosis that is intermediate between normal BP and hypertension.

What are the potential consequences of hypertension?

Hypertension can be regarded (rather dramatically) as a silent killer as it is almost always asymptomatic. End-organ damage may eventually arise and cause symptoms or even death. Consequences are:
• **Cardiac** – ischaemic heart disease, LVH, systolic and diastolic heart failure, arrhythmias (atrial fibrillation).
• **Vascular** – stroke, aortic dissection.
• **Renal** – chronic renal failure.
• **Ocular** – hypertensive retinopathy.

For every 20 mmHg systolic or 10 mmHg diastolic increase in blood pressures above 115/75 mmHg, the mortality rate from both ischemic heart disease and stroke doubles.

His in-depth physical examination, blood and urine tests are all normal. He purchases a home monitoring blood pressure machine. After a month of successive readings above the normal range, despite ongoing exercise, healthy diet, weight loss and abstinence from alcohol, he agrees to start medical therapy.

What would you prescribe him?

Not all hypertensive patients are the same. Some patients are more likely to respond to particular classes of drugs. There are a few general issues to consider.
• Treatment for isolated systolic hypertension is the same as for combined systolic and diastolic hypertension.
• Beta blockers have recently been shown to be slightly less effective than other classes of drug, so are now rarely used as first choice. Exceptions are young, pregnant patients or young patients intolerant of ACE inhibitors.
• African and Caribbean patients do not respond well to ACE inhibitors.
• Patients <55 years of age probably do best with an ACE inhibitor.
• Patients >55 years of age are probably best starting a calcium-channel blocker or thiazide-type diuretic.
• It is not unusual to need more than one drug. If the first choice is a diuretic or calcium-channel blocker, add in an ACE inhibitor.

Table 24.2 Prescription key points

Offer patients with isolated systolic hypertension (systolic blood pressure more than 160mmHg) the same treatment as patients with both raised systolic and diastolic blood pressure

Offer patients older than 80 years the same treatment as other patients aged 55 years or older. Take account of any comorbidity and other drugs they are taking

Prescribe drugs taken only once a day if possible

Prescribe non-proprietary drugs if these are appropriate and minimise cost

Give information about the benefits and side-effects of drugs so that patients can make informed choices

Table 24.2 gives some further prescription advice.

He is started on bendroflumethiazide 2.5mg od. After 3 months he still has a blood pressure >140/90mmHg. Ramipril 2mg bd is started and after 2 weeks increased to 5mg bd.

What potential side-effects are there from his medication?

Bendroflumethiazide is a thiazide diuretic. Side-effects postural hypotension and mild GI effects; impotence; hypokalaemia, hypomagnesaemia, hyponatraemia, hypercalcaemia, hypochloraemic alkalosis, hyperuricaemia, gout, hyperglycaemia, and altered plasma lipid concentration.

Ramipril is an ACE inhibitor. Side-effects include profound hypotension, renal impairment and a persistent dry cough. They can also cause angioedema, rash, pancreatitis and upper respiratory-tract symptoms as well as GI effects.

He continues on medical therapy and returns for a clinic visit 3 months later. His blood pressure is recorded as being 195/125mmHg.

What should you do?

There is obvious concern that he has a hypertensive crisis (previously called malignant or accelerated hypertension). The definitions regarding this potential emergency differ and in fact it should be the patient rather than the numbers that guide treatment and urgency. Very elevated blood pressure can be subdivided into hypertensive emergencies (severe elevation with signs and symptoms), hypertensive urgencies (severe elevation without signs or symptoms) and uncontrolled hypertension. The most common clinical presentations of hypertensive emergencies are cerebral infarction (24.5%), pulmonary oedema (22.5%), hypertensive encephalopathy (16.3%) and congestive heart failure (12.0%). Less common presentations include intracranial haemorrhage, aortic dissection and eclampsia. The 1-year mortality rate for an untreated hypertensive emergency is 79%. They are more common in males and the elderly. Most patients who develop hypertensive emergencies have a history of inadequate hypertensive treatment or an abrupt discontinuation of their medications.

- Ask about symptoms:
  - Headache, breathlessness, oedema and epistaxis may be signs of uncontrolled hypertension.
  - Shortness of breath, chest pain, nocturia, dysarthria, weakness and altered consciousness are much more worrying and signs of a hypertensive emergency.
- Ask about treatment compliance.
- Look for physical signs:
  - Evidence of target organ damage (kidneys, heart, retinopathy) is concerning, although note that fundoscopy is not a good way of distinguishing emergencies from urgencies.
  - Encephalopathy, pulmonary oedema, renal failure, cerebrovascular accident and ACSs are all signs of a hypertensive emergency.
  - Although blood pressure values are not good guides, anything over 180/100mmHg is uncontrolled and anything >220/140mmHg needs urgent assessment and treatment.

He has had a few headaches and has noticed ankle swelling over the past 2 weeks. He has been breathless on climbing stairs and hills. He is alert and orientated with no neurological signs. He has mild pitting oedema at ankle level and a few sparse inspiratory crackles at both lung bases.

What action should be taken?

Hypertensive urgencies can be treated with oral therapy and may be managed in a closely monitored outpatient setting. Hypertensive emergencies need prompt hospital admission and treatment. He has some symptoms and soft signs so needs further hospital assessment (including urgent blood tests to assess renal function and ECG to look for LVH and strain and evidence of ischaemia).

Hypertensive emergencies require continuous blood pressure monitoring and intravenous medication in a high-dependency unit setting. The initial goal of therapy is to reduce mean arterial blood pressure by no more than 25% (within minutes to 1 hour), then if stable, to 160/100–110 mmHg within the next 2–6 hours. Excessive falls in pressure that may precipitate renal, cerebral, or coronary ischaemia should be avoided. If this level of blood pressure is well tolerated and the patient is clinically stable, further gradual reductions toward a normal blood pressure can be implemented in the next 24–48 hours.

Drugs that may be used in emergencies include intravenous sodium nitroprusside, GTN and hydralazine (all vasodilators) or labetolol, esmolol or phentolamine (adrenergic inhibitors). Labetolol is probably the most commonly used, although it should be avoided if there is heart failure (use GTN or i.v. enalapril)

Hypertensive urgencies may be managed with an oral, short-acting agent such as captopril, labetalol, or clonidine, followed by several hours of observation. Patients may also benefit from adjustment in their antihypertensive therapy, particularly the use of combination drugs, or reinstitution of medications if non-compliance is a problem. Close outpatient monitoring is recommended.

He is admitted to hospital as an emergency and responds well to treatment with intravenous GTN and the introduction of an ACE inhibitor.

Once under control, how often should he have medical follow-up?

Patients diagnosed with hypertension should have an annual medical follow-up to review their blood pressure readings, medications, assess for potential complications and address life-style issues. In between visits it may be helpful for patients to have nurse-led blood pressure checks every 3–4 months, or acquire a home-monitoring blood pressure machine to monitor their progress.

When should patients diagnosed with hypertension in primary care be referred to secondary care for specialist opinions?

Secondary care referrals may be required for the following reasons:
• Hypertensive urgency or emergency (urgent referral).
• Suspected phaeochromocytoma, suggested by labile blood pressure, headaches, pallor, sweating and palpitations (urgent referral).
• Unusual signs or symptoms.
• Secondary hypertension is suspected.
• Management depends upon an accurate diagnosis and additional resources, such as ambulatory blood pressure monitoring are required.
• Symptomatic postural hypotension.

CASE REVIEW

This asymptomatic 60-year-old man was found to have a high blood pressure measurement at a screening examination. Hypertension was confirmed with three successive elevated blood pressure readings over the next 2 months. Like many patients, he was reluctant to acknowledge the diagnosis and raised the possibility of white coat hypertension. After failing to respond to life-style changes he started treatment with a thiazide diuretic. When reassessed, he had deteriorated further with a very high blood pressure and symptoms consistent with a hypertensive emergency.

KEY POINTS

- Approximately 20% of the UK population have hypertension. The prevalence of hypertension increases with age and is more common in men than women. Isolated systolic hypertension is the most common form in people >50 years of age and in this age group is more prognostically significant than the diastolic blood pressure.
- Hypertension is diagnosed after three successive measurements record a systolic blood pressure >140 mmHg or diastolic blood pressure >90 mmHg.
- Treatment should be started in low-risk individuals with systolic blood pressure recordings >160 mmHg or diastolic measurements >100 mmHg. High-risk individuals need treatment is the blood pressure is >140 mmHg systolic or >90 mmHg diastolic. The aim of treatment is to reduce blood pressure to <140/90 mmHg.
- As the majority of patients with hypertension are asymptomatic they need to be educated regarding the importance of preventing end-organ damage.
- Life-style changes are important, as is addressing cardiovascular risk factors.
- If a secondary cause of hypertension is suspected, referral to a specialist for further investigation is recommended.
- Hypertensive drug therapy needs to be tailored to the individual. In patients older than 55 years or any black (African or Caribbean descent) patient with hypertension, the initial drug should be a calcium-channel blocker or thiazide-type diuretic. In non-black patients <55 years of age the first choice drug should be an ACE inhibitor.
- In hypertensive patients, a 5–6 mmHg reduction in systolic blood pressure will reduce the stroke risk by 42% and reduce the cardiovascular risk by 14%.
- Hypertensive emergencies manifest as severe hypertension with evidence of target organ damage and require prompt treatment in minutes to hours. Hypertensive urgencies manifest as severe hypertension without target organ involvement and require treatment within days.
- In hypertensive emergencies blood pressure should be lowered gradually (although rapid treatment may be indicated in acute myocardial infarction, aortic dissection and pulmonary oedema). In hypertensive urgencies this may be done with oral therapy as a closely monitored outpatient.
- Good long-term control of hypertension is the best method for prevention of acute hypertensive emergencies. Patient education and close follow-up in patients who have had a hypertensive crisis are essential to prevent recurrence.

Case 25 A 24-year-old woman with visual loss and dysphasia

A 24-year-old woman is referred to A&E following an acute onset of difficulty in speaking. She has transient dysphasia, which recovers as she is being assessed. She tells you that 2 days earlier she had transient visual loss in her right eye ('like a black curtain coming down over the eye') which lasted for a few minutes before recovering.

Ten days ago she returned from a 2-week holiday in Goa, India. She is normally fit, well and has no past medical history of note. She takes the oral contraceptive pill.

What additional questions need to be asked?

• Are there any other **neurological signs or symptoms**? Has she had headaches, a seizure, a change in gait or conscious level? It is important to establish whether this is a primarily neurological problem (e.g. cerebral tumour, epilepsy, cerebral infection) or a consequence of a cardiac or systemic illness.

• Does she have a fever or symptoms of **infection**, either cerebral or cardiac (particularly bearing in mind her foreign travel)?

• Has she used any **illicit drugs**?

• Is there a **family history** of stroke or transient ischaemic attack? Is there a family history of clotting disorders or hypercoagulable states?

• Are there any other **cardiovascular symptoms**, in particular irregular palpitations that may suggest atrial fibrillation (causing cerebral thromboembolism) or valve disease?

She has felt slightly unwell since her return from India. She had vomiting and diarrhoea on holiday and thinks she has lost weight. Although she felt sweaty at night on holiday

she has not been aware of this since her return. She feels alert and orientated. Her grandmother died of a stroke in her 60s and her mother is a diabetic. She has not experienced any palpitations, breathlessness or chest pain.

On physical examination her temperature is 37.2 °C; blood pressure 105/75 mmHg; pulse 80 bpm, regular. The JVP is not raised. Her apex beat is not displaced. Her heart sounds are normal with a wide split of the second heart sound. There is possibly a faint systolic murmur heard at the left sternal edge. All peripheral pulses are normal and there are no bruits. The lung fields are clear. Abdominal examination is unremarkable with no hepatosplenomegaly. A neurological examination reveals an upper right quadrantanopia in the visual fields but no other abnormality. There are no sensory or coordination abnormalities. She is right handed.

What are your differential diagnoses?

She was unwell in a foreign country, raising the possibility of a tropical infection; however, her neurological symptoms have been focal and transient and she is alert, orientated and not feverish. Her description sounds like transient neurological events, each one affecting a different territory. Her quadrantanopia is consistent with a neurological lesion in the left temporal lobe; however, the transient loss of vision in the right eye is consistent with a right retinal artery embolism (amaurosis fugax) and the expressive dysphasia would fit with a left frontal lobe lesion in a right-handed person. Her family history and oral contraceptive pill may point towards a vascular or hypercoagulation cause. The possible heart murmur may be a flow murmur or represent significant valve disease or infection.

As each of her symptoms or signs involves a different area of the brain over a very short period of time the most likely diagnosis is multiple cerebral emboli. Possible sources include:

Cardiology: Clinical Cases Uncovered. By T. Betts, J. Dwight and S. Bull. Published 2010 by Blackwell Publishing.

Carotid artery stenosis

To produce the bilateral cerebral symptoms she would need bilateral stenoses. Not only is she extremely young to have carotid atheroma, she has no carotid bruits on examination and all other pulses are normal.

Left atrial thrombus due to atrial fibrillation

Left atrial appendage thrombus may develop in the fibrillating atrium and subsequently be expelled, particularly if the appendage starts contracting again with the return to sinus rhythm. The risk of thromboembolism is related to other comorbidities and age. She is in sinus rhythm, which would mean that any atrial fibrillation would be paroxysmal. She has no symptoms of palpitations; however, in a minority of people, atrial fibrillation can be asymptomatic.

Left ventricular mural thrombus

Left ventricular mural thrombus may be found in the setting of cardiomyopathies with severely dilated, non-contractile or aneurismal segments of the left ventricle, whether in sinus rhythm or atrial fibrillation.

Emboli from an infected aortic or mitral heart valve

Bacterial endocarditis may present with thromboembolism in 20–30% of cases. There is usually a history of malaise, fevers or night sweats and anorexia. There is typically an audible murmur, either from the underlying valve defect or from destruction of the valve by infection. She has a history of recent GI infection and there is possibly a heart murmur.

What additional examinations need to be performed? What tests will you do?

Her age and appearance would suggest that bacterial endocarditis is the most likely diagnosis:

• If not done already, the **nail beds** on the fingers and toes should be inspected for splinter haemorrhages (which can accompany endocarditis). Fundoscopy should be performed to look for Roth spots and the palate inspected for petechiae.

• Her **temperature** should be retaken at 4-hourly intervals to look for fever.

• **Blood tests** for FBC, ESR, C-reactive protein and biochemistry. Endocarditis is accompanied by a normocytic, normochromic anaemia in 70–90%, a raised WCC in 20–30% and typically a high ESR and C-reactive protein.

• A **clotting screen**, including factor V Leiden, lupus anticoagulant and protein C and S, to look for a hypercoagulable state.

• **Urinalysis** for microscopic haematuria and proteinuria.

• **Blood cultures** (three sets from three sites) to look for bacteraemia.

• **CT brain scan** to look for evidence of embolic events and exclude a primary neurological cause.

• **ECG monitoring** for atrial fibrillation or flutter (Holter or telemetry).

• **Transthoracic echocardiogram** to look for valve disease and or evidence of a cardiomyopathy.

There are no peripheral stigmata of endocarditis. She has 24 hours of close monitoring. She is apyrexial. Her FBC is normal with no anaemia, a normal WCC, ESR and C-reactive protein. The clotting screen is normal. Her urinalysis is normal. Her blood cultures come back with no growth. A 12-lead ECG is reported as showing sinus rhythm (Figure 25.1). She is placed on telemetry which records sinus rhythm for the next 48 hours. A CXR shows no signs of infection and a normal CTR. The CT scan of her brain shows a small ischaemic infarct in the left temporal lobe. A transthoracic echocardiogram has good echo windows and shows normal aortic, mitral, tricuspid and pulmonary valve appearances and function. There are no visible vegetations. The left ventricle has normal systolic function. The right ventricle is slightly enlarged.

Her oral contraceptive pill is stopped and she is started on aspirin. A carotid Doppler scan and 24-hour Holter monitor are booked as outpatient investigations and she is discharged home to be followed up in a clinic.

However, 1 week later she returns to A&E with symptoms and signs of a left-sided hemiparesis. Again, a full recovery occurs over a 24-hour period. A CT brain scan confirms a right internal capsule infarct. She says that she has been feeling more breathless over the last few days.

What are the differential diagnoses?

She is continuing to have neurological events despite aspirin, and a cardiac source is very likely. Obvious endocarditis and severe cardiomyopathy with left ventricular thrombus have already been excluded. The differential diagnoses are listed below.

Bacterial endocarditis

Bacterial endocarditis with an atypical organism not grown on standard cultures and small vegetations not seen

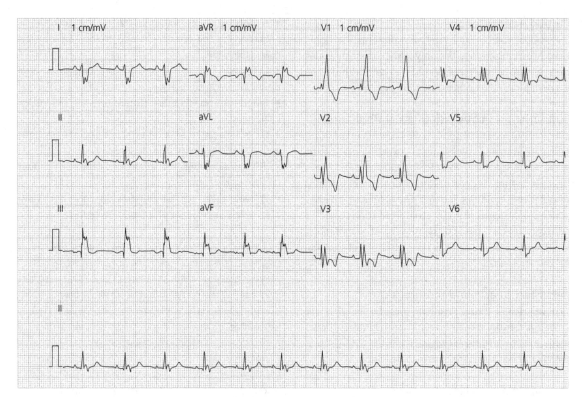

Figure 25.1 12-lead ECG showing sinus rhythm, a rightward axis and right bundle branch block (RBBB).

on transthoracic echocardiography: This remains unlikely due to the normal inflammatory markers, the lack of a pyrexia on close monitoring and that emboli are more often associated with large vegetations that should be easy to see on someone with good echocardiogram windows.

Cardiac myxoma

This is the most common cardiac tumour. Approximately 90% are solitary and pedunculated and 75–85% occur in the left atrium. They can grow to a large size, filling much of the chamber and often obstructing the mitral valve, causing symptoms of breathlessness and syncope and a diastolic tumour 'plop' on auscultation. There are frequently systemic symptoms of malaise and low-grade fever. Systemic embolism is often seen.

Paradoxical emboli through a right-left shunt

Blood clots from the venous circulation can pass to the systemic, arterial circulation through right-to-left shunts. The most common is a patent foramen ovale (present in 20–30% of individuals, although ASDs, VSDs and a PDA can also provide a conduit. A VSD or PDA would nor-

mally be detected on physical examination and transthoracic echocardiography but can occasionally be missed.

Paroxysmal atrial fibrillation with left atrial thrombus

Paroxysmal atrial fibrillation with left atrial thrombus has not yet been absolutely excluded.

What test is required? How soon should it be done?

A **transoesophageal echocardiogram** should be done urgently as the management of the four suspected conditions is quite different and it is important to prevent another neurological event. A transthoracic echocardiogram does not have a high enough resolution to detect left atrial thrombus or small vegetations. Transthoracic echocardiography may infrequently miss myxomas. It is not usually possible to see ASDs (although there may be signs of right heart volume overload such as right ventricular dilatation) and PFOs cannot be seen. A bubble study (an injection of agitated saline or contrast bubbles into a vein) may show flow of bubbles from right to left

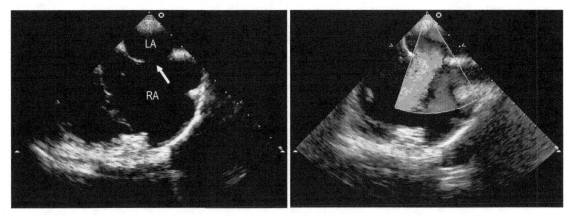

Figure 25.2 A transoesophageal echocardiogram image of a large secundum atrial septal defect (ASD). In the left image the left atrium (LA) and right atrium (RA) are labelled and the septal defect indicated by the arrow. In the right image colour Doppler has been turned on with the blue and yellow colour representing shunting from the left to right atrium.

on a transthoracic echocardiogram with an ASD or VSD, and if a Valsalva manoeuvre is performed during the injection, may unmask a PFO. A transoesophageal echocardiogram is the most sensitive imaging modality to look for left atrial thrombus, examine the atrial septum and look for a myxoma.

The transoesophageal echocardiogram shows a secundum ASD. A bubble study shows right-to-left shunting across the defect (Figure 25.2). The right ventricle is moderately dilated. There is no left atrial thrombus and no myxoma.

How should these findings be interpreted? What other test is required?

An intra-atrial communication is present, making the diagnosis of paradoxical embolism likely. Paradoxical emboli arise from venous thromboses that cross from right to left into the systemic circulation and most probably result from PFOs which open during Valsalva-type manoeuvres, although persistent communications such as ASDs may also be at fault. To diagnose paradoxical emboli as a cause of stroke a venous source of emboli needs to be confirmed, so lower limb venous Doppler scans should be performed. Having recently travelled to India she may have developed an asymptomatic DVT that has subsequently embolised.

Her ECG (right-axis deviation, incomplete RBBB), soft systolic pulmonary flow murmur and mild right

> ### Box 25.1 Atrial septal defects (ASDs)
>
> ASDs may be divided into secundum ASDs (the most common type), primum ASDs, sinus venosus defects and coronary sinus septal defects (unroofed coronary sinus). The common secundum ASD occurs in the fossa ovalis region due to inadequate formation of the septum secundum. Isolated ASDs account for 7% of isolated congenital heart defects (Table 25.1) and 5–6 occur per 10 000 live births. There is a female-to-male ratio of 2:1. Occasionally, a familial inheritance is demonstrated. There are some rare associated syndromes, e.g. Holt-Oram syndrome (autosomal dominant, upper limb developmental defects, ranging from radial thumb anomalies to phocomelia).
>
> Typically, ASDs produce little or no clinical signs in infants, unless very large or associated with other congenital heart defects. An isolated ASD rarely causes significant symptoms in children although large ones occasionally result in failure to thrive. However, by adult life the effect of continuous left-to-right shunting (the right heart being thinner, more compliant and lower pressure) may lead to right heart dilatation through volume overload. There may be a pulmonary valve systolic flow murmur, and a widely split second heart sound due to delayed closure of the pulmonary valve relative to the aortic valve. If pulmonary hypertension develops due to the high pulmonary flow, right ventricular hypertrophy will cause a parasternal heave from the prominent right ventricular impulse. Atrial arrhythmias, typically atrial fibrillation, are more common in people with ASDs.

Table 25.1 Common congenital heart defects

Defect	Clinical signs in adulthood*	Basic investigations*
ASD (secundum): • 1–2 per 1000 live births • >7% congenital heart defects	• No cyanosis • Pulmonary systolic flow murmur • RV heave • Fixed wide splitting of S2 • Tricuspid diastolic flow murmur	ECG: • Right-axis deviation • rsR pattern in lead V1 • P pulmonale • 1st degree heart block CXR: • RA and RV dilatation • Pulmonary artery dilatation • Increased pulmonary vascular markings
VSD: • 2–6 per 1000 live births • 20% congenital heart defects	• No cyanosis[†] • Pansystolic murmur at left sternal edge, sometime with thrill • Loud pulmonary component to S2	ECG: • Often normal • LVH and RVH if volume overload CXR: • May be normal • RV hypertrophy • Markedly prominent main pulmonary artery and adjacent vessels
PDA: • 2–4 per 1000 live births • 8–12% congenital heart defects	• No cyanosis[†] • Wide pulse pressure, prominent pulses • Systolic thrill • Continuous machinery murmur upper left sternum/clavicle	ECG: • Usually normal • Rarely LVH CXR: • May be normal • Prominent main pulmonary artery • Cardiomegaly if heart failure
Coarctation of the aorta: • 1–2 per 1000 live births • 5–8% congenital heart defects	• Hypertension • Radial–femoral delay • Arm BP >20 mmHg more than leg BP • Systolic murmur left clavicle and scapula • Continuous murmur from collaterals	ECG: • LVH • LV strain CXR: • Cardiomegaly • Rib notching

*Some findings will only become apparent if the defect is severe and there is a large shunt.
[†]Unless Eisenmenger's syndrome develops with subsequent right-to-left shunting.
ASD, atrial septal defect; BP, blood pressure; CXR, chest X-ray; ECG, electrocardiogram; LVH, left ventricular hypertrophy; PA, pulmonary artery; PDA, patent ductus arteriosus; RA, right atrial; RV, right ventricular; RVH, right ventricular hypertrophy; VSD, ventricular septal defect.

heart dilatation on echo are consistent with a secundum ASD (see Box 25.1).

Note that over the past week she has become very breathless and the right heart has dilated significantly. It is very likely that she has had a pulmonary embolus, also arising from a DVT. It is important to request an urgent CT pulmonary angiogram or ventilation/perfusion (V/Q) scan. Arterial blood gases should be per-formed, although a low pO$_2$ is not specific for pulmonary embolism and the pO$_2$ may be normal with smaller pulmonary embolisms. D-dimers are not sensitive or specific enough to rule in or rule out pulmonary embolism in this situation.

What is the appropriate treatment?

Immediate treatment should be with heparin and warfarin to prevent further emboli and treat the potential pulmonary embolus. ASDs should be closed if paradoxical emboli have occurred. Other indications for closure include symptoms (fatigue, breathlessness, recurrent respiratory infection) and developing right heart failure or pulmonary hypertension secondary to right heart volume overload. Surgical closure has a low mortality (<1%); however, recently percutaneous closure using catheter delivery of an Amplatzer® device has become a viable alternative for secundum ASDs. Closure in teenage years or later does not appear to protect against the development of atrial arrhythmias.

She also requires basic investigations to determine whether she has an increased susceptibility to DVT. Blood tests for a hypercoagulable state, underlying malignancies, factor C or S deficiency, factor V Leiden (resistance to activated protein C), and prothrombin mutations should all be performed at the appropriate time (which may be dependent on anticoagulation and the presence of thrombus).

CASE REVIEW

This 24-year-old woman presented with transient neurological symptoms consistent with embolic events following travel to the Indian subcontinent. The disparate nature of the symptoms made a primary neurological diagnosis very unlikely and a infective and/or cardiac source were sought. Initial investigations, including transthoracic echocardiography, were unremarkable. She was started on aspirin, but then represented with a further neurological event and increasing breathlessness. A transoesophageal echocardiogram revealed an ASD (and therefore the possibility of paradoxical emboli) and signs of right heart strain consistent with pulmonary embolism. The likely source of the emboli is as DVT, perhaps a consequence of her long-haul flight. Formal anticoagulation was started and closure of the ASD was recommended.

KEY POINTS

- Emboli from a cardiac source account for 15% of all strokes. The most common cardiac source of cerebrovascular events is left atrial thrombus resulting from atrial fibrillation; however, this arrhythmia is rare in young adults and, even if present, the annual stroke risk is usually <1%.
- Bacterial endocarditis and myxoma may cause emboli. They are often accompanied by other systemic symptoms, particular clinical signs and would be seen on transthoracic echocardiography.
- Every young patient with cerebral infarction or transient ischaemic attacks should have a transoesophageal echocardiogram performed to look specifically for intracardiac shunts, particularly ASDs and PFOs.
- The physical signs of ASDs may be subtle, particularly if the shunt is very small. Many adults are asymptomatic, at least until atrial fibrillation develops. The ECG and CXR changes are also subtle and may be missed. PFOs have no clinical signs or ECG or CXR abnormalities.

- Paradoxical emboli (venous thrombosis, air, tumour, fat or amniotic fluid embolising across an interatrial or interventricular cardiac defect into the systemic circulation) are one of the most common causes of stroke in young, otherwise healthy, individuals. Paradoxical embolus is confirmed by the presence of thrombus within an intracardiac defect on contrast echocardiography or at autopsy. Paradoxical embolus can be presumed in the presence of arterial embolism with no evidence of left-sided circulation thrombus, DVT with or without pulmonary embolism, and right-to-left shunting through an intracardiac communication (commonly a PFO).
- DVT may not be detected clinically in >50% of pulmonary emboli or paradoxical emboli. Pulmonary embolism has been demonstrated in as many as 85% of diagnosed cases of paradoxical embolism.

A 59-year-old woman with low blood pressure and breathlessness

A 59-year-old woman is brought in by ambulance to A&E having collapsed at home. She has a 24-hour history of feeling very unwell, nauseated, upper epigastric/retrosternal discomfort, breathlessness and dizzy spells.

Her immediate brief examination shows her to be dyspnoeic at rest but managing short sentences. She is orientated and fully conscious. She is pale, clammy and cold to touch, especially at the peripheries. Her blood pressure is 72/50 mmHg; pulse 112 bpm, regular and weak; O_2 saturations 89% on 4 L/min O_2 via a face mask. Her JVP is +4 cm, and auscultation reveals a gallop rhythm with a soft systolic murmur and a few inspiratory crackles at her lung bases.

What is your immediate impression and differential diagnoses?

She looks shocked (Box 26.1). The causes of shock may be divided into the following:
• **Cardiogenic** (low cardiac output due to pump failure).
• **Sepsis** (vasodilatation +/– reduced myocardial contractility).
• **Hypovolaemia** – low circulating blood volume, usually as a consequence of sudden severe bleeding.
Sinus tachycardia is a natural physiological response to hypotension and shock. If the heart rate is inappropriately fast or there is a pathological arrhythmia (atrial fibrillation, supraventricular tachycardia [SVT] or ventricular tachycardia) it may be the cause of the hypotension and needs to be addressed immediately. In developing shock, the drop in systolic blood pressure may appear quite late on in its progression, particularly in young people, whereas an increased pulse and respiratory rate and decreased perfusion may be early signs that indicate a serious situation.

What questions and aspects of the physical examination are important to achieve a diagnosis?

A brief history and examination is important, specifically:
• Is she known to have heart disease? Has she had cardiac-sounding chest pain indicating myocardial infarction?
• Does she have symptoms or signs of acute heart failure and low cardiac output (cold, clammy peripheries, gallop rhythm, new murmurs, etc.)?
• Has she had a fever, rigors, confusion or disorientation, suggesting infection? What is her temperature? Does she have lymphadenopathy or other signs of infection (e.g. signs of lung consolidation due to pneumonia)? Early sepsis has profound vasodilatation and a high cardiac output state with warm peripheries. As sepsis progresses, the cardiac output falls and the peripheries shut down
• Has she had haematemesis, melaena or any other signs of blood loss? Is there acute abdominal pain and tenderness (ruptured abdominal aortic aneurysm?)

She denies any symptoms of infection. There is no history of dark stools or haematemesis. She has been diabetic for 16 years and hypertensive for 12 years but has not had chest pain before. The epigastric/retrosternal discomfort is dull in nature and nausea started 24 hours ago. There have not been any palpitations and the dizziness and near collapse occurred with trying to stand. She did not lose consciousness. Her temperature is 36.5 °C; her abdomen is soft and not tender.

Based on the above, what is the most likely mechanism of her shock? Within that mechanism, what are the potential causes and what are the key features of each?

The most likely mechanism is cardiogenic shock due to low cardiac output. She is poorly perfused with a gallop rhythm, a raised JVP and early signs of pulmonary oedema.

Cardiology: Clinical Cases Uncovered. By T. Betts, J. Dwight and S. Bull. Published 2010 by Blackwell Publishing.

Table 26.1 Cardiovascular causes of shock

Acute myocardial infarction with extensive left ventricular damage

Acute post-infarction ventricular septal defect (VSD)

Acute severe mitral regurgitation (MR) (papillary muscle rupture)

Right ventricular infarction

Ventricular free wall rupture

Cardiac tamponade

Complete heart block

Tachyarrhythmias

Box 26.1 Definition of shock

Low blood pressure (<90 mmHg systolic) with evidence of poor perfusion.

Her epigastric discomfort may be cardiac pain, which does not always manifest as classic chest tightness radiating to the jaw and arm. Inferior myocardial infarctions may produce upper abdominal discomfort. Diabetics may have 'silent' myocardial infarction. There are no symptoms or signs to suggest infection. There no obvious bleeding history and her JVP is raised, ruling out hypovolaemia.

Cardiogenic shock (Table 26.1) may be defined as a systolic blood pressure <90 mmHg for more than 30 minutes with signs of a low cardiac output (hypoperfusion) in the presence of adequate filling (pre-load, i.e. circulating blood volume). It may occur for the following reasons:

- **Acute myocardial infarction** is the most common cause, with shock developing in 8% of ST-elevation myocardial infarction (STEMI) patients. It may manifest when >40% of the ventricular myocardium is damaged and is the leading cause of death in myocardium infarction patients who make it as far as hospital admission. Shock usually develops between 2 and 48 hours after the onset of infarction. It carries a very high early mortality (>50%, compared to 7% of non-shock myocardial infarction patients).
- **Right ventricular infarction** may cause hypotension and shock through a different mechanism. It usually occurs in the setting of inferior myocardial infarction, typically involving the right coronary artery (RCA). If the right ventricle is severely injured it is unable to pump blood to the lungs and fill the left side of the heart. A dilated right ventricle may push the septum into the left ventricle cavity, reducing its volume. There may also be associated bradycardia. This lack of filling (reduced pre-load) leads to a low cardiac output. Typically the JVP is very high, sometimes with Kussmaul's sign and pulsus paradoxus and, importantly, in isolated right ventricular infarction the lungs are clear (no pulmonary oedema).
- **Ventral septal defects (VSDs), papillary muscle rupture causing acute mitral regurgitation (MR) or myocardial rupture** may all occur 2–3 days after an acute myocardial infarction, causing a sudden deterioration, often with acute heart failure. With MR or a VSD a new systolic murmur should be present. Myocardial rupture may cause acute tamponade (see below).
- **Cardiac tamponade** is the haemodynamic result of excessive fluid accumulation in the pericardial space, causing an increase in pericardial pressure to the point it compresses the thin-walled right heart and prevents adequate ventricular filling. It can result from a sudden acute bleed (rupture following myocardial infarction, trauma), in which case it is sudden and only a small amount of fluid has a dramatic effect, or it can develop gradually with large effusions that collect over days or weeks (malignancy, infections and rheumatoid diseases). Patients are typically breathless and fatigued with engorged neck veins, Kussmaul's sign, hypotension, pulsus paradoxus and quiet heart sounds. The lung fields are clear. The diagnosis is made with imaging (principally echocardiogram; however, CT and MRI may show fluid collections).
- Although not strictly 'cardiogenic', other differential diagnoses would include **aortic dissection** and acute **pulmonary embolism**.

What simple investigations would you request immediately?

- **12-lead ECG** to look for signs of acute myocardial infarction and to check the rhythm.
- **Chest X-ray (CXR)** to look for cardiomegaly, pulmonary oedema, pneumonia, etc.
- **Blood tests**: samples for full blood count (FBC) (particularly haemoglobin (Hb) and WCC), biochemistry for renal function and cardiac enzymes. Blood cultures if sepsis suspected.
- At this stage a **transthoracic echocardiogram** would be extremely useful to assess cardiac function and identify the cause of cardiogenic shock.

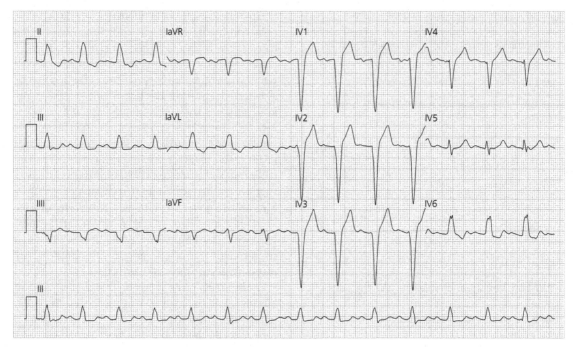

Figure 26.1 12-lead ECG of sinus rhythm with left bundle branch block (LBBB).

Her 12 -lead ECG is shown in Figure 26.1. What does it show and how does this help the diagnosis and management?

The 12-lead ECG shows sinus rhythm with left bundle branch block (LBBB). The QRS complexes are broad, measuring more than three small squares or 0.12 seconds. In lead V1 there is a deep Q wave and ST-segment elevation, in lead V6 there is a positive QRS, shaped like the letter M.

There are no old ECGs for comparison. LBBB may be a consequence of acute myocardial infarction (usually a large anteroseptal myocardial infarction) and its presence carries a worse prognosis, regardless of whether it is old or new. Its characteristic appearance means that STEMI cannot be diagnosed using the usual ECG criteria. It does indicate significant underlying cardiovascular disease, increasing the likelihood of a cardiac cause of her shock.

Her troponin is >50 μg/L, indicating a myocardial infarction >12 hours ago. Her Hb is 12.5 g/dL. She is transferred to the CCU.

A transthoracic echocardiogram is performed, demonstrating a dilated left ventricle with akinesia of the anterior wall and septum. There is mild, central MR. The right heart appears normal and contracts well (ruling out significant right ventricular infarction). There is no sign of a VSD and no pericardial effusion.

What is your management plan? Would you give her thrombolysis or other reperfusion therapy?

Her history, the cardiac enzymes and the ECG suggest a large myocardial infarction 24 hours earlier. She has subsequently developed cardiogenic shock and pulmonary oedema but is pain free. Initial management should include:

- **Invasive monitoring:**
  - Arterial pressure monitoring. This allows instant recognition of improvement or deterioration when initiating therapies, or the haemodynamic consequence of arrhythmias. Arterial blood gases may be drawn regularly to assess oxygenation and acid–base balance.
  - Central venous pressure (CVP) monitoring to aid assessment of filling pressures. A CVP line may also be used to administer inotropes.
  - Urinary catheter. The hourly urine output is a good way to assess vital organ perfusion.

○ Oxygen saturation monitor.

○ Swan-Ganz pulmonary artery catheters have fallen out of favour in recent years. They can be used to estimate cardiac output, pre-load (the pulmonary artery wedge pressure is indicative of the left atrial and left ventricle end-diastolic pressures) and systemic vascular resistance, thus helping to distinguish between right ventricle infarction and left ventricle infarction, high output failure (in septic shock) and guiding fluid replacement or diuresis more accurately than a CVP measurement.

- **Maximise oxygenation:**
  ○ High flow oxygen via a face mask.
  ○ There should be a low threshold for continuous positive airways pressure (CPAP) or intubation and ventilation, especially if pulmonary oedema is present.

- **Adequate filling and fluid balance:**
  ○ To optimise pre-load, cautious fluid replacement may be required to get a CVP of 10–14 mmHg or pulmonary capillary wedge pressure of 18–20 mmHg. If pulmonary oedema is present, fluid should not be given.
  ○ Diuretics should be given if there is pulmonary oedema or the CVP is high (and right ventricle infarction has been excluded).

- **Optimise electrolytes and blood glucose.**

- **Vasodilators:**
  ○ Intravenous GTN may reduce pre-load and afterload and increase coronary artery perfusion; however; it should only be given if the systolic blood pressure is >100 mmHg, so it should not be used in the setting of cardiogenic shock.

- **Inotropes** (Table 26.2):
  ○ Intravenous inotropes (e.g. dobutamine) have traditionally been used to increase cardiac contractility through beta-receptor stimulation and therefore cardiac output. The problem is that they increase myocardial oxygen demand and result in tachycardia and sometimes arrhythmias. Noradrenaline (norepinephrine) and dopamine are also vasopressor agents that

act as peripheral vasoconstrictors, reducing peripheral perfusion and distributing blood preferentially to vital organs. Vasoconstrictors increase afterload.

Her chest pain symptoms were 24 hours earlier and have now diminished. Although LBBB in the setting of acute myocardial infarction is an indication for thrombolysis or other forms of reperfusion, she is a delayed presentation, therefore thrombolysis is not appropriate.

On arrival at the CCU she is started on CPAP, a CVP line is inserted (CVP 19 mmHg), an arterial line and urinary catheter are inserted and she is started on a dopamine infusion at 2.5 μg/kg/min. Her systolic blood pressure remains at 80/60 mmHg with a pulse of 110 bpm. She remains pale, cool and clammy with a urine output of 5–10 mL/h.

Is there anything else that can be done?

The prognosis for medically treated cardiogenic shock is very poor, with a mortality approaching 80%. Recent studies suggest that an aggressive invasive approach, performed as early as possible after the onset of shock, may reduce mortality to 30–50%. Immediate transfer to a centre where urgent coronary angiography and revascularisation (either by percutaneous intervention or coronary artery bypass surgery) can be performed is vital.

As a short-term measure, the patient's haemodynamic status may be improved using intra-aortic balloon pumps. These devices are inserted through the femoral artery and are positioned in the descending aorta. They inflate and deflate with the cardiac cycle, increasing coronary artery perfusion and reducing afterload. There use is usually confined to centres that undertake coronary intervention and cardiac surgery.

The local cardiothoracic centre is called and they agree to accept her transfer. An emergency ambulance is requested. The alarm on her cardiac monitor suddenly sounds. The patient has slumped in her bed and is unresponsive and is not making any respiratory effort. Her arterial pressure trace is flat.

Table 26.2 Inotropes

Blood pressure (BP) <80 mmHg	BP 80–90 mmHg Signs and symptoms of shock	BP 80–90 mmHg No signs or symptoms of shock	BP >90 mmHg after dopamine or noradrenaline started
Noradrenaline 0.5–30 μg/kg/min	Dopamine 0.5–15 μg/kg/min	Dobutamine 2–20 μg/kg/min	Dobutamine 2–20 μg/kg/min to allow reduction of dopamine

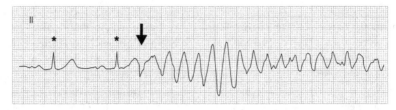

Figure 26.2 Ventricular fibrillation. There are two beats of sinus rhythm (*) followed by a ventricular ectopic (arrow) that occurs during the preceding T wave, initiating ventricular fibrillation.

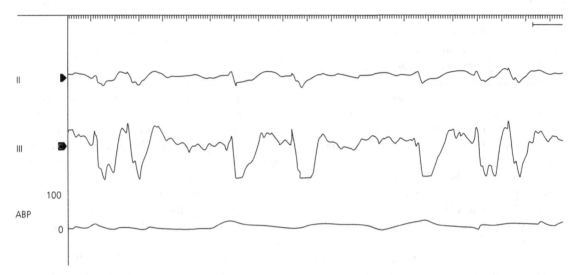

Figure 26.3 Tracing of pulseless electrical activity (PEA) with flat arterial blood pressure (ABP) tracing.

What does the monitor show?

The monitor (Figure 26.2) shows that two beats of sinus rhythm, followed by a ventricular ectopic that occurs during the preceding T wave, initiate ventricular fibrillation.

How should this be treated?

The immediate treatment is prompt external defibrillation. Using paddles placed or stuck on the sternum and apex a single 150–200 J shock from a biphasic defibrillator (or 360 J shock from a monophasic defibrillator) should be administered. It does not need to be synchronised. Although basic cardiopulmonary resuscitation (CPR) with chest compressions may be initiated while waiting to set up the defibrillator, this should not delay defibrillation. After the first shock, CPR with 30 chest compres-

sions should be continued before reassessing the rhythm. In this situation the invasive arterial pressure monitoring and the telemetry ECG will show whether this is necessary. If ventricular fibrillation persists, a second shock is administered. If ventricular fibrillation persists after the second shock, 1 mg of i.v. adrenaline should be administered (and repeated every 3–5 minutes thereafter). After 2 minutes of CPR, if ventricular fibrillation persists, a third shock may be given and CPR recommenced. If ventricular fibrillation persists despite three shocks, i.v. amiodarone 300 mg should be administered as a bolus. Repeated shocks may be administered after every 2 minutes of CPR.

After three shocks, her rhythm changes to that shown in Figure 26.3. There is no recordable pulse or blood pressure.

Table 26.3 Causes of pulseless electrical activity (PEA) in a cardiac arrest situation

Cardiac tamponade

Cardiac rupture

Large pulmonary embolism

Tension pneumothorax

Large myocardial infarction

Hypovolaemia

Hypothermia

Hyperkalaemia

Drug overdose (tricyclic antidepressants, digoxin, beta blockers, calcium-channel blockers)

Post-defibrillation (usually recovers by 60 seconds, so continue resuscitation for at least 1–2 minutes)

What is the rhythm and what treatment is required?

The rhythm is PEA (pulseless electrical activity) (Table 26.3). The treatment is continuing CPR with i.v. adrenaline 1 mg administered every 2 minutes. If the electrical rate is <60 bpm atropine 3 mg may be administered as a one-off dose. The prognosis is now very bleak. Rarely, PEA may result from sudden cardiac tamponade or a tension pneumothorax, so an urgent echocardiogram or blind pericardiocentesis could be considered, but, considering the patient's initial presentation and poor prognosis at this stage, it is appropriate to terminate resuscitation and pronounce the patient dead.

CASE REVIEW

This 59-year-old woman presented late after a large myocardial infarction with cardiogenic shock. Although her chest discomfort was not typical, the history, clinical findings of volume overload and lack of evidence of infection all point to cardiogenic cause, which carries a poor prognosis. A transthoracic echocardiogram revealed poor left ventricular systolic function, confirming the diagnosis. Invasive monitoring to guide fluid balance management and intravenous inotropic support were initiated. The late presentation means there is no role for thrombolytic therapy; however, immediate coronary angiography and percutaneous coronary angioplasty and stent insertion may improve cardiac function and mortality and also allow for insertion of an intra-aortic balloon pump. Her cardiac arrest from ventricular fibrillation was treated promptly with immediate defibrillation; however, her myocardial function was so poor that she died from PEA (electromechanical dissociation).

KEY POINTS

- Shock may be due to low cardiac output from a cardiovascular cause, a normal or high cardiac output with severe vasodilatation in the setting of septicaemia, or severe hypovolaemia.
- Simple imaging with transthoracic echocardiography is required early on to reach a diagnosis and identify potentially reversible causes.
- Supportive measures include oxygenation, adequate volume loading or diuresis as required, inotropic support and intra-aortic balloon pumps.
- Invasive monitoring with a CVP line, arterial line and urinary catheter help plan and monitor treatment.

- In the setting of acute myocardial infarction, urgent transfer to the catheter laboratory and revascularisation may improve prognosis by allowing an early invasive approach using percutaneous coronary intervention or bypass surgery.
- The decision to abandon resuscitation should be determined by the likelihood of being able to restore a normal rhythm and the subsequent chances of short-term survival. This is usually dictated by the circumstances and pathology underlying the cardiac arrest, the duration of resuscitation and the patient's age and comorbidities.

MCQs

For each situation, choose the single option you feel is most correct.

> **1** A 31-year-old woman is brought to A&E having collapsed unconscious at work. She tells you she was standing listening to a presentation when she began to feel nauseated, faint and lost her vision before losing consciousness. She has lost consciousness only once before, when having blood taken.

What is the most likely diagnosis?
a. Ventricular tachycardia.
b. Hypoglycaemia.
c. Epilepsy.
d. Neurocardiogenic syncope.
e. Complete heart block.

> **2** A 67-year-old man is referred to A&E by his GP after a 12-lead ECG performed at the surgery shows atrial fibrillation. The resting ventricular rate is 130 bpm. He reports no symptoms and said he had just gone for a blood pressure check.

What is the most appropriate treatment?
a. Immediate external DC cardioversion.
b. Oral beta blockers.
c. Intravenous amiodarone.
d. Oral amiodarone.
e. Oral flecainide.

> **3** A 78-year-old male presents to A&E with palpitations, breathlessness and near syncope. His heart rate is 160 bpm and regular. A 12-lead ECG shows a regular broad-complex tachycardia (QRS duration 140 ms).

Which one of the following is most likely to point to a diagnosis of ventricular tachycardia?
a. A history of prior myocardial infarction.
b. A systolic blood pressure of <90 mmHg.
c. A heart rate greater than 200 bpm.
d. A history of blackouts.
e. Chest pain during tachycardia.

> **4** A 65-year-old male is admitted to the CCU after undergoing after primary angioplasty for an acute anterior myocardial infarction. His blood pressure is recorded as 80/50 mmHg.

Which of the following signs is *not compatible* with a diagnosis of cardiogenic shock?
a. A urine output of 10 mL/h.
b. Cold, clammy peripheries.
c. Inspiratory crackles at both lung bases.
d. Sinus bradycardia of 50 bpm.
e. An elevated JVP.

Cardiology: Clinical Cases Uncovered. By T. Betts, J. Dwight and S. Bull. Published 2010 by Blackwell Publishing.

5 *An 80-year-old woman reports a 2-week history of extreme fatigue, breathlessness and mild dizzy spells. Her resting pulse is regular and 40 bpm.*

Which one of the following is inconsistent with a diagnosis of complete heart block?
a. Cannon waves in her JVP waveform.
b. An increase in her heart rate to 60 bpm when walking up stairs.
c. A blood pressure of 180/100 mmHg.
d. No history of syncope.
e. An ECG showing dissociation between P waves and QRS complexes.

6 *A 35-year-old male with no previous cardiac history presents to A&E with a 4-hour history of rapid, irregular palpitations, mild chest discomfort, breathlessness and dizziness. His ECG shows atrial fibrillation with a ventricular rate of 120 bpm, his blood pressure is 110/70 bpm and his O₂ saturations on room air are 99%.*

What is the most appropriate treatment?
a. 300 mg oral flecainide.
b. Urgent external DC cardioversion.
c. Oral amiodarone 200 mg three times a day.
d. Intravenous digoxin 500 μg over 1 hour.
e. Oral nifedipine 10 mg once.

7 *A 67-year-old woman is seen at her local surgery for the first time in many years for a repeat prescription for asthma inhalers. As part of an overall check-up, her resting blood pressure is recorded as 175/85 mmHg at the beginning and end of the 5-minute consultation. She is otherwise fit and well.*

Which of the following is the most appropriate course of action?
a. Prescribe a thiazide diuretic.
b. Organise 24-hour ambulatory blood pressure monitoring.
c. Request a renal ultrasound scan.
d. Repeat her blood pressure measurement in 1 month's time.
e. No action is required.

8 *A 32-year-old male attends the cardiology clinic complaining of palpitations.*

Which one of the following would not support a diagnosis of benign ectopic beats?
a. Symptoms that get worse during exercise.
b. A sensation of missed beats and slow heavy thumping.
c. A normal physical examination and echocardiogram.
d. A resting heart rate of 50 bpm with sinus arrhythmia.
e. Symptoms that occur almost every day for the past 2 weeks.

9 *A 30-year-old woman is referred to the cardiology clinic as her 25-year-old sister died suddenly and unexpectedly. The sister's post-mortem did not find any abnormalities and the coroner recorded 'sudden cardiac death' as the cause of death.*

Which of the following conditions is *not* a cause of sudden cardiac death that is usually familial?
a. HOCM.
b. LQTS.
c. Brugada syndrome.
d. Arrhythmogenic right ventricular cardiomyopathy.
e. Wolff-Parkinson-White syndrome.

10 *A 67-year-old man with previous myocardial infarctions, heart failure and an ICD is rushed to A&E having received four shocks from his ICD in 1 hour. On arrival he has another episode of ventricular tachycardia at 220 bpm with near syncope that is successfully treated with another ICD shock.*

Which of the following is incorrect?
a. There is no role for intravenous amiodarone if he is taking regular oral amiodarone.
b. Increasing the bradycardia pacing rate to 100 bpm may suppress further ventricular tachycardia.
c. Sedation, or even intubation and ventilation, may be a helpful therapeutic option.
d. Additional beta blockers should be given as long as there is no overt heart failure.
e. A pacing magnet placed over the ICD will temporarily disable shock treatments.

11 *A 34-year-old male presents to A&E with a 45-minute history of rapid, regular palpitations, chest pain and shortness of breath. His blood pressure is 75/50 mmHg; pulse 220 bpm and regular. He has a regular broad-complex tachycardia (QRS duration 150 ms).*

Which of the following is true?

a. A pulse rate >200 bpm and low blood pressure indicate a diagnosis of ventricular tachycardia.
b. The most appropriate initial treatment is intravenous adenosine.
c. The most appropriate initial treatment is intravenous amiodarone.
d. The most appropriate initial treatment is intravenous verapamil.
e. External cardioversion should not be performed until he has been fasted for 8 hours

12 *A 77-year-old diabetic woman is discovered to have atrial fibrillation at a routine blood pressure check at her GP surgery. She has no symptoms and her resting pulse rate is 75 bpm. Her GP asks for advice regarding anticoagulation.*

Which of the following is true?

a. This woman should be anticoagulated with warfarin if there are no major bleeding risks.
b. Anticoagulation with warfarin is only required if she is symptomatic.
c. Anticoagulation with warfarin is only required if the atrial fibrillation is persistent.
d. Over the age of 75 years the bleeding risks of warfarin always outweigh the benefits.
e. Arranging an elective external DC cardioversion would avoid the need for anticoagulation with warfarin.

13 *A 62-year-old male attends the A&E with a 6-week history of malaise, weight loss, occasional mild sweats and fevers and deceased appetite. Over the past 2 weeks he has become increasingly breathless on exertion and at night when trying to sleep.*

Which of the following is true?

a. A transoesophageal echocardiogram is more sensitive at detecting heart valve vegetations than a transthoracic echocardiogram.
b. If there is no audible heart murmur, bacterial endocarditis is ruled out.
c. Antibiotic therapy must be started immediately.
d. Every patient with bacterial endocarditis will require heart valve replacement.
e. Most patient with bacterial endocarditis have had previous heart valve replacement surgery.

14 *A 23-year-old male undergoes an insurance medical and is found to have a loud pansystolic murmur heard best at the left sternal edge. He is fit and well.*

Which of the following is true?

a. The murmur may be due to flow across an ASD.
b. The murmur is typical of a PDA.
c. The loud murmur and a palpable thrill is compatible with a small VSD.
d. The lack of cyanosis rules out congenital heart disease.
e. A weak right radial pulse would support the diagnosis of coarctation of the aorta.

15 *A 55-year-old Asian woman is due to undergo elective cholecystectomy. Her pre-operative blood pressure is consistently recorded as 195/115 mmHg. She denies any symptoms other than those from her gall bladder.*

Which of the following is incorrect?

a. She should have fundoscopy performed immediately.
b. Her operation should be cancelled.
c. She requires urgent intravenous labetolol.
d. She should have an ECG and renal function checked.
e. Oral beta blockers are the most appropriate single drug therapy agent to be discharged home with.

16 A 61-year-old man is admitted via A&E with a 1-hour history of cardiac-sounding chest pain at rest. On the basis of the history and ECG he is thought to have a non-ST-elevation ACS.

Which of the following is not required to assess his TIMI risk score?
a. Elevated cardiac biomarkers.
b. ST depression >0.5 mm.
c. Age >65 years.
d. Aspirin use within the past 7 days.
e. T-wave inversion in more than two leads.

17 A 45-year-old man is admitted with an ACS with a troponin rise.

Which of the following agents has not been proven in randomised clinical trials to improve prognosis in this condition?
a. Clopidogrel.
b. Aspirin.
c. IIb/IIIa antagonists.
d. Nifedipine.
e. Low-molecular-weight heparin.

18 Which of the following is not a cause of ST elevation on an ECG?

a. Coronary artery occlusion.
b. LVH.
c. Early repolarisation.
d. Hyperkalaemia.
e. Brugada syndrome.

19 60-year-old man is admitted with a 4-hour history of chest pain. He is a smoker with a 30-pack year history and suffers from non-insulin dependent diabetes. His ECG shows ST elevation of 2 mm in leads V1–V3.

Which of the following statements is true for the treatment of myocardial infarction with thrombolysis when compared to primary angioplasty?
a. Improved vessel patency.
b. Increased risk of haemorrhagic stroke.
c. Reduction in risk of embolic stroke.
d. Improved ST-segment resolution.
e. Reduced readmission rate for recurrent ACSs.

20 Which of the following are not associated with acute occlusion of the RCA?

a. ST elevation on the ECG in leads II, III and aVF.
b. Inferior myocardial infarction.
c. Complete heart block.
d. Right ventricular infarction.
e. Rupture of the anterior wall of the left ventricle.

21 A 70-year-old hypertensive man is admitted with severe central chest pain of sudden onset radiating to the back. On examination, his blood pressure is 200/70 mmHg in the right arm and there is a pressure difference of 40 mmHg between the right and left arms. On auscultation of his heart a soft early diastolic murmur is heard. He is felt to have an aortic dissection.

Which of the following statements concerning aortic dissection in this man are likely to be true?
a. Neurological features may be present in up to 20% of cases.
b. This is likely to be a type A dissection and is best treated conservatively.
c. Inferior myocardial infarction due to involvement of the RCA occurs in 50% of type A aortic dissections.
d. The CXR is abnormal in approximately 20% of cases.
e. Involvement of the aortic valve by the aortic dissection has led to a wide pulse pressure due to the development of AS.

22 *A 40-year-old woman presents with a 24-hour history of breathlessness and pleuritic chest pain. She gives a history of a hysterectomy performed 1 week previously. She is thought to have a pulmonary embolism.*

Which of the following statements concerning her investigation and treatment are likely to be correct?
a. A troponin rise indicates a relatively good prognosis.
b. If abnormal, her arterial gases will reveal type 1 respiratory failure with a decreased A–a gradient.
c. The diagnosis is usually made on the basis of a positive D-dimer.
d. The ECG will show a deep S wave in lead I, Q wave in lead III and T wave in lead III in over 80% of cases.
e. Anticoagulation should be commenced with low-molecular-weight heparin rather than warfarin in the first instance.

23 *A 40-year-old man undergoes an exercise test as part of an insurance medical.*

Which of the following are criteria for a positive exercise ECG, indicating a high probability of severe ischaemic heart disease?
a. Upsloping ST depression of 0.5 mm.
b. Termination of the test due to breathlessness.
c. A rise in systolic blood pressure of only 20 mmHg during the test.
d. ST-segment depression of >3 mm in multiple leads.
e. Atrial arrhythmias.

24 *In which of the following situations would an exercise myoview scan (isotope scan) be more appropriate to diagnose coronary artery disease than an exercise ECG?*

a. A resting ECG demonstrating partial RBBB.
b. Patients with a poor exercise tolerance.
c. A resting ECG demonstrating of left ventricular strain.
d. Patients in atrial fibrillation treated with beta blockade.
e. Patients with severe AS.

25 *A 40-year-old woman presents with a 5-day history of breathlessness following a viral upper respiratory tract infection. A CXR demonstrates an enlarged cardiac outline.*

Which of the following suggest a diagnosis of cardiac tamponade as opposed to left ventricular failure?
a. Pulsus paradoxus of 30 mmHg.
b. Pulsus alternans.
c. Quiet heart sounds.
d. An elevated JVP.
e. Increased voltages on the 12-lead ECG.

26 *A 40-year-old woman present with breathlessness. She has a BMI of 30 and is an ex-smoker. She suffers from hypertension and diabetes.*

Which of the following findings make a diagnosis of heart failure very unlikely?
a. A normal CXR.
b. A normal ejection fraction on echocardiography.
c. An elevated serum BNP.
d. The presence of a third heart sound.
e. A normal ECG.

27 *A 58-year-old man present to the outpatient clinic with a history of breathlessness. He is known to have COPD but his GP has noted a pansystolic murmur audible at the apex consistent with a diagnosis of mitral regurgitation.*

Which of the following clinical features suggest that his MR is severe and therefore likely to contribute significantly to his breathlessness?
a. An opening snap.
b. A mid-systolic click with a late systolic murmur.
c. The presence of Kerley B lines and upper lobe blood diversion on the CXR.
d. A resting O_2 saturation of 94%
e. An Austin Flint murmur.

28 *In a patient with AR, which, if any, of the following statements are true?*

a. The murmur is decrescendo in character occurring just after the first heart sound.
b. The condition is associated with a small aortic root.
c. The apex beat is characteristically displaced laterally.
d. A systolic murmur always indicates the presence of additional AS.
e. If the AR is severe, the valve should be replaced provided the left ventricular function is normal even if the patient is asymptomatic.

29 *A 40-year-old man presents with a 2-month history of breathlessness, orthopnoea and leg oedema. On examination, he is breathless at rest and has clinical features of left ventricular failure and he has oedema to his waist and ascites. He is already taking furosemide 80 mg twice daily. An echocardiogram demonstrates global left ventricular systolic dysfunction with a left ventricular ejection fraction of 30%. He is admitted to hospital.*

Which if any of the following statements are true concerning the management of his heart failure?
a. If his estimated GFR is <60 mL/min, ACE inhibitors should not be used.
b. Oral diuretics are likely to be less effective due to reduced GI absorption.
c. The beneficial effect of beta blockade will be a class effect and independent of the agent used.
d. In hospitalised patients, a fluid balance chart is preferable to daily weights in monitoring the effects of diuretic therapy.
e. Hyponatraemia should be treated by withdrawal of his diuretic therapy.

30 *A 40-year-old man who has been in the CCU for 3 days following an anterior myocardial infarction develops acute pulmonary oedema that is confirmed on CXR. His ward observations are as follows: pulse 150 bpm; blood pressure 110/70 mmHg; O_2 saturations 98% on 2 litres of O_2. He has been anuric for the past 3 hours.*

Which of the following statements concerning his management are incorrect?
a. Acute deterioration due to the onset of atrial flutter should be considered.
b. Intravenous nitrates should not be given since he is not hypertensive.
c. An echocardiogram should be performed as soon as possible to exclude papillary muscle rupture.
d. CPAP should be part of the first-line management.
e. A fluid challenge of 500 mL should be given to restore his blood pressure and prevent the onset of acute tubular necrosis.

EMQs

1 Causes of syncope

a. Hypoglycaemia.
b. *Grand mal* seizure.
c. Sinus arrest.
d. Complete heart block.
e. Ventricular tachycardia.
f. Vasovagal (neurocardiogenic) syncope.
g. AS.
h. Atrial myxoma.
i. Transient ischaemic attack.
j. MS.
k. Aortic dissection.

For each of the patients below choose the most likely cause of their loss of consciousness.

1. An 80-year-old male with breathlessness, fatigue and exertional syncope. A quiet systolic murmur is heard on examination.
2. A 25-year-old woman witnesses a car accident. There is a 2-minute prodrome of feeling nauseated, pale and clammy before collapsing.
3. A 74-year-old type 2 diabetic on metformin with a past history of myocardial infarctions, coronary artery bypass surgery and left ventricular ejection fraction of 25%. Syncope occurs while sitting with no warning and with a quick recovery after 20 seconds.
4. A 65-year-old woman with previous aortic valve replacement surgery, a blood pressure of 200/100 mmHg, sinus rhythm, PR interval 0.25 seconds, RBBB and left-axis deviation, has syncope without warning.
5. A 78-year-old woman with paroxysmal atrial fibrillation, recently started on sotalol, has a 20-minute episode of irregular palpitations which ends with a sudden 5-second loss of consciousness resulting in a collapse.

2 ECG interpretation

a. Acute anterior STEMI.
b. Acute inferior STEMI.
c. ACS (non-STEMI) due to likely plaque rupture in the LAD artery.
d. Acute pericarditis.
e. Acute pulmonary embolism.
f. Left ventricular hypertrophy due to hypertrophic cardiomyopathy.
g. Supraventricular tachycardia with RBBB.
h. Atrial flutter with LBBB.
i. Monomorphic ventricular tachycardia.
j. Single chamber ventricular pacing with underlying sinus rhythm.
k. LQTS.
l. Atrial fibrillation.
m. Complete heart block.

Choose the most accurate interpretation of the following ECGs.

Cardiology: Clinical Cases Uncovered. By T. Betts, J. Dwight and S. Bull. Published 2010 by Blackwell Publishing.

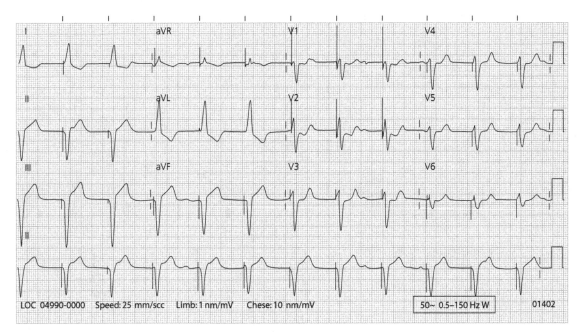

Figure EMQ 2.1

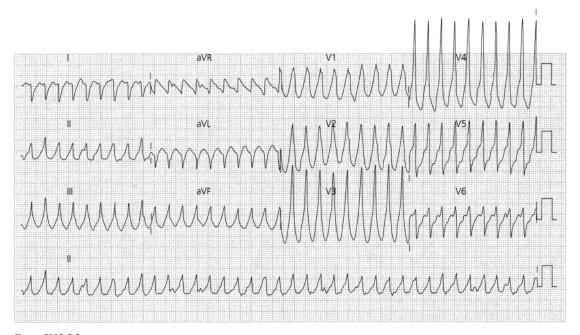

Figure EMQ 2.2

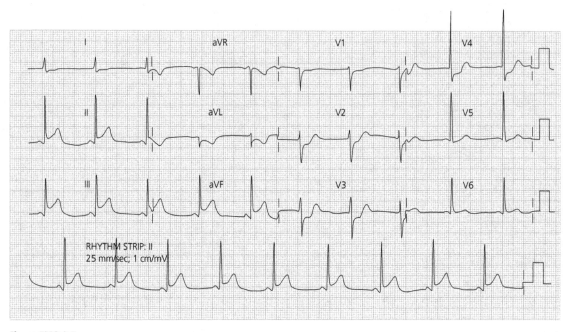

Figure EMQ 2.3

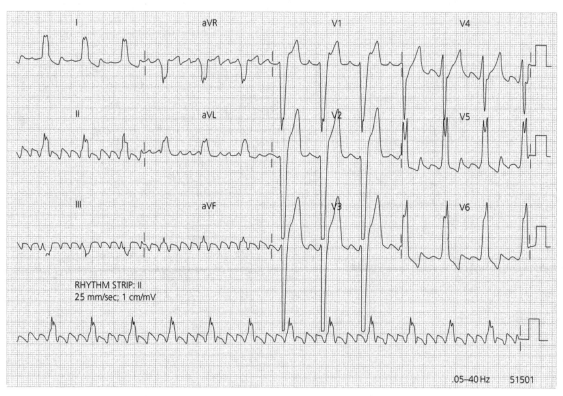

Figure EMQ 2.4

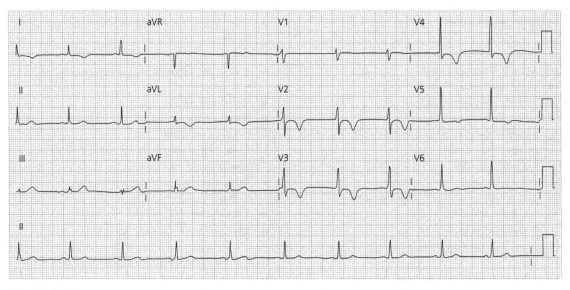

Figure EMQ 2.5

3 Palpitations

a. Ectopic beats.
b. Sinus rhythm.
c. Sinus tachycardia.
d. Atrial fibrillation.
e. Atrial flutter.
f. Automatic atrial tachycardia.
g. Wolff-Parkinson-White syndrome.
h. Mobitz 1 (Wenckebach) second-degree heart block.
i. AV-nodal reciprocating tachycardia.
j. Ventricular tachycardia.
k. Torsades de pointes.

For each of the following, choose the most likely heart rhythm.

1. A cause of syncope or sudden cardiac death in patients with congenital or acquired LQTS.
2. A regular rhythm at 150 bpm, associated with hypertension and increasing age and a risk factor for thromboembolic stroke.
3. Found in 1 in 1000 people, usually causing a sudden-onset regular tachycardia but may also rarely result in ventricular fibrillation.
4. A common form of palpitation, usually worse at times of rest, causing a heavy thumping or sensation of 'missed beats'.
5. A sudden-onset, rapid, regular rhythm at 170 bpm, presenting for the first time in a 25-year-old woman, terminated with carotid sinus massage, with a normal 12-lead ECG appearance during sinus rhythm.

4 Cardiac investigations

a. 12-lead ECG.
b. Cardiac troponin measurement.
c. Serum BNP measurement.
d. Transthoracic echocardiogram.
e. Transoesophageal echocardiogram.
f. Treadmill exercise stress test.
g. Myocardial perfusion scan (technetium).
h. 24-hour Holter monitor.
i. 7-day loop recorder.
j. Thoracic CT scan.
k. Electrophysiological studies (ventricular tachycardia stimulation protocol).
l. Flecainide/ajmaline drug challenge.
m. Head-up tilt table test.

For each of the following situations, choose the most appropriate investigation for the suspected condition.

1. A 42-year-old male smoker who has a 4-week history of exertional central chest pains when walking up hills.
2. A 68-year-old male with hypertension who has a 1-hour history of sudden-onset severe chest and interscapular back pain with a systolic blood pressure of 180 mmHg in his right arm and 90 mmHg in his left arm.
3. A 48-year-old woman receiving chemotherapy for breast cancer who presents with a 10-day history of increasing breathlessness and now 24 hours of severe dyspnoea, postural dizziness and a blood pressure of 80/55 mmHg. Her pulse cannot be felt during inspiration.
4. A 72-year-old diabetic male with a history of prior myocardial infarction, below-knee amputation and LBBB presenting with a 2-month history of exertional retrosternal pain, occasionally relieved with sublingual GTN spray.
5. A 19-year-old woman with short-lived episodes of nausea and pre-syncope, accompanied by palpitations, occurring every 10–14 days.

5 Physical signs

a. A collapsing 'waterhammer' pulse.
b. An irregularly irregular pulse.
c. An ejection systolic murmur radiating to the carotid arteries.
d. A mid-systolic click and late-systolic murmur loudest at the apex.
e. Fixed splitting of the second heart sound.
f. A fall in blood pressure of >10 mmHg during inspiration.
g. A pericardial rub.
h. Fine inspiratory crackles at both lung bases.
i. Radial–femoral delay.
j. A low, rumbling mid-diastolic murmur, loudest when lying on the left hand side.
k. A palpable thrill over the left sternal edge.
l. Central cyanosis.
m. A pulsatile liver.
n. Pitting oedema in the lower limbs.

Which of the above physical signs are typical of the cardiac conditions listed below?

1. Viral pericarditis.
2. A small VSD.
3. Mitral valve prolapse with moderate MR.
4. Atrial fibrillation.
5. Severe TR.

6 Causes of a systolic murmur

a. Severe AS.
b. MR.
c. VSD.
d. Innocent murmur.
e. Aortic coarctation.
f. Mitral valve prolapse.
g. HOCM.
h. Bicuspid aortic valve (mildly stenosed).
i. TR.
j. Functional MR due to a dilated cardiomyopathy.

For each of the patients below choose the most likely cause for their systolic murmur.

1. A 32-year-old woman presents with palpitations, which she describes as having a pause and thump pattern. She is otherwise well and plays squash on a regular basis without limitation. On examination, she looks well. Her pulse is normal in character and volume. Blood pressure is 110/70 mmHg. JVP is not elevated. Apex beat is normal. There is a mid- to late-systolic murmur, heard best at the apex.
2. A 72-year-old man presents with breathlessness on exertion after 100 m. He has a history of hypertension treated with enalapril 20 mg po bd.

On examination, he has a small volume pulse, blood pressure is 100/80 mmHg, his JVP is visible mid-neck. The apex beat is easily palpable but not displaced. Auscultation reveals a systolic murmur heard throughout the precordium and which radiates to the neck. The second sound is inaudible.

3. A 50-year-old woman presents with breathlessness and leg oedema. Her sister and father also have 'breathing problems' felt to be heart related. On examination, she is overweight; she has a tachycardia of 100 bpm in atrial fibrillation with a small volume pulse. Blood pressure is 90/70 mmHg. The JVP is elevated to the angle of the jaw. The apex beat is displaced to the anterior axillary line. On auscultation, the heart sounds are soft, there is a soft apical pansystolic murmur and an added third heart sound. The liver is palpable but not pulsatile. She has oedema to the knees.

4. A 20-year-old woman is referred by her GP having been found to have a murmur when being examined for an exacerbation of her asthma. She is well. Pulse is normal; blood pressure is 110/70 mmHg; JVP is not elevated. The apex beat is not displaced. There is a mid-systolic murmur, heard best at the left sternal edge with the patient lying flat; the murmur does not radiate. The rest of the clinical examination is normal. Her ECG shows a sinus bradycardia of 55 bpm but is otherwise normal.

5. A 5-year-old boy is seen in A&E with a fractured humerus. On auscultation, he has a loud pansystolic murmur, heard best at the left sternal edge. There are no other abnormal physical signs. His parents report that he was noted to have a murmur at birth and they were told it would probably go when he got older.

7 Causes of left hemiparesis

a. Infective endocarditis.
b. Left ventricular mural thrombus.
c. Carotid artery stenosis.
d. Paroxysmal atrial fibrillation.
e. Left atrial myxoma.
f. Paradoxical embolism.
g. Decompression sickness.
h. Haemorrhagic stroke.
i. Cerebral secondaries.
j. Subdural haematoma.

For each of the patients below give the most likely cause of their left hemiparesis.

1. A 60-year-old diabetic man with a 30-pack year history of smoking who describes waking up at night very short of breath and 'tight chested' a week before. He presents with a sudden onset of a left hemiparesis and the ECG shows Q waves in the anteroseptal leads.

2. A 45-year-old man gives a history of being generally unwell over the past 3 weeks. He has lost 1 kg in weight. On examination, there are no peripheral stigmata of endocarditis. He looks anaemic and is pyrexial at 38°C. Pulse is 100 bpm in sinus rhythm and collapsing in nature; blood pressure is 180/40 mmHg. Auscultation reveals an early diastolic murmur, heard best in inspiration at the left sternal edge.

3. A 78-year-old man with a 30-pack year history of smoking and a past history of a left femoropopliteal bypass operation presents with a week's history of intermittent weakness affecting the left arm. His wife notices that the left side of his face droops with each episode and lasts approximately 30 minutes. On examination, his pulse is 70 bpm and regular; blood pressure is 130/70 mmHg; heart sounds are normal. Both carotids are palpable and there are no carotid bruits. He has bilateral femoral artery bruits and his pulses are absent below the femoral arteries.

4. A 69-year-old woman gives a long-standing history of poorly controlled hypertension. She presents with a sudden onset of left-sided weakness. On examination, pulse is 120 bpm in atrial fibrillation; blood pressure is 200/120 mmHg; heart sounds are normal. A CT scan performed within 2 hours of the onset of symptoms is reported as normal.

5. A 50-year-old man presents to the vascular surgeons with a painful cold right foot. He has been previously quite fit but on questioning gives a history of two episodes of syncope over the past 2 weeks. He has no cardiovascular risk factors and is very fit and well. He undergoes a successful removal of a large left femoral embolus; however, 3 days later he develops a sudden onset of a left hemiparesis. On examination, he is apyrexial; pulse 70 bpm with normal character; blood pressure 130/90 mmHg. The apex is not displaced. Heart sounds reveal an apical diastolic 'plop'. Blood tests have revealed a normochromic normocytic anaemia and an ESR of 100 mm/h.

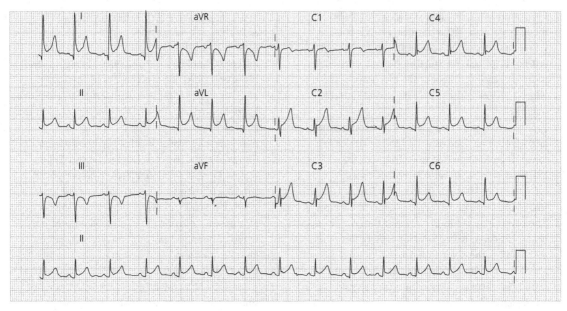

Figure EMQ 8.1

8 Causes of an elevated troponin

a. Pericarditis.
b. Non-STEMI.
c. Pulmonary embolism.
d. Hypertensive crisis.
e. Myocarditis.
f. Ischaemic cardiomyopathy with acute left ventricular failure.
g. Septic shock.
h. Amyloid heart disease.
i. Cardiac arrest.
j. Tachyarrhythmia.
k. Cardiac contusion.

For each of the patients below give the most likely cause of their elevated troponin.

1. A 40-year-old woman presenting with central chest pain. Clinical examination is normal. ECG on presentation is shown in Figure EMQ 8.1.
2. A 50-year-old man with a history of alcohol abuse presents having collapsed at home. He lives alone. On arrival he is delirious. He is warm peripherally. O_2 saturations on air are 86%. Pulse 120 bpm; blood pressure 80/30 mmHg; JVP is just visible lying flat. Heart sounds cannot be heard as a result of coarse breath sounds. His ECG shows a sinus tachycardia and a CXR shows bilateral airspace shadowing with air bronchograms.
3. An 18-year-old man presents with a history of breathlessness chest pain and fatigue over the past 3 days. On examination, he is apyrexial. He looks unwell slightly jaundiced and is cool peripherally. Pulse is 120 bpm in sinus rhythm; blood pressure 90/70 mmHg with no paradox; JVP elevated to the angle of the jaw with a normal wave form. The apex beat is displaced to the anterior axillary line. Auscultation reveals third and fourth heart sounds and a soft apical systolic murmur. Auscultation of the chest reveals crepitations to the mid-zones and he has bilateral pitting oedema. His ECG demonstrates non-specific ST abnormalities in the lateral chest leads.
4. A 60-year-old woman presents 5 days following a total knee replacement with breathlessness. She arrests in the ambulance and is resuscitated. On examination, her pulse is 120 bpm in sinus rhythm; blood pressure 60/40 mmHg, O_2 saturations on air 90%. Heart sounds are normal and chest is clear. The ECG is shown in Figure EMQ 8.2.
5. A 40-year-old man with an ECG shown in Figure EMQ 8.3 after an aortic aneurysm repair.

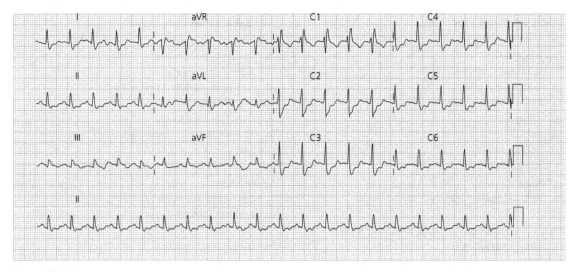

Figure EMQ 8.2

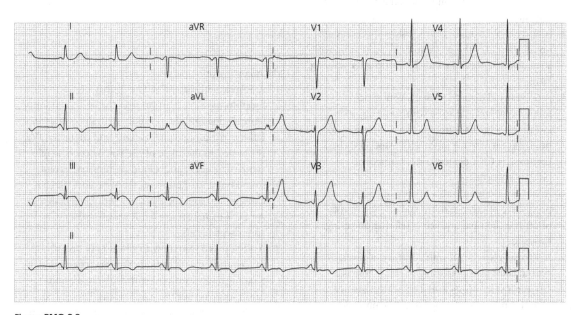

Figure EMQ 8.3

9 Causes of chest pain

a. Aortic dissection.
b. Pericarditis.
c. Pulmonary embolism.
d. Oesophageal reflux.
e. ACS – unstable angina.
f. Paroxysmal SVT.
g. Pleurisy.
h. Musculoskeletal.
i. Gall stones.
j. Stable angina.
k. ACS – myocardial infarction.

What is the most likely cause of chest pain for the following presentations?

1. A 70-year-old man presenting with severe central chest pain of sudden onset. On examination he has a right hemiparesis. Blood pressure is 180/80 mmHg. On auscultation he has an early diastolic murmur.

2. A 40-year-old woman with a history of chest pain on exertion over the past 3 months presenting with a sudden deterioration and chest pain after walking 10 m.

3. A 60-year-old diabetic presents with syncope followed by breathlessness with vomiting and sweating on the background of a 6-month history of declining exercise tolerance with associated chest tightness. A CXR demonstrates features of pulmonary oedema.

4. A 20-year-old man with a history of cough productive of green sputum and a 3-day history of central chest pain, which is relieved on sitting forwards.

5. A 40-year-old woman with a history of severe central chest pain presenting at rest. There is a 10-year history of nocturnal chest pain last up to 1 hour. An ECG performed during pain is normal.

10 Cardiac causes of dyspnoea

a. Diastolic heart failure.
b. Ischaemic heart disease.
c. Acute myocardial infarction.
d. Paroxysmal atrial fibrillation or flutter.
e. Valvular heart disease.
f. Dilated cardiomyopathy.
g. Mobitz type 2 second-degree or third-degree heart block.
h. Sustained atrial fibrillation or flutter.
i. Pericardial tamponade.
j. Constrictive pericarditis.
k. Restrictive cardiomyopathy.
l. Pulmonary embolism.
m. Pulmonary hypertension.
n. Congenital heart disease.
o. Uncontrolled hypertension.
p. Sinus node disease with bradycardia.
q. HOCM.

What is the most likely cardiac cause of dyspnoea for the following presentations?

1. A 50-year-old woman with a history of breathlessness on exertion over the past 12 months. On examination, she is mildly centrally cyanosed. Pulse is 80 bpm, normal volume and character. JVP is elevated to the angle of the jaw. There is a right ventricular heave and a loud pulmonary second sound but auscultation is otherwise normal. Her chest is clear and she has mild peripheral oedema. An ECG demonstrates tall R waves in the anteroseptal leads.

2. A 40-year-old woman with a history of breast cancer, treated with radiotherapy and chemotherapy 6 months previously, presents with fatigue and breathlessness over the past 3 weeks. There is no cardiac history and she has no risk factors for cardiac disease. On examination, she is cool peripherally. Pulse is 100 bpm in atrial fibrillation; blood pressure 100/80 mmHg; JVP is elevated to the angle of the jaw. Heart sounds are quiet and the apex beat is impalpable. An ECG demonstrates small complexes. CXR shows a globular cardiac outline.

3. A 60-year-old diabetic woman with a long-standing history of hypertension presents with increasing breathlessness on exertion over the past 2 years. Her exercise tolerance is now 20 m but she is not

breathless at rest. Her cardiac examination is normal with the exception of a soft fourth heart sound. Blood pressure is 140/80 mmHg on medication. Her chest is clear. An ECG demonstrates left ventricular hypertrophy and strain and a stress echocardiogram reveals normal wall motion at rest and stress. BNP is elevated.

4. A 45-year-old man with a history of hypertension presents with a history of four episodes of acute breathlessness over the past 6 months. The episodes occur predominantly at rest and last between 15 and 20 minutes. Between these episodes he has a normal exercise tolerance and he plays tennis on a regular basis to a high standard. Cardiac examination is normal. An echocardiogram demonstrates normal left ventricular function; the left atrium is reported as dilated.

5. A 48-year-old woman presents with fatigue and breathlessness, which has progressed over the past 6 months. She is usually quite sedentary but now has an exercise tolerance of less than 50 m. She has had three episodes of acute dyspnoea at night. There are no risk factors for cardiac disease other than a family history of early cardiac death on her father's side. On examination, she has a pulse of 80 bpm in sinus rhythm with a small volume; blood pressure is 110/70 mmHg; JVP is elevated to the middle of the neck. The apex beat is displaced to the anterior axillary line. Auscultation is normal. She has pitting oedema to the mid-calf. Her ECG demonstrates non-specific ST changes in the lateral chest leads.

1 *A 25-year-old football player collapses during a match. A paramedic crew successfully resuscitate him from ventricular fibrillation using external defibrillation. He is admitted to the local CCU. A 12-lead ECG shows sinus rhythm with large voltages in chest leads. A transthoracic echocardiogram shows asymmetrical LVH with a ventricular septal thickness of 3.2 cm. On closer questioning, he reports a maternal uncle who died 30 years ago in his 20s of a 'heart attack'.*

a. What is the most likely diagnosis? (*1 mark*)
b. Is this an inherited or acquired condition? (*1 mark*) Name two other inherited conditions that pose a risk for cardiac arrests. (*2 marks*)
c. What is the most appropriate treatment to prevent further cardiac arrests? (*1 mark*)
d. What are the five generally accepted risk factors in this condition for sudden cardiac death? (*5 marks*)

2 *A 38-year-old male is referred urgently by his GP with a 3-month history of intermittent episodes of sweating, headaches, palpitations and a blood pressure recording in the GP surgery of 200/110 mmHg. When seen the following day in the cardiology clinic his blood pressure is 110/75 mmHg. During physical examination he develops symptoms and his blood pressure increases to 220/120 mmHg.*

a. What is the diagnosis? (*1 mark*)
b. How is the diagnosis confirmed? (*2 marks*)
c. What are the immediate and subsequent treatments? (*3 marks*)

Cardiology: Clinical Cases Uncovered. By T. Betts, J. Dwight and S. Bull. Published 2010 by Blackwell Publishing.

d. What is the '10% rule'? (*1 mark*)
e. List three other causes of secondary hypertension. (*3 marks*)

3 *A 77-year old woman has a 6-month history of intermittent rapid irregular palpitations, occurring every 2–3 days for 20 minutes at a time. She has a history of a previous small myocardial infarction, asthma, hypertension and diabetes. A Holter monitor records a 15-minute episode of rapid, irregular narrow-complex tachycardia with no discernable P waves.*

a. What is the rhythm abnormality? How should it be classified? (*1 mark*)
b. How common is this condition in this age group? (*1 mark*)
c. What are the possible harmful consequences of this arrhythmia? (*2 marks*)
d. What is the CHADS2 score? (*1 mark*) What is the appropriate action? (*1 mark*)
e. What drug treatment options are there for her symptoms? (*2 marks*). If the drugs are ineffective, what else could be offered? (*2 marks*)

4 *An 84-year-old woman with a 5-year history of permanent atrial fibrillation has three episodes of pre-syncope, one when standing and two when sitting, over a 2-week period. Her resting pulse is 40–50 bpm and irregular.*

a. What is the most likely cause of her pre-syncope? (*1 mark*)
b. What are the key points in the history that help make the diagnosis? (*2 marks*)
c. What tests could be used to confirm the diagnosis? (*2 marks*)

d. What contributory causes need to be excluded?
(*2 marks*)

e. What therapeutic intervention is likely to help?
(*1 mark*) What 'prescription' would be most
appropriate in this setting? (*1 mark*)

f. She is due an MRI scan of her hip. What advice
would you give her? (*1 mark*)

---

5 *A 49-year-old male has a routine 12-lead ECG as
part of an insurance medical. The ECG is shown in
Figure SAQ 5.1.*

a. What are the abnormalities? (*1 mark*)

b. List four possible causes? (*4 marks*)

c. What are the key questions that need to be asked?
(*3 marks*)

d. What investigations may be helpful, particularly if
questioning reveals cause for concern? (*2 marks*)

---

6 *A 44-year-old banker presents with a 3-month history
of breathlessness on exertion, ankle swelling and
palpitations. He has been previously fit and well. There is
no history of hypertension or vascular disease. He is a
non-smoker. There is no family history of cardiac disease.
On examination, he is in atrial fibrillation at a rate of
100 bpm; blood pressure 100/70 mmHg. JVP is elevated
to mid-neck with a prominent 'V' wave. On cardiac
auscultation, the apex beat is displaced and he has a third
heart sound. Examination of the chest reveals bibasal
crackles. A diagnosis of heart failure is made.*

a. Give two other symptoms are associated with this
syndrome? (*2 marks*)

b. What other aspect of the history may be important?
(*1 mark*)

c. What three initial investigations would you perform
in the GP surgery (excluding FBCs, electrolytes and
renal function)? (*3 marks*)

d. Name three classes of drugs that are proven to
reduce mortality in this condition? (*3 marks*)

e. What is the cause of the finding on examination of
the JVP and how would you confirm it clinically?
(*1 mark*)

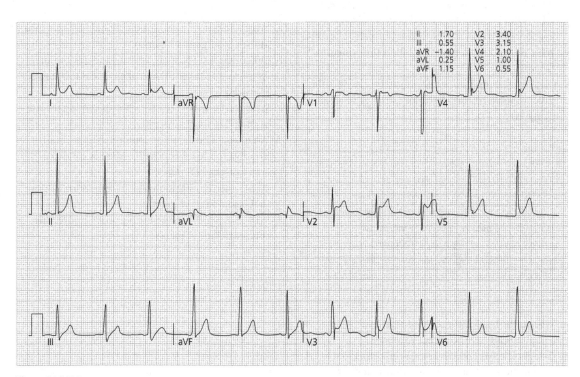

Figure SAQ 5.1

7 *A 65-year-old woman is assessed for a right hemicolectomy and is found to have a pansystolic murmur. She reports breathlessness when climbing stairs but has no other symptoms. She is a non-smoker and does not drink alcohol. There is no history of rheumatic fever. On examination, pulse is 70 bpm, good volume and normal character; blood pressure 140/70 mmHg; JVP is elevated to mid-neck. The apex beat is displaced 2 cm laterally and does not feel hypertrophied. The murmur is heard throughout the precordium and radiates to the axilla; there is a third heart sound. An ECG is normal. The CXR shows cardiomegaly. An echocardiogram is performed, which demonstrates good left ventricular function with an ejection fraction of 50%; the ventricle is moderately dilated. There is an eccentric jet of MR, which is graded as severe. The pulmonary artery pressure estimated from the tricuspid regurgitant jet is significantly elevated at 50 mmHg. There are no other valvular abnormalities.*

a. Give two other common differential diagnoses for a patient with a systolic murmur. (*2 marks*)
b. Give three features on clinical examination that make this murmur more likely to be due to MR than AS. (*3 marks*)
c. What is the cause of the third heart sound? (*1 mark*)
d. Why is this patient breathless despite an ejection fraction that is only slightly below normal? (*1 mark*)
e. What is the likely cause of the MR in this patient? (*1 mark*)
f. Give two features in this case which indicate that the patient should be considered for mitral valve repair. (*2 marks*)

8 *A 28-year-old basketball player is admitted via A&E with a history of a sudden onset of severe central chest pain while training. He has previously been fit and well. He is a non-smoker and does not drink alcohol. During examination, he becomes pale and confused with a markedly elevated JVP. His pulse is 120 bpm; blood pressure is 100/60 mmHg. On examination, he has a soft and brief early diastolic murmur. He arrests with PEA 10 minutes later.*

a. What is the likely diagnosis and what two complications have occurred? (*3 marks*)
b. Give three other clinical features on history and examination that can point to this diagnosis at presentation? (*3 marks*)

c. What is the most likely underlying pathology? (*1 mark*)
d. Which would be your investigation of choice to confirm the diagnosis in this case? (*1 marks*)
e. How should the patient be managed at this point? (*2 marks*)

9 *A 65-year-old woman with severe osteoarthritis presents to her GP's surgery with a history of exertional chest pain, particularly when climbing stairs. There have been no episodes of chest pain at rest. She is known to be hypertensive and suffers from emphysema. She is on treatment with nifedipine 20 mg orally bd, bendroflumethiazide 2.5 mg po od and a salbutamol inhaler prn. She is a non-smoker and does not drink alcohol. She weighs 90 kg. On cardiovascular examination, pulse is 50 bpm; blood pressure 170/80 mmHg; soft ejection systolic murmur; the left ventricle is clinically hypertrophied. There is no clinical evidence of heart failure. Her ECG shows LBBB, which is long standing. Her fasting lipid profile measured 1 month previously was as follows: total cholesterol 6.8 mmol/L; HDL cholesterol 1.4 mmol/L; triglyceride 6 mmol/L. Urine analysis is negative.*

a. What additional investigations should be performed in the GP surgery? (*3 marks*)
b. Other than a GTN spray, what treatments can the GP institute for her presumed angina at this stage? (*3 marks*)
c. What advice should the GP give concerning the use of the GTN spray (*1 mark*)
d. What would be the most appropriate non-invasive investigation to assess whether she has coronary artery disease? (*1 mark*)
e. What other investigation should be performed prior to this and why? (*1 mark*)
f. What is a possible cause for the raised triglyceride concentration? (*1 mark*)

10 *A 70-year-old man is admitted to hospital with a history of heart failure and long-standing atrial fibrillation due to a previous myocardial infarction. He is treated with intravenous diuretics for 3 days and responds well with a 4 kg weight loss. On the fourth day he collapses on the way to the bathroom. By the time the arrest team arrives he has been given a short period of CPR and 500 mL of normal saline. His observations are as follows: pulse 100 bpm in atrial fibrillation; blood pressure 80/50 mmHg; JVP is elevated to the earlobes; heart sounds are normal and his chest is clear. O₂ saturations are 92% on 10 litres of O₂ via a face mask. His ECG shows atrial fibrillation and new-onset RBBB. A portable CXR shows cardiomegaly; there is an area of plate atelectasis at the right base.*

a. What is the most likely diagnosis? (*1 mark*)
b. Give three alternative diagnoses that should be considered. (*3 marks*)
c. Given the diagnosis, what is the likely finding on the arterial blood gases? (*1 mark*)
d. Give three additional clinical signs should be looked for on examination in this condition. (*3 marks*)
e. If the patient is not sufficiently stable to go for CT pulmonary angiography, what alternative investigation may be performed? (*1 mark*)
f. Assuming the diagnosis is confirmed, what is the most appropriate treatment? (*1 mark*)

1. d	11. b	21. a
2. b	12. a	22. e
3. a	13. a	23. d
4. d	14. c	24. c
5. b	15. c	25. a
6. a	16. e	26. e
7. d	17. d	27. c
8. b	18. b	28. c
9. e	19. b	29. b
10. a	20. e	30. a

Cardiology: Clinical Cases Uncovered. By T. Betts, J. Dwight and
S. Bull. Published 2010 by Blackwell Publishing.

PART 3: SELF-ASSESSMENT

EMQ answers

1
1.1 g
1.2 f
1.3 e
1.4 d
1.5 c

2
2.1 j
2.2 i
2.3 b
2.4 h
2.5 c

3
3.1 k
3.2 e
3.3 g
3.4 a
3.5 i

4
4.1 f
4.2 j
4.3 d
4.4 g
4.5 i

5
5.1 g
5.2 k
5.3 d
5.4 b
5.5 m

6
6.1 f
6.2 a
6.3 j
6.4 d
6.5 c

7
7.1 b
7.2 a
7.3 c
7.4 d
7.5 e

8
8.1 a
8.2 g
8.3 e
8.4 c
8.5 b

9
9.1 a
9.2 e
9.3 k
9.4 b
9.5 d

10
10.1 m
10.2 i
10.3 a
10.4 d
10.5 f

Cardiology: Clinical Cases Uncovered. By T. Betts, J. Dwight and S. Bull. Published 2010 by Blackwell Publishing.

1

a. HOCM. (*1 mark*)

b. This is usually a familial condition that is inherited in a dominant fashion. (*1 mark*) Other inherited conditions that can cause cardiac arrest are the channelopathies LQTS, Brugada syndrome and/or catecholaminergic polymorphic ventricular tachycardia. (*1 mark each, maximum 2 marks*)

c. Any patient with HOCM who survives a cardiac arrest should be offered an ICD for secondary prevention. (*1 mark*)

d. Gross hypertrophy (wall thickness >30 mm), syncope, non-sustained VT, family history of sudden cardiac death and flat or falling blood pressure during exercise. (*1 mark each, maximum 5 marks*) The presence of two or more of these risk factors is generally considered enough to offer a primary prevention ICD. Some authorities believe that one risk factor is enough.

2

a. Phaeochromocytoma. This is a rare, catecholamine-secreting tumour, usually in the adrenal glands. (*1 mark*) They are found in 0.05–0.2% of hypertensive individuals.

b. 24-hour urinary collection for catecholamines and metanephrines has a sensitivity of 87.5% and a specificity of 99.7% (*1 mark*). Plasma metanephrine levels are more sensitive but less specific. Cross-sectional imaging of the abdomen, specifically to look at the adrenal glands. (*1 mark*) MRI is more sensitive than CT. A MIBG scan (with iodine I^{131}-labelled metaiodobenzylguanidine) is only performed if a phaeochromocytoma is confirmed biochemically but CT scanning or MRI do not show a tumour.

Cardiology: Clinical Cases Uncovered. By T. Betts, J. Dwight and S. Bull. Published 2010 by Blackwell Publishing.

c. Immediate treatment should be alpha-receptor blockade such as phenoxybenzamine, (*1 mark*) followed by beta-receptor blockade to control sinus tachycardia. (*1 mark*) Beta blockers should only be started after adequate alpha blockade is achieved, otherwise they might precipitate a hypertensive crisis. Definitive treatment is surgical resection of the tumour, (*1 mark*) but not until 7–10 days after alpha- and beta-blockade has been achieved.

d. 10% is the proportion of phaeochromocytomas that are (i) bilateral; (ii) extra-adrenal; (iii) malignant; (iv) familial; (v) recur; (vi) occur in children; (vii) occur as part of the multiple endocrine neoplasia (MEN) syndrome; or (viii) have stroke as the presenting symptom. (*1 mark*)

e. Renal artery stenosis, Conn's syndrome (primary hyperaldosteronism), renal disease (hydronephrosis, polycystic kidney disease, glomerulonephritis, etc.), Cushing's syndrome, coarctation of the aorta, drugs (oral contraceptive, liquorice-based laxatives). (*1 mark each, maximum 3 marks*)

3

a. Paroxysmal atrial fibrillation. (*1 mark*)

b. Approximately 10% of men aged 75 years and older and 5.6% in women aged 75 years and older have documented atrial fibrillation. The actual incidence (including asymptomatic and undocumented atrial fibrillation) is probably much higher. (*1 mark*)

c. Other than symptoms, atrial fibrillation increases the risk of thromboembolic stroke by 3–5 times. (*1 mark*) The other harmful consequence, which can only occur in persistent atrial fibrillation with a rapid ventricular rate, is tachycardia cardiomyopathy. (*1 mark*)

d. The CHADS2 score is a means of assessing the risk of thromboembolic stroke in people with paroxysmal, persistent or permanent atrial fibrillation. Her CHADS2 score is 3 for age, diabetes and hypertension. (*1 mark*) She should be anticoagulated with warfarin. (*1 mark*)

e. A rhythm-control strategy could be attempted, using amiodarone. (*1 mark*) Sotalol is relatively contraindicated due to her asthma, and flecainide is contraindicated due to her ischaemic heart disease. A rate-control strategy could be attempted with a calcium-channel blocker. (*1 mark*) Again, beta blockers are contraindicated and digoxin is less effective although may be combined with another agent. If drugs fail, alternative non-pharmacological treatments include AV-node ablation and pacemaker implant (*1 mark*) or left atrial ablation. (*1 mark*) For this woman, her age and comorbidities would be relative contraindications to left atrial ablation.

4

a. A slow ventricular response to her atrial fibrillation resulting in long pauses (*1 mark*). Pauses of >3 seconds while awake are considered pathological and an indication for pacemaker implant.

b. The fact that two episodes occurred when sitting make postural (orthostatic) hypotension unlikely. (*1 mark*) The slow but irregular rate despite not taking any medications indicate AV-node disease, (*1 mark*) but is different from atrial fibrillation with complete heart block, which would have a regular escape rhythm.

c. A 12-lead ECG with a rhythm strip is unlikely to record for long enough to uncover a 3 second pause; however, the presence of bifascicular block or LBBB would indicate conduction system disease, adding strength to the possible diagnosis. (*1 mark*) A 24-hour Holter monitor should be performed. (*1 mark*) Ideally, there would be symptoms that correlate with a long pause.

d. AV-node-blocking drugs (e.g. beta blockers, including eye drops, calcium-channel blockers, digoxin, etc.). (*1 mark*) Hypothyroidism. (*1 mark*)

e. A permanent pacemaker. (*1 mark*) The most appropriate system would be single chamber with rate response (ventricular inhibited rate responsive, VVIR). (*1 mark*)

f. Patients with metal implants, including pacemakers, should not go into MRI scanners. (*1 mark*) She should have CT scanning instead.

5

a. There is marked ST elevation in leads V1–V4 with slight ST elevation in V5, V6 and I. (*1 mark*)

b. Acute STEMI, acute pericarditis, 'benign' early repolarisation, left ventricular aneurysm, Brugada syndrome. (*1 mark each, maximum 4 marks*)

c. Has he got, or ever had, chest pains or a known heart attack? Has he ever had a blackout? Is there a family history of heart disease or sudden death? (*1 mark each, maximum 3 marks*)

d. A transthoracic echocardiogram would show any structural heart disease, such as prior myocardial infarction and left ventricular aneurysm. (*1 mark*). An exercise stress test may show normalisation of the ST segments with benign early repolarisation or increasing ST-segment elevation with an aneurysm. (*1 mark*) A drug challenge with ajmaline or flecainide would increase the ST-segment elevation and change it to convex rather than concave in Brugada syndrome. (*1 mark each, maximum 2 marks*) If the individual had presented with severe chest pain, whether it was acute myocardial infarction or myopericarditis, cardiac enzymes may be elevated and coronary angiography may be required for a definitive diagnosis.

6

a. Orthopnoea and paroxysmal nocturnal dyspnoea are the most specific symptoms for heart failure but are only present in a minority of patients. Fatigue, anorexia, abdominal discomfort and sleep disturbance are common but less specific. (*1 mark each, maximum 2 marks*)

b. In patients of this age presenting with a history of heart failure in conjunction with atrial fibrillation, a history of alcohol intake is important. A history of alcohol consumption equivalent to a bottle of wine a day makes a diagnosis of alcoholic cardiomyopathy likely. (*1 mark*)

c. An ECG (*1 mark*) and thyroid function tests (*1 mark*) would be appropriate initial investigations. A CXR (*1 mark*) may be helpful in confirming heart failure; however, a normal CXR does not exclude the diagnosis. In a patient presenting with these physical findings the diagnosis of heart failure is confirmed and a BNP measurement is unlikely to add to the diagnostic accuracy.

d. ACE inhibitors, angiotensin II blockers, beta blockers and aldosterone antagonists are all proven to reduce mortality in heart failure. (*1 mark each, maximum 3 marks*) Diuretics will be required in the treatment of this patient; however, there are no randomised control trials of their impact on mortality. Digoxin may be of help symptomatically, especially as the patient is in atrial fibrillation but again does not improve prognosis.

e. The presence of a prominent 'V' wave suggests a diagnosis of TR, which is associated with the finding of a pulsatile liver on abdominal examination. (*1 mark*)

7

a. AS and an innocent flow murmur, both of which are ejection in nature. (*1 mark each*) Alternatives such as a VSD (pansystolic) and HOCM (ejection systolic) are less common.

b. The pulse is of normal character, (*1 mark*) whereas that due to AS is slow rising. The left ventricle is dilated rather than hypertrophied. (*1 mark*) The murmur is pansystolic rather than ejection systolic and radiates to the mitral area, as opposed to the carotids. (*1 mark*)

c. A third heart sound is the sound created by filling of the ventricle in early diastole. (*1 mark*) Although it can be a normal finding in young people, at this age it is pathological. In this patient the third sound is created by an increased rate of filling in diastole, together with changes in left ventricular compliance brought on by chronic volume overload. A third sound is one of the features of left ventricular failure.

d. In MR, left ventricular function on echocardiography can be misleading. Because the ventricle is offloaded by emptying blood into the left atrium, which is at lower pressure than the aorta, the ejection fraction measured on echocardiography remains normal until late in the disease process. The patient is breathless because the left atrial pressure is elevated on exercise due to regurgitation of blood through the mitral valve. (*1 mark*)

e. Mitral valve prolapse. (*1 mark*) An echocardiography report will normally give an indication of the probable cause of the MR where the image quality is adequate. In mitral valve prolapse either the anterior or, more commonly, the posterior valve leaflet can be seen to prolapse into the left atrium, giving rise to an eccentric jet of MR. The valve leaflets may be reported as floppy or containing redundant tissue and the chordae may be stretched. In chordal rupture the valve leaflet may be described as flail and the ruptured chordae may be visible. Ischaemic papillary muscle rupture is usually diagnosed on the basis of the history of a recent myocardial infarction and the findings of a flail mitral valve. Rheumatic MR is often accompanied by MS, the valve leaflets are usually thickened and the subvalvular apparatus may be involved. In MR secondary to a cardiomyopathy and annular dilatation due to dilatation of the left ventricle, the jet of MR is usually central and is accompanied by gross ventricular dilatation and impaired left ventricular function. The presence of an eccentric jet in the absence of a history of rheumatic fever, severe ventricular dilatation or a history of ischaemic heart disease suggests that mitral valve prolapse is the likely cause.

f. Although the threshold for mitral valve repair in patients with MR is falling, it is generally accepted that severe MR alone does not make mitral valve repair mandatory. The features in this case that would support surgical intervention would be the presence of symptoms of breathlessness, the slight depression of left ventricular function, and an elevated pulmonary artery pressure. (*1 mark each, maximum 2 marks*)

8

a. The most likely diagnosis is aortic dissection. (*1 mark*) Although myocardial infarction remains a possibility in a patient this young, without a history of cardiovascular risk factors this would be unlikely. The presence of hypotension and a markedly elevated JVP indicate that the dissection has dissected back into the pericardial sac, giving rise to tamponade. (*1 mark*) The aortic valve has become involved and has become incompetent. (*1 mark*)

b. Other clinical features include: (*1 mark each, maximum 3 marks*)

   i.   An instantaneous onset of severe chest pain (unlike myocardial infarction, which takes a few minutes to reach maximum).

ii. Radiation through to the back or pain that travels from the anterior chest to the back.
iii. Syncope.
iv. Inequality of blood pressure in the upper limbs.
v. Neurological signs or symptoms, e.g. hemiparesis associated with involvement of the carotid arteries, or paraparesis associated with spinal artery involvement.
vi. Loss of lower limb pulses.

c. The most likely pathology is cystic medical necrosis seen in Marfan's syndrome. (*1 mark*) Aortic dissection is the major cause of mortality in patients with Marfan's syndrome and frequently occurs at a young age. Always be aware of the possibility in tall individuals with a history of chest pain and look for other features, such as a high-arched palate. Hypertension associated with aortic root dilatation, coarctation and bicuspid aortic valves are also associated with aortic dissection but are unlikely in this case.

d. CT angiography, MRI and transthoracic or trans-oesophageal echocardiography can all be used to confirm the diagnosis. (*1 mark for any of these*) A CXR may suggest the diagnosis but is not reliable. In a patient this unwell, urgent bed-side echocardiography is the most practical initial approach.

e. If the patient has arrested then percutaneous pericardial drainage is the only option unless a cardiothoracic surgeon is in attendance; however, the prognosis is very poor. For type A dissection with aortic valve involvement and evidence of tamponade, the cardiothoracic surgeons should be called and the patient taken directly to theatre for surgery. (*1 mark*)

9

a. The following would be appropriate: (*1 mark for each, maximum 3 marks*)
i. FBC to exclude anaemia.
ii. Urea and electrolytes – the patient is on diuretics.
iii. Thyroid function tests – hyperthyroidism can trigger angina and hypothyroidism is associated with coronary artery disease.
iv. Fasting blood sugar.

b. The GP can introduce aspirin, a statin and a nitrate on the basis that the patient has a high probability of having angina. (*1 mark for each*) A beta-blocker is contraindicated by the presence of a combination of bradycardia and LBBB; there is also a relative contraindication in the context of COPD, although significant reversibility would seem unlikely in this case.

c. The patient should take the GTN spray at the onset of pain and repeat at 5-minute intervals if the pain does not resolve. If the pain persists for more than 15 minutes, an ambulance should be called. (*1 mark*) Patients with rest pain with a pre-existing history of angina should be advised to seek medical advice, even if the pain resolves with the use of GTN.

d. A pharmacological stress Myoview scan. (*1 mark*) A standard exercise test is not possible in the context of her arthritis and will not be interpretable in the context of LBBB. Pharmacological stress echocardiography is an alternative; however, in the context of emphysema the image quality is likely to be poor. CT coronary angiography is available in some centres but is primarily a rule out test for coronary disease.

e. A transthoracic echocardiogram (*1 mark*) should be performed to exclude significant aortic stenosis since the patient has an ejection systolic murmur.

f. Hypothyroidism. (*1 mark*) High triglycerides can be associated with obesity, alcohol, nephrotic syndrome and hypothyroidism. She does not drink alcohol and has a normal urinary analysis. In the context of a bradycardia and obesity, hypothyroidism should be excluded.

10

a. Acute massive pulmonary embolism. (*1 mark*) The diagnosis is supported by the finding of hypotension, hypoxaemia and an elevated JVP in the context of a CXR that does not show pulmonary oedema, despite a 500-mL fluid challenge.

b. Postural hypotension (*1 mark*) due to over-diuresis, myocardial infarction (*1 mark*) or cardiac arrhythmia (other than atrial fibrillation, *1 mark*) should be considered.

c. Type 1 respiratory failure, i.e. a low or normal pCO_2 in the context of a low pO_2. (*1 mark*)

d. A right ventricular heave (*1 mark*) and loud pulmonary second (*1 mark*) sound may be present as a result of raised pulmonary artery pressures. There may be clinical evidence of a DVT. (*1 mark*)

e. Transthoracic echocardiography may be used. (*1 mark*) However, it is most useful in patients without a history of left ventricular disease. The finding of normal left ventricular function and a dilated right heart with an elevated pulmonary artery pressure in the context of a shocked patient is highly suggestive of pulmonary embolism. A D-dimer is of no use – it will be elevated in almost all patients who are this unwell, from whatever cause.

f. Thrombolysis is indicated. (*1 mark*) The patient is severely hypotensive and has already arrested.

Index of cases by diagnosis

Index

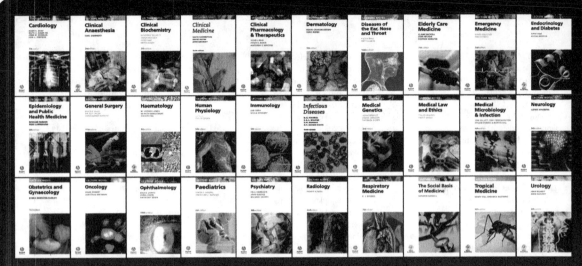

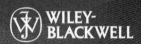
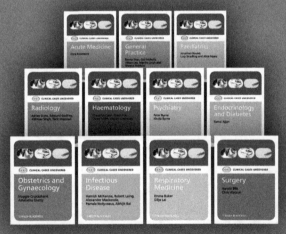
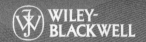